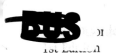
... or
1st Edition
Genetic Disor...
2nd Edition
Head Trauma Sourcebook
Headache Sourcebook
Health Insurance Sourcebook
Health Reference Series Cumulative
  Index 1999
Healthy Aging Sourcebook
Healthy Children Sourcebook
Healthy Heart Sourcebook for Women
Heart Diseases & Disorders
  Sourcebook, 2nd Edition
Household Safety Sourcebook
Immune System Disorders Sourcebook
Infant & Toddler Health Sourcebook
Injury & Trauma Sourcebook
Kidney & Urinary Tract Diseases &
  Disorders Sourcebook
Learning Disabilities Sourcebook,
  1st Edition
Learning Disabilities Sourcebook,
  2nd Edition
Liver Disorders Sourcebook
Leukemia Sourcebook
Lung Disorders Sourcebook
Medical Tests Sourcebook
Men's Health Concerns Sourcebook
Mental Health Disorders Sourcebook,
  1st Edition
Mental Health Disorders Sourcebook,
  2nd Edition
Mental Retardation Sourcebook
Movement Disorders Sourcebook
Obesity Sourcebook
Ophthalmic Disorders Sourcebook,
  1st Edition
Oral Health Sourcebook
Osteoporosis Sourcebook
Pain Sourcebook, 1st Edition
Pain Sourcebook, 2nd Edition
Pediatric Cancer Sourcebook
Physical & Mental Issues in Aging
  Sourcebook

... Sourcebook
... y & Birth Sourcebook
... Cancer
... ealth Sourcebook
Reconstructive & Cosmetic Surgery
  Sourcebook
Rehabilitation Sourcebook
Respiratory Diseases & Disorders
  Sourcebook
Sexually Transmitted Diseases
  Sourcebook, 1st Edition
Sexually Transmitted Diseases
  Sourcebook, 2nd Edition
Skin Disorders Sourcebook
Sleep Disorders Sourcebook
Sports Injuries Sourcebook, 1st Edition
Sports Injuries Sourcebook, 2nd Edition
Stress-Related Disorders Sourcebook
Stroke Sourcebook
Substance Abuse Sourcebook
Surgery Sourcebook
Transplantation Sourcebook
Traveler's Health Sourcebook
Vegetarian Sourcebook
Women's Health Concerns Sourcebook
Workplace Health & Safety Sourcebook
Worldwide Health Sourcebook

Teen Health Series

Diet Information for Teens
Drug Information for Teens
Mental Health Information
  for Teens
Sexual Health Information
  for Teens
Skin Health Information
  for Teens
Sports Injuries Information
  for Teens

Childhood
Diseases and
Disorders
SOURCEBOOK

Health Reference Series

First Edition

Childhood Diseases and Disorders SOURCEBOOK

*Basic Consumer Health Information about Medical
Problems Often Encountered in Pre-Adolescent Children,
Including Respiratory Tract Ailments, Ear Infections, Sore
Throats, Disorders of the Skin and Scalp, Digestive and
Genitourinary Diseases, Infectious Diseases,
Inflammatory Disorders, Chronic Physical and
Developmental Disorders, Allergies, and More*

*Along with Information about Diagnostic Tests,
Common Childhood Surgeries, and Frequently
Used Medications, with a Glossary of Important Terms
and Resource Directory*

Edited by
Chad T. Kimball

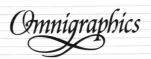

615 Griswold Street • Detroit, MI 48226

Bibliographic Note

Because this page cannot legibly accommodate all the copyright notices, the Bibliographic Note portion of the Preface constitutes an extension of the copyright notice.

Edited by Chad T. Kimball

Health Reference Series

Karen Bellenir, Managing Editor
David A. Cooke, MD, Medical Consultant
Elizabeth Barbour, Permissions Associate
Dawn Matthews, Verification Assistant
Laura Pleva Nielsen, Index Editor
EdIndex, Services for Publishers, Indexers

* * *

Omnigraphics, Inc.

Matthew P. Barbour, Senior Vice President
Kay Gill, Vice President-Directories
Kevin Hayes, Operations Manager
Leif Gruenberg, Development Manager
David P. Bianco, Marketing Consultant

* * *

Peter E. Ruffner, Publisher

Frederick G. Ruffner, Jr., Chairman

Copyright © 2003 Omnigraphics, Inc.

ISBN 0-7808-0458-9

Library of Congress Cataloging-in-Publication Data

Childhood diseases and disorders sourcebook : basic consumer health information about medical problems often encountered in pre-adolescent children, including respiratory tract ailments, ear infections, sore throats, disorders of the skin and scalp, digestive and genitourinary diseases, infectious diseases, inflammatory disorders, chronic physical and developmental disorders, allergies, and more; along with information about diagnostic tests, common childhood surgeries, and frequently used medications, with a glossary of important terms and resource directory / edited by Chad T. Kimball. -- 1st ed.
    p. cm. -- (Health reference series)
  Includes index.
  ISBN 0-7808-0458-9 (lib. bdg. : alk. paper)
   1. Pediatrics. 2. Children--Health and hygiene. 3. Children--Diseases. I. Kimball, Chad T. II. Health reference series (unnumbered)

RJ61.C5427 2003
618.92--dc21

                                                   2003049785

Table of Contents

Part V: Skin and Scalp Ailments

Part VI: Other Infectious Diseases

Part VII: Chronic Conditions

Part VIII: Allergies

Part IX: Additional Help and Information

Preface

About This Book

In the United States, childhood death rates have declined significantly over the past several decades, and statistics compiled by the federal government suggest that most children are in good health; however, a need for continued vigilance persists. Vaccine-preventable diseases occur much less frequently than they once did, but several, including measles, mumps, rubella, hepatitis, and influenza, still pose a threat to children's health. Asthma, the most common chronic childhood illness, affects nearly five percent of American children. Major causes of hospitalization include metabolic diseases, infectious and parasitic diseases, mental disorders, diseases of the skin and subcutaneous tissue, diseases of the digestive system, and respiratory diseases. Cancer and congenital disorders continue to be two of the leading causes of death in children under the age of 14.

This *Sourcebook* provides parents and caregivers with information about some of the most commonly encountered childhood ailments, including asthma, influenza, bronchitis, ear infections, sore throats, impetigo, urinary tract infections, hernias, allergies, and many other infectious diseases and inflammatory disorders. It also offers basic facts about cancer, sickle cell disease, diabetes, and other chronic conditions in children. Frequently used diagnostic tests, surgeries, and medications are described, and facts about long-term care for seriously ill children are presented. A glossary and resource directory provide additional help and information.

Some concerns related to the topics in this book are addressed in greater detail in other volumes of the *Health Reference Series*. Parents seeking further information may find the following books helpful:

Adolescent Health Sourcebook

Allergies Sourcebook

Asthma Sourcebook

Attention Deficit Disorder Sourcebook

Colds, Flu, and Other Common Ailments Sourcebook

Congenital Disorders Sourcebook

Diabetes Sourcebook

Genetic Disorders Sourcebook

Infant and Toddler Health Sourcebook

Learning Disabilities Sourcebook

Mental Health Disorders Sourcebook

Mental Retardation Sourcebook

Pediatric Cancer Sourcebook

How to Use This Book

This book is divided into parts and chapters. Parts focus on broad areas of interest. Chapters are devoted to single topics within a part.

Part I: Introduction to Child Health provides an overview of the general health status of America's children. It describes common medical tests, explains how to take a child's temperature, and discusses concerns related to giving medication to children.

Part II: Common Respiratory Tract Ailments begins with a detailed discussion of asthma. Other individual chapters provide information about such disorders as bronchitis, croup, influenza, pneumonia, and tuberculosis.

Part III: Ailments of the Head, Throat, and Mouth presents facts about ear infections, labyrinthitis, sinusitis, gum disease, and cold sores. One chapter discusses special concerns related to headaches in children. Chapters pertaining to tonsil and adenoid problems are also included.

Part IV: Digestive and Genitourinary Diseases and Disorders offers information about vomiting and diarrhea as well as a variety of digestive disorders caused by bacteria, viruses, and parasites. It also discusses constipation, incontinence, and hernias.

Part V: Skin and Scalp Ailments provides information about disorders such as impetigo, tinea infections, warts, scabies, and fifth disease. The care of bites, scratches, and stings is discussed, and a chapter on head lice will help readers recognize the symptoms produced by these common pests.

Part VI: Other Infectious Disorders describes vaccine-preventable disorders, such as chickenpox, hepatitis, measles, mumps, rubella, and tetanus, and many other disorders caused by infectious agents.

Part VII: Chronic Conditions begins with a chapter providing information about how to care for a seriously ill child. It discusses specific illnesses and conditions with long-term care implications, such as autism, cancer, cerebral palsy, diabetes, epilepsy, and sickle cell disease.

Part VIII: Allergies provides detailed information about children's allergies to airborne substances, insects, food, and drugs. It also describes various methods of allergy testing.

Part IX: Additional Help and Information includes a glossary of terms related to childhood diseases, suggestions for additional reading, and a resource directory.

Bibliographic Note

This volume contains documents and excerpts from publications issued by the following U.S. government agencies: Centers for Disease Control and Prevention (CDC); Federal Interagency Forum on Child and Family Statistics; National Cancer Institute (NCI); National Diabetes Education Program (NDEP); National Digestive Diseases Information Clearinghouse (NDDIC); National Heart, Lung, and Blood Institute (NHLBI); National Information Center for Children and Youth with Disabilities; National Institute of Allergy and Infectious Diseases (NIAID); National Institute of Arthritis and Musculoskeletal and Skin Diseases (NIAMS); National Institute of Child Health and Human Development (NICHD); National Institute of Diabetes and Digestive and Kidney Diseases (NIDDK); National Institute of Mental Health (NIMH); National Institute of Neurological Disorders and Stroke (NINDS); National Institute on Deafness and Other Communication Disorders (NIDCD); National Institutes of Health (NIH);

National Kidney and Urologic Diseases Information Clearinghouse (NKUDIC); U.S. Environmental Protection Agency (EPA); and the U.S. Food and Drug Administration (FDA).

In addition, this volume contains copyrighted documents from the following organizations: A.D.A.M., Inc.; About.com, Inc.; American Academy of Allergy, Asthma, and Immunology; American Academy of Child and Adolescent Psychiatry; American Academy of Dermatology; American Academy of Family Physicians; American Academy of Otolaryngology–Head and Neck Surgery; American College of Chest Physicians; American Council for Headache Education; American Institute of Preventive Medicine; British Hernia Centre; California Poison Control System; Canadian Paediatric Society; Children's Hospital of the King's Daughters; Cincinnati Children's Hospital Medical Center; Cleveland Clinic; Community Health Services Department of the County of Lambton; Consumer Health Interactive, Inc.; Cooley's Anemia Foundation, Inc.; Epilepsy Foundation, Inc.; Illinois Department of Public Health; Iron Disorders Institute; Keep Kids Healthy, LLC; Lippincott, Williams, and Wilkins; Mamashealth.com; Medical College of Wisconsin; MedicineNet.com; Merck and Co., Inc.; Muscular Dystrophy Association; National Alliance for the Mentally Ill (NAMI); National Jewish Medical and Research Center; New Mexico AIDS InfoNet, University of New Mexico; Ohio State University Extension, Family and Consumer Sciences; Smiles4Ever; Texas Pediatric Surgical Associates; The Nemours Foundation (KidsHealth); Tufts University; and the University of Iowa, Virtual Children's Hospital.

Acknowledgements

Special thanks go to the many organizations, agencies, and individuals who have contributed material for this *Sourcebook* and to managing editor Karen Bellenir, verification assistant Dawn Matthews, and permissions specialist Liz Barbour.

Note from the Editor

This book is part of Omnigraphics' *Health Reference Series*. The series provides basic information about a broad range of medical concerns. It is not intended to serve as a tool for diagnosing illness, in prescribing treatments, or as a substitute for the physician/patient relationship. All persons concerned about medical symptoms or the possibility of disease are encouraged to seek professional care from an appropriate health care provider.

Our Advisory Board

The *Health Reference Series* is reviewed by an Advisory Board comprised of librarians from public, academic, and medical libraries. We would like to thank the following board members for providing guidance to the development of this series:

Dr. Lynda Baker,
Associate Professor of Library and Information Science,
Wayne State University, Detroit, MI

Nancy Bulgarelli,
William Beaumont Hospital Library, Royal Oak, MI

Karen Imarisio,
Bloomfield Township Public Library, Bloomfield Township, MI

Karen Morgan,
Mardigian Library, University of Michigan-Dearborn,
Dearborn, MI

Rosemary Orlando,
St. Clair Shores Public Library, St. Clair Shores, MI

Medical Consultant

Medical consultation services are provided to the *Health Reference Series* editors by David A. Cooke, MD. Dr. Cooke is a graduate of Brandeis University, and he received his M.D. degree from the University of Michigan. He completed residency training at the University of Wisconsin Hospital and Clinics. He is board-certified in Internal Medicine. Dr. Cooke currently works as part of the University of Michigan Health System and practices in Brighton, MI. In his free time, he enjoys writing, science fiction, and spending time with his family.

Health Reference Series *Update Policy*

The inaugural book in the *Health Reference Series* was the first edition of *Cancer Sourcebook* published in 1989. Since then, the *Series* has been enthusiastically received by librarians and in the medical community. In order to maintain the standard of providing high-quality health information for the layperson the editorial staff at Omnigraphics felt it was necessary to implement a policy of updating volumes when warranted.

Medical researchers have been making tremendous strides, and it is the purpose of the *Health Reference Series* to stay current with the most recent advances. Each decision to update a volume will be made on an individual basis. Some of the considerations will include how much new information is available and the feedback we receive from people who use the books. If there is a topic you would like to see added to the update list, or an area of medical concern you feel has not been adequately addressed, please write to:

Editor
Health Reference Series
Omnigraphics, Inc.
615 Griswold Street
Detroit, MI 48226
E-mail: editorial@omnigraphics.com

Part One

Introduction to Child Health

Chapter 1

General Health Status of America's Children

Health Indicators

- Children living in poverty tend to be in poorer health than children living in higher-income families. Nevertheless, this gap narrowed between 1984 and 2000. In 1984, 62 percent of children living in poverty and 83 percent of children living at or above poverty were reported to be in very good or excellent health. By 2000, 70 percent of children living in poverty and 85 percent of children living at or above poverty were in very good or excellent health.

- While the infant mortality rate did not decline in 1998, there was a significant drop in 1999, to 7 deaths per 1,000 live births.

- Mortality for children ages 5 to 14 declined between 1998 and 1999. However, there was no significant change in mortality rates for children ages 1 to 4, or for adolescents ages 15 to 19.

Nutrition

- In 2000, 0.8 percent of children lived in households reporting child hunger, down from 1.0 percent in 1998. In 2000, 18 percent

This chapter contains text from "America's Children: Key National Indicators of Well-Being, 2002," Federal Interagency Forum on Child and Family Statistics, 2002. Available online at http://www.childstats.gov/ac2002/highlight.asp and http://www.childstats.gov/ac2002/hea.asp.

of children lived in households reporting any level of food insecurity, down from 20 percent in 1998. Children in families below the poverty line were nearly three times more likely to experience food insecurity and hunger than children in families with incomes above the poverty line.

• According to the Healthy Eating Index, the proportion of children ages 2 to 5 with good diets improved from 21 percent to 27 percent between 1996 and 1998, reversing the decline from 1995 and 1996. However, the diet quality of children ages 6 to 9 changed little between 1996 and 1998. Children in families living in poverty were less likely than higher-income children to have a diet rated as good. In 1998, for children ages 2 to 5, 22 percent of those living in poverty had a good diet, compared with 29 percent of those living above the poverty line.

General Health Status

• The health of children and youth is basic to their well-being and optimal development. Parental reports of their children's health provide one indication of the overall health status of the Nation's children. This indicator measures the percentage of children whose parents report them to be in very good or excellent health.

• In 2000, about 82 percent of children were reported by their parents to be in very good or excellent health.

• Children under age 5 are slightly more likely to be in very good or excellent health than are children ages 5 to 17 (85 and 81 percent, respectively).

• White non-Hispanic children were more likely than black non-Hispanic and Hispanic children to be in very good or excellent health. In 2000, 86 percent of white non-Hispanic children were reported to be in very good or excellent health, compared with 74 percent of black non-Hispanic children and 75 percent of Hispanic children.

• Child health varies by family income. Children living below the poverty line are less likely than children in higher-income families to be in very good or excellent health. In 2000, about 70 percent of children in families below the poverty line were in very good or excellent health, compared with 85 percent of children in families living at or above the poverty line.

- Each year, children at or above the poverty line were substantially more likely to be in very good or excellent health than were children whose families were below the poverty line. However, the health gap between children below and those at or above the poverty line decreased slightly between 1984 and 2000.

Activity Limitation

- Having chronic conditions can limit a child's ability to participate in activities such as going to school, playing, and many other activities of children. Children whose activities are limited by one or more chronic health conditions may need more specialized health care than children without such limitations. Their medical costs are generally higher; they are more likely to miss days from school; and they may require special education services. Chronic conditions (such as asthma, hearing impairment, or diabetes) included in this measure usually have a duration of more than 3 months.

- In 2000, 7 percent of children ages 5 to 17 were limited in their activities because of one or more chronic health conditions, compared with 3 percent of children younger than 5. Children and youth ages 5 to 17 have much higher rates of activity limitation than younger children, partly because some chronic conditions are not diagnosed until children enter school and because the number of activities that children participate in increases with age.

- Children and youth in families of lower socioeconomic status (as measured by parental education and family income) have significantly higher rates of activity limitation than children in higher-status families. Among children and youth ages 5 to 17, 8 percent of children whose parents had less than a high school education had activity limitations due to chronic conditions in 2000, compared with 5 percent of children living with at least one parent who finished college.

- The difference in activity limitation by socioeconomic status is also present among preschool-age children. Children under age 5 in families below poverty had a higher rate of activity limitation than children in families at or above poverty.

- Males ages 5 to 17 were more likely than females in the same age group to have activity limitations (9 percent of boys compared with 5 percent of girls in 2000).

5

Childhood Immunization

- Adequate immunization protects children against several diseases that killed or disabled children in past decades. Rates of
  childhood immunization are one measure of the extent to which
  children are protected from serious vaccine-preventable illnesses.

- In 2000, 76 percent of children ages 19 to 35 months had received the recommended combined series of vaccines (often referred to as the 4:3:1:3 combined series).

- Children with family incomes below the poverty level had lower
  rates of coverage with the combined series than children with
  family incomes at or above the poverty line—71 percent of children below poverty compared with 78 percent of higher-income
  children.

- Rates of coverage with the full series of vaccines (4:3:1:3) were
  higher among white non-Hispanic children than among black
  non-Hispanic or Hispanic children. Seventy-nine percent of
  white non-Hispanic children ages 19 to 35 months received
  these immunizations compared with 71 percent of black non-
  Hispanic children and 73 percent of Hispanic children.

- Overall and for children living above and below the poverty
  level, coverage with the combined series remained relatively
  stable between 1999 and 2000, as did the gap in coverage between children in families living above and below the poverty
  level.

- Coverage with three or more doses of Hib vaccine among children ages 19 to 35 months remained relatively stable at 93 percent.

- In addition to the combined series of vaccines, there are other
  important immunizations such as those for Hib and varicella
  (chicken pox). Coverage with three or more doses of hepatitis B
  vaccine among children ages 19 to 35 months increased from 88
  percent in 1999 to 90 percent in 2000.

- Coverage with varicella (chicken pox) vaccine among children
  ages 19 to 35 months continued to increase from 58 percent in
  1999 to 68 percent in 2000. Gains in coverage for varicella vaccine were seen among all children regardless of race or ethnicity

and poverty level; however, children living at or above the poverty line had higher coverage levels.

Child Mortality

- Child death rates are the most severe measure of ill health in children. These rates have generally declined over the past two decades. Deaths to children ages 1 to 4 are calculated separately from those for children ages 5 to 14 because causes and death rates vary substantially by age.

- In 1999, the death rate for children ages 1 to 4 was 35 per 100,000 children.

- Between 1980 and 1999, the death rate declined by almost half for children ages 1 to 4.

- Among children ages 1 to 4, black children had the highest death rate in 1999, at 59 per 100,000 children. Asian/Pacific Islander children had the lowest death rate, at 23 per 100,000.

- Among children ages 1 to 4, unintentional injuries were the leading cause of death at 13 per 100,000, followed by birth defects at 4 per 100,000 and cancer at 3 per 100,000 children.

- Most unintentional injury deaths among children result from motor vehicle traffic crashes. Use of child restraint systems, including safety seats, booster seats, and seat belts, can greatly reduce the number and severity of injuries to child occupants of motor vehicles. In 1999, 47 percent of child occupants ages 1 to 4 who died in crashes were unrestrained.

- Death rates for children ages 5 to 14 are lower than those for children under age 5. The leading cause of death for children at this age remains unintentional injuries, but some other causes of death, such as birth defects, are less common among children ages 5 to 14 than among children ages 1 to 4.

- The death rate in 1999 for children ages 5 to 14 was 19 per 100,000 children.

- Between 1980 and 1999, the death rate declined by almost one-third, from 31 to 19 deaths per 100,000 children ages 5 to 14.

- Similar to mortality patterns for children under the age of 5, among children ages 5 to 14, black children had the highest death rates in 1999 at 29 deaths per 100,000, and Asians/Pacific Islanders had the lowest death rate at 12 per 100,000.

• Among children ages 5 to 14, unintentional injuries were the leading cause of death, followed by cancer, birth defects, and homicides.

• The majority of unintentional injury deaths among children ages 5 to 14 result from motor vehicle traffic crashes. More than 65 percent of children ages 5 to 14 who died in traffic crashes in 1999 were not wearing a seatbelt or other restraint.

Chapter 2

Common Medical Tests

Chapter Contents

Section 2.1

Understanding Medical Tests

The information in this section is reprinted with permission from *The Merck Manual of Medical Information—Home Edition*, pp. 1374-1380, edited by Mark H. Beers and Robert Berkow. Copyright 1997 by Merck & Co., Inc., Whitehouse Station, NJ; reprinted with permission. Available online at http://www.merck.com/pubs/mmanual_home.

A large number of laboratory tests are widely available. Many tests are specialized for a particular group of diseases. Many tests are used commonly in many specialties and in general practice.

Screening tests are used to try to detect a disease when there is little or no evidence that a person has the disease. For example, measuring cholesterol levels helps identify the risk of cardiovascular disease, but these tests are performed for people who have no symptoms of cardiovascular disease. To be useful, screening tests must be accurate, be relatively inexpensive, pose little risk, and cause little or no discomfort.

Diagnostic tests, on the other hand, are used when a disease is suspected. For example, a doctor who suspects serious heart disease might recommend cardiac catheterization. This test would not be a good screening test because it is expensive, can produce side effects, and is uncomfortable. However, all of these drawbacks are outweighed by the need for this test when disease must be evaluated.

Every test, whether used for screening or diagnosis, has some risk. The risk may be only the need for further testing if the result is abnormal, or it may be the possibility of injury during the test. Doctors weigh the risk of a test against the usefulness of the information it will provide.

No test is completely accurate. Sometimes a test result is incorrectly abnormal in a person who doesn't have the disease (a false-positive result). Sometimes a test result is incorrectly normal in a person who has the disease (a false-negative result). Tests are rated in terms of their sensitivity (the probability that their results will be positive when a disease is present) and their specificity (the probability that their results will be negative when a disease is not present). A very sensitive test is unlikely to miss the disease in people who have it. However, it may falsely indicate disease in healthy people. A very specific test is unlikely to indicate disease in healthy people. However, it may miss the disease in some who have it. Problems with sensitivity and specificity can be largely overcome by using several different tests. For example, a person who tests positive for AIDS with a very sensitive test is retested with another more specific one.

Routine blood testing is often misleading and may cause unnecessary anxiety and expense. When automated analyzers such as the Sequential Multiple Analyzer (SMA) are used to perform several blood tests, false-positive results are very common. By chance alone, at least one false-positive result is expected in almost half the people having 12 tests (SMA-12) and in two thirds of those having 20 tests (SMA-20). Because a doctor can't be sure whether a result in a particular person is false or true, a person with an abnormal result may need to be retested or undergo other tests.

Normal test result values are expressed as a range, which is based on the average values in a healthy population; 95 percent of healthy people have values within this range. These values vary somewhat among laboratories.

Table 2.1. Common Medical Tests (*continued on next page*)

Procedure	Body Area Tested	Description
Amniocentesis	Fluid from the sac surrounding the baby	Analysis of fluid to detect an abnormality in the fetus
Arteriography (angiography)	Any artery in the body; commonly in the brain, heart, kidneys, aorta, or legs	X-ray study to detect a blockage or defect of an artery
Audiometry	Ears	Assessment of the ability to hear and distinguish sounds at specific pitches and volumes
Auscultation	Heart	Listening with a stethoscope for abnormal heart sounds
Barium x-ray studies	Esophagus, stomach, duodenum, intestine	X-ray study to detect ulcers, tumors, or other abnormalities

Table 2.1. Common Medical Tests (*continued from previous page*)

Procedure	Body Area Tested	Description
Biopsy	Any tissue in body	Examination of tissue specimen under a microscope for cancer or another abnormality
Blood pressure measurement	Usually an arm	Test for high or low blood pressure
Blood tests	Usually a blood sample from an arm	Measurement of substances in the blood to evaluate organ function and to help diagnose and monitor various disorders
Bone marrow aspiration	Hipbone or breastbone	Examination of marrow under a microscope for abnormalities of blood cells
Bronchoscopy	Airways of the lungs	Direct visual inspection for a tumor or other abnormality
Cardiac catheterization	Heart	Study of heart function and structure
Chorionic villus sampling	Placenta	Examination of a sample under a microscope for an abnormality in the fetus
Chromosomal analysis	Blood	Examination under a microscope to detect a genetic disease or to determine a fetus' sex
Colonoscopy	Large intestine	Direct visual inspection for a tumor or other abnormality
Colposcopy	Cervix	Direct visual examination of the cervix with a magnifying lens
Computed tomography (CT)	Any part of body	Computer-enhanced x-ray study to detect structural abnormalities
Conization	Cervix	Removal of a cone-shaped piece of tissue for biopsy
Dilatation and curettage (D and C)	Cervix and uterus	Examination of a sample under a microscope for an abnormality of the uterine lining
Echocardiography	Heart	Study of heart structure and function using sound waves

Table 2.1. Common Medical Tests (*continued on next page*)

Procedure	Body Area Tested	Description
Electrocardiography (ECG)	Heart	Study of the heart's electrical activity
Electroenceph-alography (EEG)	Brain	Study of brain electrical function
Electromyography	Muscles	Recording of a muscle's electrical activity
Electrophysiologic testing	Heart	Test to evaluate rhythm or electrical conduction abnormalities
Endoscopic retrograde cholangiopancreatography (ERCP)	Biliary tract	X-ray study of the biliary tract after injection of a radiopaque substance using a fiber-optic tube
Endoscopy	Digestive system	Direct visual examination of internal structures using a fiber-optic tube
Fluoroscopy	Digestive system, heart, lungs	A continuous x-ray study that allows a doctor to see the inside of an organ as it functions
Hysteroscopy	Uterus	Direct visual examination of the inside of the uterus with a fiber-optic tube
Intravenous urography	Kidneys, urinary tract	X-ray study of the kidneys and urinary tract after intravenous injection of a radiopaque substance
Laparoscopy	Abdomen	Direct visual inspection for diagnosis and treatment of abnormalities in the abdomen
Magnetic resonance imaging (MRI)	Any part of body	Magnetic imaging test for any structural abnormality
Mammography	Breasts	X-ray study for breast cancer
Mediastinoscopy	Chest	Direct visual examination of the area of the chest between the lungs
Myelography	Spinal column	X-ray or computed tomography (CT) of the spinal column after injection of a radiopaque substance

13

Table 2.1. Common Medical Tests (*continued from previous page*)

Procedure	Body Area Tested	Description
Occult blood test	Stool	Test for blood in the stool
Ophthalmoscopy	Eyes	Direct visual inspection to detect abnormalities at the back of the eye
Papanicolaou (Pap) test	Cervix	Examination under a microscope of cells scraped from the cervix to detect cancer
Paracentesis	Abdomen	Insertion of a needle into the abdominal cavity to remove fluid for examination
Percutaneous transhepatic cholangiography	Liver, biliary tract	X-ray study of the liver and biliary tract after injection of a radiopaque substance into the liver
Positron emission tomography (PET)	Brain and heart	Radioactive imaging to detect abnormality of function
Pulmonary function tests	Lungs	Tests to measure the lungs' capacity to hold air, to move air in and out of the body, and to exchange oxygen and carbon dioxide
Radionuclide imaging	Many organs	Radioactive imaging to detect abnormalities of blood flow, structure, or function
Reflex tests	Tendons	Tests for abnormalities of nerve function
Retrograde urography	Bladder, ureters	X-ray study of the bladder and ureters after direct insertion of a radiopaque substance
Sigmoidoscopy	Rectum and lower intestine	Direct visual inspection to detect polyps or cancer
Skin allergy tests	Usually an arm or the back	Tests for allergies
Spinal tap	Spinal canal	Test for abnormalities of spinal fluid
Spirometry	Lungs	Test of lung function involving blowing into a measuring device

Table 2.1. Common Medical Tests (*continued from previous page*)

Procedure	Body Area Tested	Description
Stress test (exercise tolerance)	Heart	Test of heart function with exertion
Thoracentesis	Pleural fluid	Removal of fluid from the chest with a needle to detect abnormalities
Thoracoscopy	Lungs	Examination of the lungs through a viewing tube
Tympanometry	Ears	Measurement of the impedance (resistance to pressure) of the middle ear which helps in determining the cause of hearing loss
Ultrasonography (ultrasound scanning)	Any part of body	Ultrasound imaging to detect structural or functional abnormalities
Urinalysis	Urine	Chemical analysis of urine specimen to detect protein, sugar, ketones, and blood cells
Venography	Veins	X-ray study to detect blockage of a vein

Section 2.2

Urine Tests

Excerpted from "Urinalysis," © 1998 MedicineNet, Inc.
(http://www.medicinenet.com), reprinted with permission.

Questions and Answers about Urinalysis

What is a urinalysis?

A urinalysis is simply an analysis of the urine.

What can a urinalysis show?

Urinalysis can disclose evidence of diseases, even some that have not caused significant signs or symptoms. Therefore, a urinalysis is commonly a part of routine health screening.

Examples of diseases that can be detected by urinalysis include diabetes mellitus, kidney diseases such as glomerulonephritis, and chronic infections of the urinary tract.

What does urinalysis involve?

Urinalysis consists of macroscopic urinalysis, urine dipstick chemical analysis, and microscopic urinalysis.

What is macroscopic urinalysis?

Macroscopic urinalysis is the direct visual observation of the urine, noting its quantity, color, clarity or cloudiness, etc.

What is urine dipstick chemical analysis?

This microchemistry system permits qualitative (yes/no) and semi-quantitative analysis within a minute by simple observation. The color change occurring on each segment of a dipstick is read by being compared to a color chart.

Dipsticks can, for example, be used to determine the urine's pH (acidity), specific gravity (density), protein content, glucose, ketones, nitrite content, and to determine an estimate of the number of white blood cells in the urine.

What are the pros and cons of dip sticks?

Dipsticks, whether they be paper or plastic, have many advantages. They are simple, fast, convenient, easy to use, and they are the most cost-effective way to screen urine.

However, what can be learned from a dipstick is limited by the design of the dipstick.

What is microscopic urinalysis?

The microscopic urinalysis is the study of the urine under the microscope. It requires only a relatively inexpensive light microscope.

How is microscopic urinalysis done?

The sample of urine is prepared in the laboratory and a drop of the urine sediment is put onto a glass slide.

First, the sediment is examined through the microscope under low-power to identify what are called casts, crystals, squamous (flat) cells, and other large objects.

Examination is then performed through the microscope at high power to further identify any cells, bacteria, and clumps of cells or debris called casts.

What kind of cells can be detected?

Epithelial (flat cells) and red and white blood cells may be seen in the urine.

What can the presence of red blood cells in the urine mean?

Red blood cells can enter the urine from the vagina in menstruation or from the trauma of bladder catheterization.

Red blood cells in the urine otherwise may be due to many causes including kidney damage, tumors eroding the urinary tract, stones, and urinary tract infections.

What can the presence of white blood cells in the urine mean?

White cells from the vagina or the opening of the urethra (in males, too) can contaminate a urine sample. Such contamination aside, the presence of abnormal numbers of white blood cells in the urine is important.

It can mean there is kidney disease or an infection of the kidney, bladder, or urinary tubes (upper or lower urinary tract). The presence of abnormal numbers of white cells in the urine is referred to as pyuria (pus in the urine).

Section 2.3

Stool Tests

"Stool Collection: Hemoccult Test," ©1998 Cincinnati Children's Hospital Medical Center; reprinted with permission. Additional information is available online from Cincinnati Children's Hospital Medical Center at http://www.cincinnatichildrens.org/Health_Topics/Your_Childs_Health.

Why Is a Stool Collection Needed?

Lab testing is done on stool to detect bacterial, parasitic, and viral infections. Stool can also be tested for blood. This testing enables the doctor to appropriately treat your child's illness. A Hemoccult test looks for hidden blood in stool samples. This test will not be painful to your child.

Procedure

- If you have a test card, collect a small amount of stool on a cotton swab and apply a thin smear to the card.

- Collect another small amount of stool on a cotton swab and apply a thin smear on the card, next to the first sample.

- Close, cover, and label specimens.

- The specimen may be collected with the aid of a container or toilet tissue.

- Keep the specimen at room temperature and bring it to the clinic or doctor's office within 14 days.

- If you do not have a test card, you must bring your child's fresh stool to the lab within 2 hours after you have taken the sample.

- Important: Please keep urine from mixing with stool.

Tips

False positive reactions can occur if your child's diet is high in red meat, processed meat and liver, and raw fruits and vegetables.

Be sure to protect your child's Hemoccult test card from light, heat, and volatile chemicals. Store completed slides at controlled room temperature (59–86° F [15–30° C]).

Section 2.4

Blood Tests

This chapter contains text from "Complete Blood Count," reviewed April 2002, and "Thyroid Blood Tests," reviewed April 2002, both © 2002 MedicineNet, Inc. (http://www.medicinenet.com); reprinted with permission.

Complete Blood Count

What is the complete blood count test?

The complete blood count is the calculation of the cellular (formed) elements of blood. These calculations are generally determined by specially designed machines that analyze the different components of blood in less than a minute.

A major portion of the complete blood count is the measure of the concentration of white blood cells, red blood cells, and platelets in the blood. The complete blood count (also called CBC) is generated by testing a simple blood sample.

What are values for a complete blood count?

The values generally included are the following:

- *White blood cell count (WBC).* The number of white blood cells in a volume of blood. Normal range varies slightly between laboratories but is generally between 4,300 and 10,800 cells per cubic millimeter (cmm). This can also be referred to as the leukocyte count and can be expressed in international units as 4.3–10.8 x 10^9 cells per liter.

- *Automated white cell differential.* A machine generated percentage of the different types of white blood cells, usually split into granulocytes, lymphocytes, monocytes, eosinophils, and basophils.

- *Red cell count (RBC).* The number of red blood cells in a volume of blood. Normal range varies slightly between laboratories but is generally between 4.2–5.9 million cells/cmm. This can also be referred to as the erythrocyte count and can be expressed in international units as 4.2–5.9 x 10^{12} cells per liter.

- *Hemoglobin (Hb).* The amount of hemoglobin in a volume of blood. Hemoglobin is the protein molecule within red blood cells that carries oxygen and gives blood its red color. Normal range for hemoglobin is different between the sexes and is approximately 13–18 grams per deciliter for men and 12–16 for women (international units 8.1–11.2 millimoles/liter for men, 7.4–9.9 for women).

- *Hematocrit (Hct).* The ratio of the volume of red cells to the volume of whole blood. Normal range for hematocrit is different between the sexes and is approximately 45–52% for men and 37–48% for women.

- *Mean cell volume (MCV).* The average volume of a red cell. This is a calculated value derived from the hematocrit and red cell count. Normal range is 86–98 femtoliters.

- *Mean cell hemoglobin (MCH).* The average amount of hemoglobin in the average red cell. This is a calculated value derived from the measurement of hemoglobin and the red cell count. Normal range is 27–32 picograms.

- *Mean cell hemoglobin concentration (MCHC).* The average concentration of hemoglobin in a given volume of red cells. This is a calculated volume derived from the hemoglobin measurement and the hematocrit. Normal range is 32–36%.

- *Red cell distribution width (RDW).* A measurement of the variability of red cell size. Higher numbers indicate greater variation in size. Normal range is 11–15.

- *Platelet count.* The number of platelets in a volume blood. Platelets are not complete cells, but actually fragments of cytoplasm from a cell found in the bone marrow called a megakaryocyte. Platelets play a vital role in blood clotting. Normal range varies slightly between laboratories but is in the range of 150,000–400,000/cmm (150–400 x 10^9/liter).

Thyroid Blood Tests

The thyroid gland produces hormones that are essential for normal body metabolism. Blood testing is now commonly available to determine the adequacy of the levels of thyroid hormones. These blood tests can define whether the thyroid gland's hormone production is normal, overactive, or underactive.

What are thyroid hormones?

Thyroid hormones are produced by the thyroid gland. This gland is located in the lower part of the neck, below the Adam's apple. The gland wraps around the windpipe (trachea) and has a shape that is similar to a butterfly—formed by two wings (lobes) and attached by a middle part (isthmus).

The thyroid gland uses iodine (mostly available from the diet in foods such as seafood, bread, and salt) to produce thyroid hormones. The two most important thyroid hormones are thyroxine (T4) and triiodothyronine (T3), which account for 99.9% and 0.1% of thyroid hormones present in the blood respectively. However, the hormone with the most biological activity is T3. Once released from the thyroid gland into the blood, a large amount of T4 is converted into T3—the active hormone that affects the metabolism of cells.

The thyroid itself is regulated by another gland that is located in the brain, called the pituitary. In turn, the pituitary is regulated in part by the thyroid (via a feedback effect of thyroid hormone on the pituitary gland) and by another gland called the hypothalamus.

The hypothalamus releases a hormone called thyrotropin releasing hormone (TRH), which sends a signal to the pituitary to release thyroid stimulating hormone (TSH). In turn, TSH sends a signal to the thyroid to release thyroid hormones. If a disruption occurs at any of these levels, a defect in thyroid hormone production may result in a deficiency of thyroid hormone (hypothyroidism).

The rate of thyroid hormone production is controlled by the pituitary gland. If there is an insufficient amount of thyroid hormone circulating in the body to allow for normal functioning, the release of TSH is increased by the pituitary gland in an attempt to stimulate more thyroid hormone production. In contrast, when there is an excessive amount of circulating thyroid hormone, TSH levels fall as the pituitary attempts to decrease the production of thyroid hormone. In persons with hypothyroidism (thyroid hormone production is below normal), there is a continuously decreased level of circulating thyroid hormones. In persons with hyperthyroidism (thyroid hormone production is above normal), there is a continuously elevated level of circulating thyroid hormones.

How is hypothyroidism diagnosed?

A diagnosis of hypothyroidism can be suspected in patients with fatigue, cold intolerance, constipation, and dry, flaky skin. A blood test is needed to confirm the diagnosis.

When hypothyroidism is present, the blood levels of thyroid hormones can be measured directly and are usually decreased. However, in early hypothyroidism, the level of thyroid hormones (T3 and T4) may be normal. Therefore, the main tool for the detection of hyperthyroidism is the measurement of the TSH, the thyroid stimulating hormone. As mentioned earlier, TSH is secreted by the pituitary gland. If a decrease of thyroid hormone occurs, the pituitary gland reacts by producing more TSH and the blood TSH level increases in an attempt to encourage thyroid hormone production. This increase in TSH can actually precede the fall in thyroid hormones by months or years. Thus, the measurement of TSH should be elevated in cases of hypothyroidism. However, there is one exception. If the decrease in thyroid hormone is actually due to a defect of the pituitary or hypothalamus, then the levels of TSH are abnormally low. As noted above, this kind of thyroid disease is known as secondary or tertiary hypothyroidism. A special test, known as the TRH (thyrotropin-releasing hormone) test, can help distinguish if the disease is caused by a defect in the pituitary or the hypothalamus. This test requires an injection of the TRH hormone and is performed by an endocrinologist (hormone specialist).

How is hyperthyroidism diagnosed?

Hyperthyroidism can be suspected in patients with tremors, excessive sweating, smooth, velvety skin, fine hair, a rapid heart rate, and an enlarged thyroid gland. There may be puffiness around the eyes and a characteristic stare due to the elevation of the upper eyelids.

Advanced symptoms are easily detected, but early symptoms, especially in the elderly, may be quite inconspicuous. In all cases, a blood test is needed to confirm the diagnosis.

The blood levels of thyroid hormones can be measured directly and are usually elevated with this disease. However, the main tool for detection of hyperthyroidism is measurement of the blood TSH level. As mentioned earlier, TSH is secreted by the pituitary gland. If an excess amount of thyroid hormone is present, TSH is down-regulated, and the level of TSH falls in an attempt to control thyroid hormone production. Thus, the measurement of TSH should result in low or undetectable levels in cases of hyperthyroidism. However, there is one exception. If the excessive amount of thyroid hormone is actually due to a TSH secreting pituitary tumor, then the levels are abnormally high. This uncommon disease is known as secondary hyperthyroidism.

Are there other tests of the thyroid gland?

The blood tests mentioned above can confirm the presence of deficiency or an excess of thyroid hormone and, therefore, be used to diagnose hypothyroidism or hyperthyroidism. They do not point to a specific cause. In order to determine a cause of the thyroid abnormality, the doctor will consider the patient's history, physical examination, and medical condition. Further testing might be used to isolate an underlying cause. These tests might include more blood testing for thyroid antibodies, nuclear medicine thyroid scanning, ultrasound of the thyroid gland, or others.

Chapter 3

Taking Your Child's Temperature

When your child is sick with an infection (caused by either bacteria or a virus), it is normal to have a fever. A fever will not hurt your child. Usually, it goes away after 72 hours (3 days).

Babies younger than 6 months old should see a doctor when they have a fever. Older children can be treated at home, as long as they get enough liquids and seem well otherwise.

There are several ways to take your child's temperature:

- Rectal method (by the rectum or 'bum')
- Oral method (through the mouth)
- Axillary method (under the armpit)
- Tympanic method (in the ear)

The right method depends on your child's age. And it's important that the measurement is accurate. For instance, taking a rectal temperature is the best way to get an exact reading for children under 2 years of age. But most children don't like to have their temperature taken this way. Although taking a temperature under the armpit isn't as precise, it will let you know whether your child has a fever. If so, you can then take a rectal temperature for the exact reading.

Excerpted from "How to Take a Child's Temperature," © 2000 Canadian Paediatric Society (http://www.caringforkids.cps.ca); reprinted with permission. The full text of this document is available online at http://www.caringfor kids.cps.ca/whensick/temperature.htm.

Table 3.1 will help you decide which method to use.

Table 3.1. Techniques for taking temperature in children.

Age	Recommended technique
Birth to 2 years	First choice: Rectum (for an exact reading)
	Second choice: Armpit (to check for fever)
Between 2 and 5 years	First choice: Rectum
	Second choice: Ear
	Third choice: Armpit
Older than 5 years	First choice: Mouth
	Second choice: Ear
	Third choice: Armpit

Temperature Taking Tips

To get an accurate reading of your child's temperature, you'll need to make sure it's done right. Here are some tips to help you.

Rectum

If you are using a glass thermometer, be sure that it is a rectal thermometer (the bulb is fatter than on an oral thermometer).

- Clean the thermometer with cool, soapy water and rinse.
- Shake it so that the mercury inside goes below 36° C (96.8° F).
- Cover the silver tip with petroleum jelly (such as Vaseline).
- Place your baby on his back with his knees bent.
- Gently insert the thermometer in the rectum, about 2.5 cm (1 inch), while holding it with your fingers.
- After at least 2 minutes, remove the thermometer and read the temperature.
- Clean the thermometer.

Mouth

Because a glass thermometer can break if a child bites down on it, this method is not recommended for children younger than 5 years old.

- Clean the thermometer with cool, soapy water and rinse.
- Shake the thermometer so that the mercury inside goes below 36° C (96.8° F).
- Carefully place the tip of the thermometer under your child's tongue.
- With your child's mouth closed, leave the thermometer in place for 3 to 4 minutes.
- Remove the thermometer and read the temperature.
- Clean the thermometer.

Armpit

This method is usually used to check for fever in newborns and young children. If your child is under 2 years of age, and you find a fever, confirm it by taking a rectal temperature.

- Use a rectal or oral thermometer.
- Clean the thermometer with cool, soapy water and rinse.
- Shake the thermometer so that the mercury inside goes below 36° C (96.8° F).
- Place the tip of the thermometer in the center of the armpit.
- Make sure your child's arm is tucked snugly against her body.
- Leave the thermometer in place for at least 4 minutes.
- Remove the thermometer and read the temperature.
- Clean the thermometer.

Ear

- Use a clean probe tip each time, and follow the manufacturer's instructions carefully.
- Gently tug on the ear, pulling it up and back. This will help straighten the ear canal, and make a clear path inside the ear to the ear drum.

- Gently insert the thermometer until the ear canal is fully sealed off.

- Squeeze and hold down the button for one second.

- Remove the thermometer and read the temperature.

What Is a Normal Temperature?

Now that you've taken the temperature, check the following chart to see whether your child has a fever. The normal temperature range varies, depending on what method you used.

Table 3.2. Temperature ranges for different measurement methods.

Measurement method	Normal temperature range
Rectum	36.6° C to 38° C (97.9° F to 100.4° F)
Mouth	35.5° C to 37.5° C (95.9° F to 99.5° F)
Armpit	34.7° C to 37.3° C (94.5° F to 99.1° F)
Ear	35.8° C to 38° C (96.4° F to 100.4° F)

Chapter 4

Your Child and Medication

If you are planning to have a doctor see your child, you should share a record of any of your child's medical problems, any medications your child is taking, including over-the-counter medications or vitamin and herbal supplements, and any allergic reactions your child has suffered. If a medication is prescribed for your child, there are certain questions you should ask. It will be helpful to take notes as it is easy to forget exactly what the doctor says.

- What is the name of the medication and how will it help my child? Is the medicine available in both brand-name and generic versions, and is it all right to use the less expensive (generic) medication? What is the name of the generic version? Is it all right to switch among brands, or between brand-name and generic forms?

- What is the proper dosage for my child? Is the dose likely to change as he or she grows?

- What if my child has a problem with the pill or capsule? Is it available in a chewable tablet or liquid form?

- How many times a day must the medicine be given? Should it be taken with meals, or on an empty stomach? Should the school give the medication during the day?

Excerpted from "Your Child and Medication," National Institute of Mental Health (NIMH), updated June 17, 2001. More information from NIMH is available online at www.nimh.nih.gov.

- How long must my child take this medication? If it is discontinued, should it be done all at once or slowly?

- Will my child be monitored while on this medication and, if so, by whom?

- Should my child have any laboratory tests before taking this medication? Will it be necessary to have blood levels checked or have other laboratory tests during the time my child is taking this medication?

- Should my child avoid certain foods, other medications, or activities while using this medication?

- Are there possible side effects? If I notice a side effect—such as unusual sleepiness, agitation, fatigue, hand tremors—should I notify the doctor at once?

- What if my child misses a dose? Spits it up?

- How well established and accepted is the use of this medication in children or adolescents?

You may think of other questions. Don't be afraid to ask. When you have the prescription filled, be sure the pharmacist gives you a flyer describing the medication, how it should be taken, and any possible side effects it may have. The label on the medication will have lots of information. Read the label carefully before giving the medication to your child. The label will give the name of the pharmacy, its telephone number, the name of the medication, the dosage, and when it should be taken. It will also tell you how many times the medication can be refilled.

If you want to learn more about your child's medication, you will find helpful books at your public library, or the reference librarian can show you how to look up the medication in the *Physicians' Desk Reference (PDR)*.

Help Your Child Take Medication Safely

- Be sure the doctor knows all medications—including over-the-counter medications and herbal and vitamin supplements—that your child takes.

- Read the label before opening the bottle. Make sure you are giving the proper dosage. If the medication is liquid, use a special measure—a cup, a teaspoon, a medicine dropper, or a syringe.

Often a measure comes with the medicine. If not, ask your pharmacist which measure is most suitable to use with the medication your child is taking.

- Always use child-resistant caps and store all medications in a safe place.

- Never decide to increase or decrease the dosage or stop the medication without consulting the doctor.

- Don't give medication prescribed for one child to another child, even if it appears to be the same problem.

- Keep a chart and mark it each time the child takes the medication. It is easy to forget.

Resources

A Guide to Children's Medications
American Academy of Pediatrics
Website: http://www.aap.org/family/medications.htm

Facts for Families
A series of informative fact sheets that include information on medications for children, health insurance, how to seek help, etc.
American Academy of Child and Adolescent Psychiatry
Website: http://www.aacap.org/publications/factsfam/index.htm

How to Give Medicine to Children
Food and Drug Administration
Website: http://www.fda.gov/fdac/features/196_kid.html

Chapter 5

Why Aspirin Should Not Be Given to Children: Reye Syndrome

Each year between March 1951 and March 1962, the Royal Alexandra Hospital for Children in New South Wales, Australia, admitted one or two children in such a critical state that most of them could not be saved, despite the most advanced medical care.

The cases had a number of unusual features in common. When admitted, all but two of the 21 children were in a coma or stupor, although their illness had started out a few days or weeks earlier with only common childhood upper respiratory symptoms—usually cough, sore throat, runny nose, or earache. Some children had even appeared to be recovering before the more serious phase of the illness began, with fever, relentless vomiting, convulsions, wild delirium, screaming, intense irritability, and violent movements.

Seventeen of the children died within an average of 27 hours after admission. At autopsy, all were found to have brain swelling, a slightly enlarged, firm and uniformly bright yellow liver, and a change in the appearance of the kidneys. Douglas Reye, M.D., the hospital's director of pathology, and his colleagues believed this set of symptoms represented a distinct disease, which they called fatty degeneration of the viscera (internal organs) of unknown cause. Though they suspected that ingestion of drugs or poisons may have been responsible

Excerpted from "Reye Syndrome, The Decline of a Disease," by Evelyn Zamula, *FDA Consumer*, Food and Drug Administration (FDA) Pub. No. 94-1172, June 1994. Updated in December 2000 by Dr. David A. Cooke, MD, Diplomate, American Board of Internal Medicine.

33

for the condition, an investigation into the children's homes revealed they had no access to these substances.

In 1963, George Johnson, M.D., and his coworkers reported an epidemic of 16 fatal cases of an encephalitis-like disease occurring within a four-month period during an outbreak of influenza B in a small North Carolina community. Although children in this group were older than those studied by Reye, and their preceding illness was flu, it was subsequently theorized from Johnson's description of the symptoms and postmortem findings that several of the children who died may have also had the syndrome described by Reye. It became known as Reye-Johnson syndrome, though it's usually referred to as Reye (pronounced rye) syndrome.

After the Reye-Johnson reports were published, numerous reports came in from the United States and other parts of the world showing that the syndrome was both more widespread and more common than was thought. Though this was not a new disease—it had been reported as early as 1929—for the first time it had been identified and characterized as a distinct entity.

During the 1960s and 70s, when regional and then national surveillance of Reye syndrome was established by the Atlanta-based Centers for Disease Control (now the Centers for Disease Control and Prevention or CDC), scientists observed that the syndrome occurred in association with outbreaks of the flu, especially influenza B. They also noted that it followed chickenpox, with children aged 5 to 15 most often affected. Less often it was associated with other viruses and acute respiratory and diarrheal illnesses.

Reye Syndrome Symptoms

In most cases, children seem to be recovering from a viral illness when the following symptoms occur:

- nausea

- vomiting, usually very severe

- fever

- lethargy

- stupor or coma, sometimes followed by convulsions

- wild delirium and unusual restlessness noted in about half of patients

How the Illness Progresses

The course of the illness is variable. Reye syndrome can be mild and self-limiting, or it can progress rapidly, causing death within hours of onset, usually from brain swelling. But the progression may also stop at any stage, with complete recovery in 5 to 10 days and the quick return of normal liver function.

Doctors classify stages of Reye syndrome based on the level of the patient's consciousness and corresponding physical signs. Stages 0 to 2 are pre-comatose, with lethargy or delirium, and sometimes combativeness, but with the child still responding to stimuli. Coma progressively deepens in stages 3 to 5; the child is unresponsive to stimuli, and heart and lung function begin to shut down.

The earlier the diagnosis and treatment, the better the chance for survival. Intense supportive care in a hospital experienced in dealing with Reye syndrome also improves odds. Children who survive but experience the most severe stages of the illness—especially infants— are sometimes left with neurological abnormalities, often mental retardation or disorders of voice and speech.

Fatality rates when national surveillance began on a regular basis in 1976 were as high as 40 percent, declined to between 20 and 30 percent from 1978 to 1987, but rose in 1988 and have stayed between 40 and 53 percent ever since. CDC experts speculate that these higher death rates despite fewer reports each year may reflect decreasing interest in the syndrome—because of its rarity—resulting in the reporting of only the most serious cases.

The Aspirin Connection

Just as Reye suspected that a drug or poison may have triggered the disease's development, investigators in the United States looked for some common factor among children who developed the syndrome. They found it in aspirin taken during flu or chickenpox.

In 1980, results of studies conducted in Ohio, Michigan, and Arizona demonstrated an association between Reye syndrome and aspirin use during a preceding respiratory tract or chickenpox infection.

"It was those initial studies that we reviewed in 1980 that first led CDC to report in its *Morbidity and Mortality Weekly Report* (*MMWR*) that there was an association," states Lawrence B. Schonberger, M.D., an epidemiologist with the agency. In 1981, CDC reported in *MMWR* results of a fourth study that revealed the same association. In 1982, the Surgeon General of the U.S. Public Health Service

35

issued a warning against giving aspirin to children with flu or chickenpox.

The public was quick to pick up on the association. "A kind of natural study was occurring, because once people heard about the results [of the studies], they started to lower the use of aspirin in their children," says Schonberger. "If aspirin had nothing to do with it [Reye syndrome], then one might anticipate that there would be no clear decrease in the incidence of Reye syndrome."

That's not what happened. Aspirin use in children under 10 declined by at least 50 percent from 1981 to 1988, and the number of Reye syndrome cases went down correspondingly. In the opinion of Peter C. Rowe, M.D., assistant professor of pediatrics, Children's Hospital of Eastern Canada, Ottawa, Ontario, the declining use of aspirin and the decreasing incidence of Reye syndrome represent a "natural ecological experiment."

When Is It Reye?

Many toxic substances (such as carbon tetrachloride, phosphorus and alcohol) and other diseases (such as acute hepatitis and viral encephalitis) can produce symptoms like Reye syndrome. Since most physicians were completely unfamiliar with the syndrome at the time, they needed to know what constituted a positive diagnosis. CDC established case definitions for regional surveillance and outbreak investigations in the late 1960s. Criteria for a case included mental status changes, such as delirium or coma, and a liver biopsy (tissue sample) showing fat accumulation in the liver (or high levels of liver enzymes and ammonia in the blood). There also needed to be no other more reasonable explanation for the brain or liver abnormalities.

Records show that Reye syndrome has affected an infant as young as 4 days old and has occurred in a 59-year-old man; however, more than 90 percent of reported cases are in children under 15. About 2 percent are in adults over 20.

Other Government Actions

The federal government made other moves. To confirm the preliminary findings of the state studies, in 1985–1986 the government sponsored the "Public Health Service Study of Reye's Syndrome and Medications." Twenty-seven children who developed Reye syndrome after a preceding respiratory illness or chickenpox were matched with 140 children who had had the same illnesses at the same time, but did not develop Reye syndrome. More than 96 percent of the Reye syndrome cases, compared with 38 percent of the controls (the children who did not develop Reye syndrome), had received aspirin (or other salicylates) to treat the preceding illness. The study was prematurely ended because not enough Reye syndrome children who had not been exposed to aspirin could be found to justify the expense of continuing the investigation, in itself an indication of a public health triumph.

In 1986, the Food and Drug Administration (FDA) adopted a preliminary rule requiring aspirin manufacturers to add warnings to product labels about the possible association between aspirin use and the development of Reye syndrome. The permanent rule became final in 1988, and the labeling reads: "Children and teenagers should not use this medicine for chicken pox or flu symptoms before a doctor is consulted about Reye syndrome, a rare but serious illness reported to be associated with aspirin."

The number of Reye syndrome cases, which reached a high in 1980 with 555 cases, has steadily decreased, compared with years in which there has been similar types of influenza activity. The decline has been most dramatic among children from 5 to 10 years of age. In fact, Reye syndrome has now become sufficiently rare that many younger pediatric intensive care physicians have never seen the disease. The reasons for this sharp drop-off in cases are not entirely known. However, public health efforts to reduce aspirin use in sick children, and improved accuracy of diagnosis have been frequently credited.

Other Factors?

Some questions about the relationship between aspirin and Reye syndrome still remain. Although figures show that 90 to 95 percent of Reye syndrome patients in the United States have taken aspirin during a preceding viral illness, it is estimated that less than 0.1 percent of children having a viral infection and treated with aspirin develop the syndrome. Are other factors involved?

Apparently so. Reye syndrome has always been a puzzling disease. Research on possible causes has been hampered because no one can come up with a simple specific diagnostic test for the syndrome. The waters are further muddied by the existence of at least 19 viruses, including the chickenpox and flu viruses, which cause infectious illnesses that can precede Reye syndrome development. Some experts have proposed that Reye syndrome develops from the interaction of a viral illness, genetic susceptibility to the disease, and exposure to chemicals, such as salicylates, pesticides, and aflatoxin. Others speculate that unidentified viruses or other infectious agents are involved. That some children may be more susceptible to Reye syndrome than others has been shown by cases appearing among children in the same family and by recurrent episodes of the illness in the same child. It is possible that more than one type of Reye syndrome exists, or that some of these cases may not be Reye syndrome at all.

Reye-Like Disorders

In the light of what we know now, it is questionable whether all of Dr. Reye's cases were true Reye syndrome. During the 1980s and 1990s, understanding of hereditary metabolic diseases, as well as the means to diagnose them, advanced dramatically. It became clear that many of these conditions could produce symptoms very similar to Reye syndrome. With new diagnostic methods, up to half of cases formerly classified as Reye syndrome were shown to have another explanation. Retrospective studies have shown that some patients treated years earlier were misdiagnosed. The original CDC criteria for diagnosis of Reye syndrome were shown to be too broad, and several new classification systems were developed.

Still, metabolic disorders do not appear to account for all of Reye syndrome diagnoses. Studies demonstrating the association of aspirin use and Reye syndrome have stood up to intense scrutiny. Most experts still believe Reye is a distinct disease, albeit now a rare one.

Someday, the controversy may be fully laid to rest. Until then, it's important to remember that aspirin use during flu or chickenpox is asking for trouble.

In Schonberger's words: "The association between aspirin and Reye syndrome is so strong that it has now become literally foolhardy to act as if no etiologic (cause-and-effect) relationship exists."

—by Evelyn Zamula

Evelyn Zamula is a freelance writer in Potomac, MD.

Chapter 6

Iron Supplements and Iron Poisoning

Iron is important for good nutrition because it is used in blood and muscle tissue. However, it is also very poisonous if too much is taken. Each year, there are over 3,500 iron poisonings in children under the age of 6 years. It is also one of the most frequent causes of poisoning death in children.

Why is iron poisoning common?

First, iron supplements are found in many homes with small children. Iron is available in numerous over-the-counter and prescription tablets and liquids, such as ferrous sulfate, ferrous gluconate and ferrous fumarate. It is also found in many multivitamin preparations for both children and adults. Finally, pregnant women are often prescribed prenatal vitamins that have high amounts of iron. Prenatal vitamins are often kept around the house after the pregnant woman stops taking them.

Second, many people are not aware that iron can be dangerous. It may be regarded as "just a vitamin" or as a nutritional product instead of a medicine.

Third, iron tablets may be attractive to a young child. This is certainly true of the chewable children's vitamins with iron that are often in cartoon shapes with various colors and fruit flavors. The much more dangerous adult formulations contain more iron and often look like brightly colored candies to young children.

What happens in an iron overdose?

When someone takes too much iron, the first effect is irritation and ulceration of the stomach lining. This results in nausea, abdominal pain, and vomiting as early as 20 minutes after the ingestion. This can be followed by an apparent recovery, which is very deceptive because a few hours later the person can go into profound shock with a severe blood chemistry imbalance. When too much iron gets into the bloodstream, it goes to all the organs and can damage the stomach, liver, kidneys, lungs, blood vessels and brain.

What should I do in case of an iron poisoning?

If there is a possibility that a child (or anyone) took too much iron, immediately contact the Poison Control Center. This is very important, even if the patient seems to be doing fine. The poison specialist will determine if treatment is necessary. You will be advised what to do for the child at home or, if necessary, you will be directed to take the child to a nearby hospital. Treatment for iron poisoning may include removing iron from the stomach, checking a blood level and, when needed, giving a chelating agent to bind up the iron in the bloodstream and help eliminate it from the body.

Part Two

Common
Respiratory Tract Ailments

Chapter 7

Asthma

Chapter Contents

Section 7.1

Asthma Basics

Excerpted from "Controlling Asthma," by Ken Flieger, *FDA Consumer*,
November 1996, http://www.fda.gov/fdac/features/996_asth.html,
revised June 2000.

Think of someone—a child or an adult—racked by uncontrolled
coughing. With a heaving, distended chest, neck muscles straining, and
eyes showing alarm verging on panic, the person can utter only a few
brief words between rasping, wheezing, frantic efforts to breathe.

The person puts a tube-like device in his or her mouth and inhales
twice. Within minutes, remarkably it seems, the crisis is over. Breathing
returns to normal. The person can go back to school or work or even
jogging—until the next attack, which might be hours or months away.

Asthma attacks are often milder than this description—just a
shortness of breath that soon passes without treatment. But they can
also be much, much worse, requiring a hurried trip to the hospital for
emergency—sometimes lifesaving—care. Even in severe cases, hospital treatment usually enables asthma patients to regain near-normal
breathing. But not always.

Inflamed Airways

Most of America's estimated 17 million people with asthma, of
whom almost 5 million are under age 18, are mildly affected. About a
quarter of asthmatic children seem to "outgrow" their disease in their
teen years or as young adults. It's not certain, however, that they are
completely free of asthma. Studies of people with late-onset asthma—
asthma that first shows up in the fifth or sixth decade of life or even
later—have found that many of them experienced asthma-like breathing difficulties as children.

There is no known cure, but asthma often can be well-controlled
by a strategy aimed at preventing acute episodes and halting those
that do occur.

This two-pronged attack is increasingly effective because scientists
are piecing together a more comprehensive picture of the nature of

asthma and gaining new insights into the cause, prevention and management of acute asthma attacks. New information is changing the way practicing physicians and the Food and Drug Administration view the role of drugs in asthma treatment and prevention.

Changing Theories

Until the 1970s and early 1980s, asthma was understood to result from over-responsiveness of the tubes (bronchi and bronchioles) that carry air to and from the lungs. People with hypersensitive airways, when exposed to certain irritants called "triggers"—such as household dust, tobacco smoke, cat fur (dander), cockroach droppings, air pollutants, even vigorous exercise or cold air—would experience "bronchospasm," a narrowing of the airways caused by contraction of the muscles that encircle the bronchial tubes.

Asthmatics also tend to produce thick, sticky mucus and have inflamed, damaged airways, both of which worsen the breathing restriction caused by bronchospasm. During an acute attack, asthmatics seem to have a hard time getting their breath. Actually they are struggling to push air out of over-inflated lungs through constricted airways.

That understanding of asthma led to treatments aimed primarily at opening up the bronchial tubes by using drugs that cause the bronchial muscles to relax their grip on air passages. Bronchodilators are still a mainstay of asthma therapy. But Robert Meyer, M.D., of the Food and Drug Administration's (FDA) Center for Drug Evaluation and Research, notes that scientists' understanding of asthma has changed significantly over the last decade or so.

He points out that since the early 1980s, increasing scientific evidence shows that inflammation is as much responsible for bronchospasm as anything else. Today, Meyer says, "putting primary emphasis on controlling bronchospasm rather than chronic airway inflammation looks like "putting the cart before the horse."

The evidence Meyer refers to strongly indicates that asthma is a chronic inflammatory disease that usually develops within the first few years of life. Much of this evidence is discussed by H.W. Kelly of the University of New Mexico College of Pharmacy in the October 1992 issue of the *Journal of Clinical Pharmacology and Therapeutics*. Kelly is a member of FDA's Pulmonary and Allergy Drugs Advisory Committee.

In people with asthma, whether mild or severe—even in asthmatics whose first acute attack occurs long after childhood—the air passages are continuously inflamed, causing them to be swollen and to react strongly to inhaled irritants. But because patients may not be aware of any symptoms, this inflammation is sometimes called "the quiet part" of asthma.

People with chronically inflamed airways may show no outward signs of asthma until the first acute attack requires urgent medical attention, often at a hospital emergency department. Emergency care physicians and nurses—who are all too familiar with acute asthma—are able to administer powerful drugs to open the patient's air passages and restore more normal breathing. They are likely to recommend the patient be seen by an asthma specialist, who can devise a combination of treatment and prevention measures aimed at avoiding or minimizing further acute asthma attacks. The first step in that process is an accurate diagnosis.

Diagnosing Asthma

The diagnosis of asthma is based on repeated, careful measurements of how efficiently the patient can force air out of the lungs and on a thorough medical history and laboratory tests to find out what triggers the patient's acute attacks.

People with asthma react to external irritants in a way that non-asthmatics don't. Many, but not all, asthmatics have allergies that cause their bodies to produce an abnormal array of chemicals in response to environmental allergens. In that sense, asthma is akin to pollen allergies, hives, and eczema. But in asthma, the allergic reaction contributes to inflammation of the airways rather than of skin, eyes, or nose and throat. An acute asthma attack may come on rapidly after exposure to an irritant or develop slowly over several days or weeks, which can complicate the job of identifying a patient's asthma triggers.

Which drugs asthma patients need, when to use them, and how much to use depend largely on the character of their illness, as shown by the degree of breathing impairment and the frequency and severity of acute attacks. Asthma experts agree, however, that the first line of defense is avoidance of whatever brings on an acute asthma episode. For many patients triggers—there are often more than one—are likely to be identified as common allergens or air pollutants. In some asthmatics, attacks can be brought on by strenuous exercise, exposure to cold outdoor air, industrial or household chemicals (cleaning fluids, for example), and food additives such as sulfites. Influenza or even cold viruses can also trigger asthma episodes. In other cases, the triggers cannot be identified, even after a thorough investigation.

Asthma Drugs

Knowing what provokes an asthma attack is critically important in prevention, but it's often difficult or impractical to avoid contact with triggering irritants. Today, however, physicians can prescribe drugs to lessen the risk of acute attacks after exposure to an offending irritant, as well as halt attacks that can't be prevented.

The drugs used to treat asthma fall into two broad categories: controllers to prevent acute attacks and relievers that check acute symptoms when they occur. Some drugs do both.

In light of mounting evidence that asthma is fundamentally an inflammatory disease, asthma authorities today regard inhaled corticosteroids—marketed under numerous brand names, including AeroBid, Azmacort, Vanceril, Flovent and Pulmicort—as the most effective agents for controlling airway inflammation and thus preventing acute asthma attacks. Corticosteroids in pill or tablet form (such as Medrol) and in liquid form for children (such as Pediapred and Prelone) are prescribed long-term for some patients with severe asthma, or short-term for patients with a serious asthma episode.

Other inhaled anti-inflammatory controller drugs include Intal (cromolyn sodium), which is useful in preventing asthma brought on by exercise, and Tilade (nedocromil sodium). A new class of oral anti-inflammatory controller drugs acts by blocking a certain part of the inflammation pathway. This class of "anti-leukotriene" drugs include Zyflo (zileuton), Accolate (zafirlukast) and Singulair (montelukast).

Bronchodilators work to help open the breathing tubes (bronchi), but do not treat the underlying inflammation. There are both short-acting and long-acting bronchodilators. Long-acting inhaled bronchodilators, such as Serevent (salmeterol), and long-acting oral bronchodilators, such as Alupent (metaproterenol), Proventil (albuterol sulfate), Theo-24 (theophylline anhydrous), and many others, are often used in conjunction with anti-inflammatory agents to control symptoms. They don't provide immediate relief of symptoms, but their preventive action persists for many hours, which makes them useful in controlling attacks that might occur during hours of sleep.

Drugs to bring quick relief in acute asthma attacks are chiefly short-acting inhaled bronchodilators that act rapidly but for a relatively brief time to relax bronchial constriction. There are many short-acting bronchodilators to choose from, including Alupent or Metaprel (metaproterenol), Brethaire (terbutaline), and Ventolin or Proventil (albuterol). Although these drugs are effective in treating asthma, there is some controversy about their safety, especially when they are overused. Scientific debate makes it clear, however, that an increasing need for inhaled bronchodilators, or a decreasing response to each dose, is a signal that the patient's asthma is not being adequately controlled. Patients who have an increasing necd for short-acting inhaled bronchodilators should be reevaluated promptly by their physicians.

Both prescription and over-the-counter (OTC) short-acting bronchodilators are available. Like the prescription drugs, the OTC drugs act only to provide symptom relief, and they are generally effective for a shorter period. They may be useful, therefore, as temporary treatment for mild asthma attacks. Ready availability in drugstores makes the OTC products potentially helpful as a "stopgap" for patients who do not have their prescription medication at hand when an asthma attack occurs. More importantly, patients who use OTC inhalers should still seek advice from a health professional about the long-term treatment of their asthma.

The key to effective, long-term treatment of asthma is finding the drugs and dosage plan most effective in dealing with or preventing acute episodes. But effective treatment depends as well on the patient and the care-giver knowing what the various anti-asthma drugs do, when and in what amount each drug should be used, when a change in symptoms or in the response to a particular drug requires a call or visit to the physician, and when to get emergency help. Physicians who specialize in treating asthmatics go over these points in detail as part of an overall treatment plan designed and, as necessary, adjusted to meet the needs of each individual patient.

A cure for asthma is judged by experts to be still a far-off possibility. But the majority of asthma sufferers can lead essentially normal, symptom-free lives by understanding and sticking to a well-planned strategy to keep clear of asthma triggers and to use the right drugs in the right way.

It isn't easy, but it works.

—by Ken Flieger

Ken Flieger is a writer in Washington, D.C.

Section 7.2

Asthma and Physical Activity in School

"Asthma and Physical Activity in the School: Making a Difference," National Heart, Lung, and Blood Institute (NHLBI), National Institutes of Health (NIH), http://www.nhlbi.nih.gov/health/public/lung/asthma/phy_astr.htm, September 1995. Updated in February 2001 by Dr. David A. Cooke, MD, Diplomate, American Board of Internal Medicine.

Introduction

Lifelong physical fitness is an important goal for all students. Yet students with asthma frequently restrict their physical activities—and about 1 child in every 15 has asthma. Much of this restriction is unnecessary—children with asthma can and should be physically active. This presents a challenge to classroom teachers, physical education teachers and coaches.

What Is Asthma?

Asthma is a chronic lung condition with ongoing airway inflammation that results in recurring acute episodes (attacks) of breathing problems such as coughing, wheezing, chest tightness, and shortness of breath. These symptoms occur because the inflammation makes the airways overreact to a variety of stimuli including physical activity, upper respiratory infections, allergens, and irritants. Exposure to these stimuli—often called triggers—creates more swelling and blocking of the airways. Asthma episodes can be mild, moderate, or even life-threatening. Vigorous exercise will cause symptoms for most students with asthma if their asthma is not well-controlled. Some students experience symptoms only when they exercise. However, today's treatments can successfully control asthma so that students can participate fully in physical activities most of the time.

Asthma varies from student to student and often from season to season. This is why physical education teachers and coaches need to understand what asthma is and what the individual needs of their students are. At times, programs for students with asthma may need

49

temporary modification, such as varying the type, length, and/or frequency of activity. At all times, students with asthma should be included in activities as much as possible. Remaining behind in the gym or library or frequently sitting on the bench can set the stage for teasing, loss of self-esteem, unnecessary restriction of activity, and low levels of physical fitness.

Helping Students Control Their Asthma

Getting control of asthma means recognizing asthma triggers (the factors that make asthma worse or cause an asthma episode), avoiding or controlling these triggers, following an asthma management plan, and having convenient access to asthma medications. It also means modifying physical activities to match the students' current asthma status.

Recognize Asthma Triggers

Asthma Triggers

- exercise—running or playing hard—especially in cold weather
- upper respiratory infections—colds or flu
- laughing or crying hard
- allergens
- pollens—from trees, plants and grasses, including freshly cut grass
- animal dander from pets with fur or feathers
- dust and dust mites—in carpeting, pillows and upholstery
- cockroach droppings
- molds
- irritants
- cold air
- strong smells and chemical sprays, including perfumes, paint and cleaning solutions, chalk dust, lawn and turf treatments
- weather changes
- cigarette and other tobacco smoke

Each student with asthma has a list of triggers that can make his or her condition worse—that is, that increase airway inflammation and/or make the airways constrict, which makes breathing difficult.

Avoid or Control Asthma Triggers

Some asthma triggers—like pets with fur or feathers—can be avoided. Others—like physical exercise—are important for good health and should be controlled rather than avoided.

Actions to Consider

Identify students' known asthma triggers and eliminate as many as possible. For example, keep animals with fur out of the classroom. Consult the students' asthma management plans for guidance.

- Use wood, tile or vinyl floor coverings instead of carpeting.

- Schedule maintenance or pest control that involves strong irritants and odors for times when students are not in the area and the area can be well-ventilated.

- Adjust schedules for students whose asthma is worsened by pollen or cold air. A midday or indoor physical education class may allow more active participation.

- Help students follow their asthma management plans. These plans are designed to keep asthma under control.

Follow the Asthma Management Plan

A student's asthma management plan is developed by the student, parent/guardian, and health care provider. Depending on the student's needs, the plan may be a brief information card or a more extensive individualized health plan (IHP). A copy of the plan should be on file in the school office or health services office, with additional copies for the student's teachers and coaches. The plan—as well as the student's asthma medications—should be easily available for all on- and off-site activities before, during and after school.

Asthma Management Plan Contents

- brief history of the student's asthma

- asthma symptoms

- information on how to contact the student's health care provider, parent/guardian

- physician and parent/guardian signature

- list of factors that make the student's asthma worse

- the student's personal best peak flow reading if the student uses peak flow monitoring

- list of the student's asthma medications

- a description of the student's treatment plan, based on symptoms or peak flow readings, including recommended actions for school personnel to help handle asthma episodes

Supporting and encouraging each student's efforts to follow his or her asthma management plan is essential for the student's active participation in physical activities. Students with asthma need understanding from both teachers and students in dealing with their asthma. If students with asthma are teased about their condition, they may be embarrassed, avoid using their medication, or cut class. If students with asthma are encouraged to "tough it out," they may risk health problems or just give up.

Actions to Consider

- Get a copy of each student's asthma management plan. Review the plan to identify the role of the teacher and coach in the student's asthma management plan.

- Teach asthma awareness and peer sensitivity. As students learn more about asthma, they can more easily offer support instead of barriers to their classmates with asthma.

Ensure That Students with Asthma Have Convenient Access to Their Medications

Many students with asthma require two different medications: one for daily control and prevention, the other to treat and relieve symptoms. These medications are usually taken by metered-dose inhaler. Preventive asthma medications are taken daily and usually can be scheduled for before and after school hours. However, some students may need to take preventive daily medication during school hours. All students with asthma need to have their medication that relieves symptoms available at school in case of unexpected exposure to asthma triggers, or an asthma episode. In addition, students with asthma often benefit from using their inhaled medication 5–10 minutes before exercise. If accessing the medication is difficult, inconvenient, or embarrassing, the student may be discouraged and fail to use the inhaler as needed. The student's asthma may become unnecessarily worse and his or her activities needlessly limited.

Actions to Consider

- Provide students with asthma convenient access to their medications for all on- and off-site activities before, during and after school. These medications prevent as well as treat symptoms and enable the student to participate safely and vigorously in physical activities.

- Enable students to carry and administer their own medications if the parent/guardian, health care provider, and school nurse so advise.

Modify Physical Activities to Match Current Asthma Status

Students who follow their asthma management plans and keep their asthma under control can usually participate vigorously in the full range of sports and physical activities. Activities that are more intense and sustained—such as long periods of running, basketball, and soccer—are more likely to provoke asthma symptoms or an asthma episode. However, Olympic medalists with serious asthma have demonstrated that these activities are possible with good asthma management.

When a student experiences asthma symptoms, or is recovering from a recent asthma episode, exercise should be temporarily modified in type, length, and/or frequency to help reduce the risk of further symptoms. The student also needs convenient access to his or her medications.

Actions to Consider

- Include adequate warm-up and cool-down periods. These help prevent or lessen episodes of exercise-induced asthma.

- Consult the student's asthma management plan, parent/guardian, or health care provider on the type and length of any limitations. Assess the student and school resources to determine how the student can participate most fully.

- Remember that a student who experiences symptoms or who has just recovered from an asthma episode is at even greater risk for additional asthma problems. Take extra care. Observe for asthma symptoms, and check the student's peak flow if he or she uses a peak flow meter. Review the student's asthma management plan if there are any questions.

- Monitor the environment for potential allergens and irritants, for example, a recently mowed field or refinished gym floor. If an allergen or irritant is present, consider a temporary change in location.

- Make exercise modifications as necessary to get appropriate levels of participation. For example, if running is scheduled, the student could walk the whole distance, run part of the distance, alternate running and walking.

- Keep the student involved when any temporary but major modification is required. Ask the student to act, for example, as a scorekeeper, timer, or equipment handler until he or she can return to full participation. Dressing for a physical education class and participating at any level is better than being left out or left behind.

Recognizing Symptoms and Taking Appropriate Action

Recognizing asthma symptoms and taking appropriate action in response to the symptoms is crucial to asthma treatment and control.

Symptoms That Require Prompt Action

Acute symptoms require prompt action to help students resume their activities as soon as possible. Prompt action is also required to prevent an episode from becoming more serious or even life-threatening. The following section lists the symptoms that indicate an acute asthma episode and the need for immediate action. The student's asthma plan and the school's emergency plan should be easily accessible so that all staff, substitutes, volunteers, and aides know what to do.

Acute Symptoms Requiring Prompt Action

- coughing or wheezing
- difficulty in breathing
- chest tightness or pressure—reported by the student

- other signs, such as low peak flow readings as indicated on the asthma management plan

Symptoms of exercise-induced asthma (coughing, wheezing, pain or chest tightness) may last several minutes to an hour or more. These symptoms are quite different from breathlessness (deep, rapid breathing) that quickly returns to normal after aerobic exercise.

Actions to Take

- Stop the student's current activity.
- Follow the student's asthma management/action plan.
- Help the student use his or her inhaled medication.
- Observe for effect.

Get Emergency Help

- if the student fails to improve
- if any of the symptoms listed on the student's asthma plan as emergency indicators are present
- If any of the following symptoms are present (consider calling 911):
  - The student is hunched over, with shoulders lifted, and straining to breathe.
  - The student has difficulty completing a sentence without pausing for breath.
  - The student's lips or fingernails turn blue.

Signs That May Indicate Poorly Controlled Asthma

Students may have symptoms that do not indicate an acute episode needing immediate treatment, but instead indicate that their asthma is not under complete control. These signs may indicate poorly controlled asthma:

- a persistent cough
- coughing, wheezing, chest tightness, or shortness of breath after vigorous physical activity, on a recurring basis
- low level of stamina during physical activity or reluctance to participate

The teachers and coaches who supervise students' physical activities are in a unique position to notice signs that a child who struggles with physical activity might in fact have asthma. Because exercise provokes symptoms in most children with poorly controlled asthma, the student may need to be evaluated by his or her health care provider. It may also be that the student simply needs to follow his or her asthma management plan more carefully.

Actions to Consider

- Share observations of the symptoms with the school nurse and the student's parents or guardians. Helping students get the medical attention they need is an important way to help children become active and take control of their condition.

- Provide students convenient access to their asthma medication.

Confusing Signs: Is It an Asthma Episode or a Need for More Support?

At some times teachers and coaches may wonder if a student's reported symptoms indicate a desire for attention or a desire not to participate in an activity. At other times it may seem that students are overreacting to minimal symptoms.

It is always essential to respect the student's report of his or her own condition. If a student regularly asks to be excused from recess or avoids physical activity, a real physical problem may be present. It also may be that the student needs more assistance and support from his or her teacher and coach in order to become an active participant.

Actions to Consider

- Talk with the student to:
  - learn his or her concerns about asthma and activity.
  - offer reassurance that you understand the importance of appropriate modifications or activity limits.
  - develop a shared understanding about the conditions that require activity modifications or medications.
- Consult with the school nurse, parent/guardian, or health care provider to find ways to ensure that the student is safe, feels safe, and is encouraged to participate actively.

- If the student uses a peak flow meter, remind him or her to use it. This may help the student appreciate his or her asthma status and appropriate levels of activity.

Peak Flow Monitoring

There are different types of peak flow meters available. A peak flow meter is a small device that measures how well air moves out of the airways. Monitoring peak flow helps a student determine changes in his or her asthma and identify appropriate actions to take.

Each student has his or her personal best peak flow reading. This number should be noted in the student's asthma plan or school health file. A peak flow reading of less than 80 percent of the student's personal best indicates the need for action. A student should avoid running and playing until the peak flow reading returns or exceeds 80 percent of the personal best.

A peak flow reading is only one indicator of asthma problems. Symptoms such as coughing, wheezing, and chest tightness are also indicators of worsening asthma. Follow the student's individual plan or the school plan if you observe any of the signs or symptoms listed in the asthma emergency section or in the student's own plan.

Using a Metered Dose Inhaler

It is important that students take their medications correctly. Many asthma medications are delivered by metered dose inhalers, which are highly effective, but they can be difficult to use.

The school nurse or health room technician should review proper use of the inhaler with the student. These instructions are provided for your information.

How to Use a Metered Dose Inhaler

1. Take off the cap. Shake the inhaler.

2. Stand up. Breathe out.

3. Use the inhaler in one of two ways:
   - Open Mouth: Hold inhaler 1 to 2 inches in front of your mouth (about the width of two fingers).
   - Spacer: Use a spacer/ holding chamber. These come in many shapes and can be useful to any patient.

4. As you start to breathe in, push down on the top of the inhaler and keep breathing in slowly for 3 to 5 seconds. Hold your breath for 10 seconds. Breathe out.

Note: Dry powder capsules are used differently. To use a dry powder inhaler, close your mouth tightly around the mouthpiece and breathe in very fast.

Chapter 8

Bronchitis, Bronchiectasis, and Bronchiolitis

Chapter Contents

Section 8.1

Childhood Bronchitis

There are 2 kinds of bronchitis:

• Acute bronchitis lasts from 3 days to 3 weeks.

• Chronic bronchitis can last up to 3 months, and come back over and over for 2 years or more.

Children usually get acute bronchitis.

Acute Bronchitis

An infection or something in the air can cause acute bronchitis. Bronchitis attacks the respiratory tract. The mucous membranes in the windpipe and lungs get red and swollen. A child can get bronchitis after a sinus infection, a cold, or other respiratory infection. Coughing is often the first sign of bronchitis. The child may also get chills, a small fever, a sore throat, and muscle aches.

Signs of Acute Bronchitis

• A dry cough

• Chills, low-grade fever; less than 101° F (38.2° C)

• Sore throat and achy muscles

• Pressure or a burning feeling in the chest

The doctor may prescribe any of these medicines:

• Bronchodilators to open up the bronchial passages in the lungs

• Antibiotics to fight infection

Chronic Bronchitis

The bronchial tubes are the airways to and from the lungs. A child can get chronic bronchitis when the bronchial tubes get irritated or infected over and over again. Tobacco smoke is the most common cause. Don't smoke near your children, and don't let them smoke. This is very important. Sometimes just quitting smoking can cure bronchitis. Allergens and air pollution are also problems. (An allergen is something your child is allergic to.) Boys get chronic bronchitis more than girls. You can't catch chronic bronchitis from someone else.

Signs of Chronic Bronchitis

- Coughing that brings up mucus or phlegm.

- Shortness of breath when the child over does it. This happens when chronic bronchitis first begins.

- Shortness of breath when the child is resting. This happens when the child has had chronic bronchitis for a while.

Treating Chronic Bronchitis

- Keep your child away from second-hand smoke.

- Try to keep your child away from air pollution and chemicals that make him or her sick.

- Keep your child out of cold, wet weather.

- Give your child a cough medicine that has an expectorant. An expectorant helps bring up phlegm.

Pediatric Bronchitis

Emergency Care

With a cough, are any of the following problems present?

- Bluish or purple color around the lips, fingernails, or skin

- Severe shortness of breath, inability to say more than 4 to 5 words between breaths, or to make sounds normally

- Inability to swallow

- Coughing up blood

- Shortness of breath at rest and at non-coughing times

- Persistent cough following an episode of choking on food or a foreign object

See Doctor

Does the cough occur in an infant or young child with any of these conditions?

- The infant is younger than three months old.

- The cough occurs with rapid breathing and sounds like a seal's bark.

With a cough, are any of these symptoms also present?

- Fever of 102° F (38.8° C) or higher
- Green, yellow, or bloody-colored mucus
- Severe or increasing chest pain
- Repeated or multiple episodes of vomiting

Call Doctor

- Did the cough occur after exposure to chemicals at school or at home, such as those in new carpet, tobacco smoke, etc.?

- Has the cough lasted longer than two weeks without getting better?

Self-Care Procedures

- Don't smoke in the house. Don't let your child smoke. It will make your child's bronchitis worse.

- Use a cool-mist vaporizer or humidifier in your child's room. Use distilled (not tap) water. Clean the vaporizer or humidifier every day.

- Give your child plenty of liquids, like water and clear soup.

- Have your child rest in bed.

- For fever and aches, give your child acetaminophen or ibuprofen. Make sure you give the right kind and dose for your child's weight. **Do not give aspirin to anyone under 19**

years old. Aspirin and other medicines that have salicylates have been linked to Reye's syndrome, a condition that is potentially fatal.

- Keep your child away from air pollution as much as you can. Use air conditioning and air filters. Have your child wear a filter mask over his or her nose and mouth, if needed, Keep your child inside when air pollution is heavy if he or she gets bronchitis easily.

- Call the doctor if your child doesn't get better in 24 hours.

Section 8.2

Bronchiectasis Can Affect Children and Adults

"Bronchiectasis" is from *Medfacts*, an educational health series, © 2002 National Jewish Medical and Research Center; reprinted with permission. For more information visit National Jewish online at www.njc.org or call the Lung-Line® at 800-222-LUNG.

Bronchiectasis (pronounced bron-kee-ek'-tas-is) is a disorder of the airways within the lungs. Inflammation and infections cause damage to the airways with alteration in the lining layer of the airways. The airways become distorted and enlarged. Enlargement can be uniform or irregular. Mucus can collect in the airways and is difficult to clear because of the damage to the normal ways the airways clear the mucus. This can lead to episodes of infection. Early diagnosis and treatment of bronchiectasis and the infections that occur are very important. You may be born with bronchiectasis, or you may acquire it as an adult or child through one or more of the following ways:

- Inadvertent inhalation of oral or stomach material into your lungs, causing chronic airway inflammation. Severe gastroesophageal reflux (heartburn), which occurs when the valve or sphincter connecting your esophagus and stomach is too relaxed, may allow a backward flow of stomach contents to enter your lungs and irritate the airways. Impaired ability to swallow may also cause saliva or food to enter the lungs.

- Having another chronic lung condition, such as cystic fibrosis, allergic aspergillosis, tuberculosis, other mycobacteria diseases such as *Mycobacterium avium-intracellulare* complex (MAI), whooping cough (pertussis), or an immune deficiency disease or severe or repeated episodes pneumonia.

- Disorders that affect the function of the cilia (small hairs that line the airways).

- Obstruction in your airways because of a growth or tumor.

- Kartagener's Syndrome, a rare inherited disease that combines bronchiectasis, loss of ability to clear mucus and chronic sinusitis.

Development of Bronchiectasis

First, inflammation to the walls of the airway occurs from any mechanism (listed in the previous section). The inflammation causes injury to the airways. The resulting loss of the normal defenses of the respiratory tract leads to the loss of ability to clear mucus, making the airways susceptible to infections. Repeated lung infections can cause worsening of the damage to the airway walls.

What are the symptoms?

Symptoms of bronchiectasis include a cough with raising mucus from the lungs. With infections the mucus may be discolored and foul smelling, sometimes containing blood. Fatigue, weight loss, shortness of breath and abnormal chest sounds can occur. Occasionally people with bronchiectasis also have chronic sinusitis that requires further evaluation since bronchiectasis and sinusitis may be due to other diseases. If bronchiectasis is not treated, you may experience increasing shortness of breath, rounding at the tips of the fingers (clubbing) from chronic lung infection and possibly heart failure.

How is bronchiectasis diagnosed?

The evaluation for bronchiectasis usually includes:

- A complete medical history and physical examination by a physician.

- A chest X-ray.

- Breathing tests, called pulmonary function tests, to determine the presence and severity of abnormal airflow out of the lungs.

- A CAT scan (a specialized X-ray which produces detailed slice-like pictures) of the lungs.

What is the treatment?

Bronchiectasis can be treated in a number of ways. Your health care provider will evaluate your case and recommend the best treatment for you.

- **Bronchodilator medicine:** A bronchodilator medicine, which opens the airways by relaxing the muscles surrounding the airways, is usually recommended. This type of medicine is available as a metered-dose-inhaler. Commonly used inhaled bronchodilators include Proventil®, Ventolin® (albuterol) and Maxair® (pirbuterol). Theophylline is an oral (tablet or capsule) bronchodilator. A steroid medicine, such as the tablet prednisone or methylprednisolone, is not usually used for chronic treatment.

- **Antibiotics:** If a specific infection, such as *Mycobacteria*, is found to be the cause of the bronchiectasis, then antibiotics are tailored to the underlying cause. Antibiotics are also used for episodes of infection. Rarely continuous treatment with an antibiotic can help bronchiectasis, but drug-resistant organisms can develop in the lungs. Therefore, your health care provider will prescribe an antibiotic based on your signs, symptoms, and appropriate sputum cultures. For example, you may need an antibiotic only when you experience increased shortness of breath, cough, blood in the mucus or an increase in the amount and thickness of the mucus.

- **Treatment of sinusitis:** Salt water nasal washes help control sinusitis, which causes drainage into the airways and subsequent infections. A prescription steroid nasal spray can decrease swelling in the nose.

- **Treatment of gastroesophageal reflux:** Elevate the head of your bed six to eight inches. Avoid consuming food, alcohol, coffee, cola, or tea for several hours before bedtime. You may need antacids or other medicines to control gastroesophageal reflux because stomach acids can irritate the lungs. If your case is severe, you may need surgery to tighten the sphincter at the base of the esophagus.

- **Techniques to clear mucus from the lungs:** Your health care provider may recommend a variety of techniques if you produce an abnormally large amount of mucus or if you are having recurrent infections. A Flutter® valve is a small device you exhale into that can help can help clear mucus from the lungs. Postural drainage and clapping, uses gravity to promote drainage of mucus from the lungs and may increase mucus clearance and reduce the risk of infection. Both techniques can be prescribed and demonstrated by your health care provider.

- Any specific condition contributing to bronchiectasis should be treated. Examples include:
  - Prompt removal of any foreign object in the lungs.
  - Treatment of immune deficiency disorders with gamma globulin if appropriate.
  - Treatment of allergic bronchopulmonary aspergillosis with steroids.
  - Treatment of chronic infections such as non-tuberculous *Mycobacteria*.
- **Surgery is occasionally indicated:** Usually only if bronchiectasis is very localized in the lung and medical treatment and other therapies are not effective.

What are your responsibilities in managing bronchiectasis?

- Quit smoking and avoid exposure to passive smoke. Ask your health care provider for techniques to help you quit smoking.
- Get a flu shot yearly and a pneumococcal vaccine every 5 or 6 years as recommended by your health care provider.
- Exercise regularly as directed by your health care provider. This helps you breathe easier by improving your muscle strength and tone and helps improve clearing the mucus from the airways.
- Eat a well-balanced diet and drink plenty of fluids.

What is the role of National Jewish?

National Jewish physicians have evaluated and treated bronchiectasis for decades. Currently, National Jewish scientists are investigating new treatments for bronchiectasis. They are also pursuing aggressive treatment programs designed to minimize or prevent the occurrence of bronchiectasis. You may call 1-800-222-LUNG to make an appointment for further evaluation of your bronchiectasis.

Note: This information is provided to you as an educational service of LUNG LINE® (1-800-222-LUNG). It is not meant to be a substitute for consulting with your own physician.

National Jewish Medical and Research Center is the nation's leading treatment center for respiratory diseases and immune disorders. National Jewish offers the following services to provide current information on respiratory, immunologic diseases and treatment options:

- LUNG LINE® 1-800-222-LUNG (5864) Monday-Friday from 8:00 AM-4:30 PM, Mountain Time. Registered Nurses can answer questions and provide educational literature on respiratory and immunologic diseases. LUNG LINE® also provides information on the treatment options available at the National Jewish Center.

- PHYSICIAN LINE 1-800-NJC-9555 Monday-Friday from 8:00 AM-5:00 PM, Mountain Time. Provides physicians direct access to National Jewish for patient referrals and medical consultations.

- CASE MANAGER LINE 1-800-573-LUNG Monday-Friday 8 AM-5 PM Mountain Time.

Section 8.3

Bronchiolitis: A Concern in Younger Children

Excerpted from "Bronchiolitis," by Donna D'Alessandro, M.D., © 2001 University of Iowa Virtual Hospital; available online at http://www.vh.org/Patients/IHB/Peds/CQQA/bronchiolitis.htm, October 2001, revised April 2002. Copyright protected material used with permission of the author and the University of Iowa's Virtual Children's Hospital, www.vh.org/VCH.

Questions and Answers about Bronchiolitis

What is bronchiolitis?

- Bronchiolitis is a lung infection caused by a virus.

- In infants it is often caused by respiratory syncytial virus, or RSV.

- Troubled breathing is caused by mucus that collects in the tiny airways of the lungs (the bronchioles).

Who can get bronchiolitis?

- Children under 2 years old can get bronchiolitis. It is most common in 6-month-old infants.

- It is more common in males.

- Infants who are around cigarette smoke or who attend daycare are more likely to get it.

- Infections are most common in the winter and early spring.

- Children who have bronchiolitis 2 or 3 times are more likely to have asthma.

What are the symptoms of bronchiolitis?

- The first symptoms are usually like a cold: stuffy nose, runny nose, and mild cough. These last 1–2 days.

- A cough, fast breathing, and wheezing usually follow.

- Your child's neck and chest may suck in with each breath.

- Your child may have a fever.

- Children who have trouble breathing may get very tired or dehydrated (not enough fluid in body).

Is bronchiolitis contagious?

- Yes. Bronchiolitis is contagious.

- It can be spread by sneezing and coughing.

- It can also be spread when the hands touch the mouth or nose after coming into contact with germs.

How is bronchiolitis treated?

- Children with bronchiolitis do not need to see the doctor unless symptoms are severe (see "What Is an Emergency?" below).

- Give your child plenty of clear fluids (such as water, juice, and gelatin-water), at least 2–3 ounces every 1–2 hours while she is awake.

- Run a cool mist vaporizer in the child's room while she sleeps. Change bedding if it gets damp. Clean the vaporizer daily with bleach and water (1 part bleach to 10 parts water).

- If your infant has a stuffy nose, saline (salt-water) nose drops might help. Drops can be found at the store. Ask the pharmacist for help.

- Use a suction bulb to clear the nose. Put 1–2 drops of saline in each nostril.

- Cleaning out the nose might help your child eat, drink, and sleep.

- Tilt your infant's mattress so her head is higher than her body.

- Acetaminophen (such as Tylenol, Tempra, or Panadol) can be used to bring down fever. Give the right amount based on your child's weight.

- Watch your child's breathing. Call the doctor if breathing is troubled.

- Do not smoke around a child with bronchiolitis.

How long does bronchiolitis last?

- Symptoms usually last for about 7 days.
- A cough can last longer.

How can bronchiolitis be prevented?

- Wash your hands often after being around an infected person.

What is an emergency?

- Breathing is very difficult or very fast.
- Your child is wheezing or very drowsy.
- Your child's stomach or between her ribs sucks in with each breath and her nostrils flare.
- Her skin is pale or gray or her lips are blue.
- Your child complains of a tight chest.

When should I call the doctor?

- Anytime your child has breathing problems.
- Your child is short of breath after coughing.
- Your child will not drink or nurse.
- Your child sleeps more than usual or sleeps through feedings.
- Your child is fussy, can't sleep, or is hard to calm.
- Your child has a fever of 102° F (38.9° C) or higher.
- Your child has not urinated in 6–8 hours or if her mouth and lips are dry.
- The soft spot on your infant's head is sunk in.

Quick Answers

- Bronchiolitis is a lung infection caused by a virus.
- It is most common in children under 2 years old, especially 6-month-old infants.
- The first symptoms are usually like a cold. A cough, fast breathing, and wheezing often follow.

- Bronchiolitis can be spread by sneezing and coughing.
- Children do not need to see the doctor unless symptoms are severe. Give plenty of fluids.
- Symptoms usually last for about 7 days. A cough can last longer.
- Wash your hands often after being around an infected person.
- If your child has very troubled breathing, call the emergency room.
- If your child's symptoms do not get better in 7 days, call the doctor.

Chapter 9

The Common Cold

Sneezing, scratchy throat, runny nose—everyone knows the first signs of a cold, probably the most common illness known. Although the common cold is usually mild, with symptoms lasting one to two weeks, it is a leading cause of doctor visits and of school and job absenteeism.

The Problem

Colds are most prevalent among children, and seem to be related to youngsters' relative lack of resistance to infection and to contacts with other children in day-care centers and schools. Children have about six to ten colds a year. In families with children in school, the number of colds per child can be as high as 12 a year. Adults average about two to four colds a year, although the range varies widely. Women, especially those aged 20 to 30 years, have more colds than men, possibly because of their closer contact with children. On average, individuals older than 60 have fewer than one cold a year.

The Causes

More than 200 different viruses are known to cause the symptoms of the common cold. Some, such as the rhinoviruses, seldom produce

A fact sheet prepared by the National Institute of Allergy and Infectious Diseases (NIAID), March 2001. For more information from NIAID, visit www.niaid.nih.gov.

serious illnesses. Others, such as parainfluenza and respiratory syncytial virus, produce mild infections in adults but can precipitate severe lower respiratory infections in young children.

The same viruses that produce colds in adults appear to cause colds in children. The relative importance of various viruses in pediatric colds, however, is unclear because of the difficulty in isolating the precise cause of symptoms in studies of children with colds.

- Rhinoviruses (from the Greek *rhin*, meaning "nose") cause an estimated 30 to 35 percent of all adult colds, and are most active in early fall, spring and summer.

- Coronaviruses are believed to cause a large percentage of all adult colds. They induce colds primarily in the winter and early spring.

- Approximately 10 to 15 percent of adult colds are caused by viruses also responsible for other, more severe illnesses: adenoviruses, coxsackieviruses, echoviruses, orthomyxoviruses (including influenza A and B viruses), paramyxoviruses (including several parainfluenza viruses), respiratory syncytial virus and enteroviruses.

- The causes of 30 to 50 percent of adult colds, presumed to be viral, remain unidentified.

Does cold weather cause a cold?

Although many people are convinced that a cold results from exposure to cold weather, or from getting chilled or overheated, National Institute of Allergy and Infectious Diseases (NIAID) grantees have found that these conditions have little or no effect on the development or severity of a cold. Nor is susceptibility apparently related to factors such as exercise, diet, or enlarged tonsils or adenoids. On the other hand, research suggests that psychological stress, allergic disorders affecting the nasal passages or pharynx (throat), and menstrual cycles may have an impact on a person's susceptibility to colds.

The Cold Season

In the United States, most colds occur during the fall and winter. Beginning in late August or early September, the incidence of colds increases slowly for a few weeks and remains high until March or April, when it declines. The seasonal variation may relate to the opening of schools and to cold weather, which prompt people to spend more time indoors and increase the chances that viruses will spread from person to person.

Seasonal changes in relative humidity also may affect the prevalence of colds. The most common cold-causing viruses survive better when humidity is low—the colder months of the year. Cold weather also may make the nasal passages' lining drier and more vulnerable to viral infection.

Cold Symptoms

Symptoms of the common cold usually begin two to three days after infection and often include nasal discharge, obstruction of nasal breathing, swelling of the sinus membranes, sneezing, sore throat, cough, and headache. Fever is usually slight but can climb to 102° F in infants and young children. Cold symptoms can last from two to 14 days, but two-thirds of people recover in a week. If symptoms occur often or last much longer than two weeks, they may be the result of an allergy rather than a cold.

Colds occasionally can lead to secondary bacterial infections of the middle ear or sinuses, requiring treatment with antibiotics. High fever, significantly swollen glands, severe facial pain in the sinuses, and a cough that produces mucus, may indicate a complication or more serious illness requiring a doctor's attention.

How Cold Viruses Cause Disease

Viruses cause infection by overcoming the body's complex defense system. The body's first line of defense is mucus, produced by the membranes in the nose and throat. Mucus traps the material we inhale: pollen, dust, bacteria and viruses. When a virus penetrates the mucus and enters a cell, it commandeers the protein-making machinery to manufacture new viruses which, in turn, attack surrounding cells.

Cold symptoms are probably the result of the body's immune response to the viral invasion. Virus-infected cells in the nose send out signals that recruit specialized white blood cells to the site of the infection. In turn, these cells emit a range of immune system chemicals such as kinins. These chemicals probably lead to the symptoms of the common cold by causing swelling and inflammation of the nasal membranes, leakage of proteins and fluid from capillaries and lymph vessels, and the increased production of mucus.

Kinins and other chemicals released by immune system cells in the nasal membranes are the subject of intensive research. Researchers are examining whether drugs to block them, or the receptors on cells to which they bind, might benefit people with colds.

How Colds are Spread

Depending on the virus type, any or all of the following routes of transmission may be common:

- Touching infectious respiratory secretions on skin and on environmental surfaces and then touching the eyes or nose.

- Inhaling relatively large particles of respiratory secretions transported briefly in the air.

- Inhaling droplet nuclei: smaller infectious particles suspended in the air for long periods of time.

Much of the research on the transmission of the common cold has been done with rhinoviruses, which are shed in the highest concentration in nasal secretions. Studies suggest a person is most likely to transmit rhinoviruses in the second to fourth day of infection, when the amount of virus in nasal secretions is highest. Researchers also have shown that using aspirin to treat colds increases the amount of virus shed in nasal secretions, possibly making the cold sufferer more of a hazard to others.

Prevention

Handwashing is the simplest and most effective way to keep from getting rhinovirus colds. Not touching the nose or eyes is another. Individuals with colds should always sneeze or cough into a facial tissue, and promptly throw it away. If possible, one should avoid close, prolonged exposure to persons who have colds.

Because rhinoviruses can survive up to three hours outside the nasal passages on inanimate objects and skin, cleaning environmental surfaces with a virus-killing disinfectant might help prevent spread of infection.

The development of a vaccine that could prevent the common cold has reached an impasse because of the discovery of many different cold viruses. Each virus carries its own specific antigens, substances that induce the formation of specific protective proteins (antibodies) produced by the body. Until ways are found to combine many viral antigens in one vaccine, or take advantage of the antigenic cross-relationships that exist, prospects for a vaccine are dim. Evidence that changes occur in common-cold virus antigens further complicate development of a vaccine. Such changes occur in some influenza virus antigens and make it necessary to alter the influenza vaccine each year.

Treatment

Only symptomatic treatment is available for uncomplicated cases of the common cold: bed rest, plenty of fluids, gargling with warm salt water, petroleum jelly for a raw nose, and acetaminophen to relieve headache or fever.

> **A word of caution:** Several studies have linked the use of aspirin to the development of Reye's syndrome in children recovering from influenza or chickenpox. Reye's syndrome is a rare but serious illness that usually occurs in children between the ages of three and 12 years. It can affect all organs of the body, but most often injures the brain and liver. While most children who survive an episode of Reye's syndrome do not suffer any lasting consequences, the illness can lead to permanent brain damage or death. The American Academy of Pediatrics recommends children and teenagers not be given aspirin or any medications containing aspirin when they have any viral illness, particularly chickenpox or influenza. Many doctors recommend these medications be used for colds in adults only when headache or fever is present. Researchers, however, have found that aspirin and acetaminophen can suppress certain immune responses and increase nasal stuffiness in adults.

Nonprescription cold remedies, including decongestants and cough suppressants, may relieve some cold symptoms but will not prevent, cure, or even shorten the duration of illness. Moreover, most have some side effects, such as drowsiness, dizziness, insomnia, or upset stomach, and should be taken with care.

Nonprescription antihistamines may have some effect in relieving inflammatory responses such as runny nose and watery eyes that are commonly associated with colds.

Antibiotics do not kill viruses. These prescription drugs should be used only for rare bacterial complications, such as sinusitis or ear infections, that can develop as secondary infections. The use of antibiotics "just in case" will not prevent secondary bacterial infections.

Does vitamin C have a role?

Many people are convinced that taking large quantities of vitamin C will prevent colds or relieve symptoms. To test this theory, several large-scale, controlled studies involving children and adults have been conducted. To date, no conclusive data has shown that large doses of vitamin C prevent colds. The vitamin may reduce the severity or duration of symptoms, but there is no definitive evidence.

Taking vitamin C over long periods of time in large amounts may be harmful. Too much vitamin C can cause severe diarrhea, a particular danger for elderly people and small children. In addition, too much vitamin C distorts results of tests commonly used to measure the amount of glucose in urine and blood. Combining oral anticoagulant drugs and excessive amounts of vitamin C can produce abnormal results in blood-clotting tests.

Does steam treatment help?

Inhaling steam also has been proposed as a treatment of colds on the assumption that increasing the temperature inside the nose inhibits rhinovirus replication. Recent studies found that this approach had no effect on the symptoms or amount of viral shedding in individuals with rhinovirus colds. But steam may temporarily relieve symptoms of congestion associated with colds.

Chapter 10

Your Child's Cough: Understanding and Treating a Problem with Many Causes

Cough Is a Common Complaint

Almost everyone coughs sometime; some people cough a lot, nearly all the time. There are many causes of cough. While cough is sometimes just a minor annoyance, it can warn of a more serious problem.

Four ways to look at cough:

- Cough helps us clear mucus and foreign material from our airways; in this respect, cough is useful and needs to be as effective as possible.

- Cough can be a symptom of a disease or of a problem, such as a peanut stuck in the airway.

- Cough spreads colds and other infections from one person to another.

- Occasionally, in certain persons with heart trouble, cough can be lifesaving by helping restore normal beating in a heart experiencing abnormal beating or rhythm.

From "Cough: Understanding and Treating a Problem with Many Causes," by the American College of Chest Physicians. This patient education guide is based on a consensus panel report on managing cough that appeared in the August 1998 issue of the journal *Chest*. © 1998 American College of Chest Physicians. Reprinted with permission.

What Makes Us Cough?

A cough probably begins with irritation of nerves in the respiratory tract. The irritation may come from a plug of mucus in the airway, for example, or from exposure to a chemical aerosol such as hair spray, or postnasal drip, or from a number of other causes.

What Makes Cough Useful and Effective?

- Normal nerve pathways in the respiratory tract, so cough can be stimulated when needed.

- Normal expiratory muscles such as the diaphragm and abdomen wall, so a strong push can be given to air in the lungs.

- Normal mucus stickiness, so mucus can be dislodged and expelled from airways by cough.

What Makes Cough Less Effective?

- Weakness or paralysis of expiratory muscles makes it difficult or impossible to push air from the lungs by coughing.

- Mucus that is abnormally thick and sticky can be difficult to remove from airways by coughing.

- Bronchial tubes that are abnormally narrowed and obstructed.

Ineffective Cough May Require Medical Treatment to Keep Airways Free of Mucus and Other Secretions

- Physical therapy can help people whose expiratory muscles have been weakened or paralyzed by disease or spinal cord injury.

- Some drugs are available that may help some patients cough up and expel abnormally thick mucus.

- Keeping airways free of mucus is important to prevent invasion of airways by bacteria that can cause serious disease.

Sometimes Cough Is Not Useful, Just Annoying

- Cough that persists and serves no apparently useful purpose can be a problem that ranges from annoying to exhausting, depending on the duration and forcefulness of the cough.

- If a physician determines that a cough serves no useful purpose, medication can be given to stop the cough.

- An example of cough that is not useful is the cough that some people experience as a side effect when taking certain drugs.

Cough Can Be Defined by How Long It Persists

- Acute cough lasts for 3 weeks or less; its most frequent cause is the common cold, but occasionally, acute cough can be due to a more serious illness such as pneumonia or congestive heart failure.

- Chronic cough lasts for 3 weeks or more; it is sometimes caused by more than one condition (most commonly in nonsmokers by post-nasal drip syndrome [PNDS], asthma, or gastroesophageal reflux disease [GERD]) and is very frequent in tobacco smokers whose smoker's cough can mask a second, more serious cause of cough.

Cough Is a Symptom

Acute cough and chronic cough are symptoms of conditions that may require medical attention. Hundreds of conditions can cause cough; about a dozen conditions are the most frequent causes.

The cause of cough may not be immediately apparent. In the case of chronic cough, more than one cause may simultaneously be at work. A full medical examination and laboratory tests may be necessary to arrive at a correct diagnosis and effective treatment. In the greatest majority of cases, the specific cause of cough can be diagnosed and successfully treated with therapy specific for the cause. Specific therapy is so often successful that there is a limited role for nonspecific medicines.

Postnasal Drip Syndrome (PNDS)

PNDS is the most frequent cause of both acute and chronic cough. PNDS plus one or two other conditions, such as GERD, are often involved in chronic cough.

In addition to cough, complaints associated with PNDS are (1) a feeling of something dripping into the throat, (2) a need to constantly clear the throat, (3) nasal congestion or discharge, and (4) hoarseness.

The person with PNDS usually has recently had a cold, or suffers from allergic rhinitis, or suffers from acute or chronic sinusitis. Treatment of cough due to PNDS is determined by the diagnosis, including diagnosis of underlying conditions such as sinusitis.

Asthma

Asthma is a common cause of chronic cough in both children and adults. In some persons, chronic cough is the only symptom of asthma. In other persons, symptoms in addition to cough include wheezing, shortness of breath, and a feeling of tightness in the chest.

Asthma is a serious medical condition that requires monitoring and treatment with carefully selected drugs. When cough is due to asthma, the cough usually goes away when the asthma is effectively treated.

Gastroesophageal Reflux Disease

GERD is caused when contents from the stomach reflux (backs up) into the esophagus. GERD is a common cause of chronic cough in adults and children. In addition to cough, serious respiratory complications of GERD include chronic bronchitis, worsening bronchial asthma, and other lung diseases.

GERD is often difficult to diagnose. More than half of the persons with cough due to GERD are unaware of reflux; they do not complain of typical gastrointestinal symptoms such as heartburn, sour taste, or regurgitation. Tests to detect GERD may include 24-hour monitoring of acidity in the esophagus with a catheter.

GERD is sometimes one of the other causes of chronic cough when chronic cough is due to more than one cause. GERD and cough also can have a self-perpetuating cycle in conjunction with another cause of cough: cough due to another cause precipitates reflux from the stomach, which in turn causes cough due to GERD, so that the patient ends up with two causes of chronic cough.

Treatment of GERD includes dietary restrictions and antireflux drugs, and occasionally, surgery. Treatment of cough due to GERD also includes treatment of any other conditions causing cough.

Chronic Bronchitis

Chronic bronchitis is a frequent cause of chronic cough, especially in smokers. Tobacco smoke causes airway inflammation, excessive mucus secretion, and impairment of normal clearance of mucus. Effective cough is important for the smoker, as it helps clear excessive mucus from the airway.

Smoking cessation is the only fully effective treatment for chronic cough due to chronic bronchitis in a smoker.

Because smokers often expect to cough, they may not seek medical attention for a cough that persists. Smokers should be aware, however, that cough is also an important symptom of lung cancer, which is primarily a disease of smokers.

Bronchiectasis

Cough is one of the most important symptoms of bronchiectasis, a lung disease in which the bronchial tree is dilated and chronically colonized by bacteria. Bronchiectasis is most likely to occur in persons with cystic fibrosis and persons who have multiple respiratory infections, especially in childhood.

Effective cough is essential for the person with bronchiectasis. Chest physiotherapy and drugs to stimulate clearance of mucus are accompanied by intermittent courses of antibiotics to keep lung infection in check.

Postinfectious Cough

Cough that persists for 3 or more weeks as the only symptom after a viral upper respiratory tract infection may be a postinfectious cough. This cough due to persisting inflammation after infection will usually go away in time, but medical treatment may ease discomfort.

Postinfectious cough is more significant if there was contact with a known case of pertussis (whooping cough). In this case, antibiotic treatment should be given to the persons with this bacterial infection and to all persons who were exposed to pertussis.

Bronchogenic Carcinoma

Bronchogenic carcinoma (lung cancer) is an uncommon cause of chronic cough in nonsmokers. The danger for smokers or recent ex-smokers is that they expect to cough, and may overlook a cough that may be symptomatic of lung cancer.

Suspicion of lung cancer is an indication for diagnostic tests including chest x-ray, bronchoscopy, and examination of sputum for presence of cancer cells.

ACE (Angiotensin-Converting Enzyme) Inhibitor-Induced Cough

Angiotensin-converting enzyme (ACE) inhibitors are blood pressure-lowering drugs that cause chronic cough as a side effect in about 10% of persons who take the drugs. The cough is typically dry and hacking. Discontinuance of the drug causes the cough to improve or resolve within a month.

Habit Cough

Habit or nervous cough is a throat-clearing noise made by a person who is nervous and self-conscious. Medical treatment is not necessary. Occasionally, habit cough overlaps with postnasal drip syndrome, which can be treated.

Psychogenic Cough

Psychogenic cough has no apparent physical cause. Emotional and psychological problems are likely causes. However, other illnesses have to be ruled out before a firm diagnosis is made.

Psychogenic cough is thought to be more common in children than in adults. A possible scenario: psychogenic cough develops in a child who has a chronically ill brother or sister.

Chronic Interstitial Pulmonary Disease

This group of lung diseases that includes idiopathic pulmonary fibrosis is characterized more by shortness of breath than by cough. Before cough is assumed to be due to interstitial pulmonary disease, the most common causes of chronic cough, such as PNDS, need to be ruled out since they may be contributing factors. Then, if cough persists despite specific treatment for the interstitial lung disease, nonspecific medication, such as codeine, may be needed to suppress coughing and ease discomfort.

Other Causes of Cough in Infants and Children

Asthma, sinusitis, and GERD are the most frequent causes of chronic cough in children. Other causes can be hard to diagnose, especially in infants and small children who cannot describe symptoms and are difficult to examine. Some of these other causes of chronic cough include:

- Congenital diseases or anomalies of the heart and lungs—that is, diseases or anatomic problems that were present at birth.

- A foreign body (a peanut or a small toy, for example) lodged in the airway.

- Chronic aspiration of milk into the airway while bottle feeding; in some infants this can be a chronic problem that needs medical attention.

- Exposure to tobacco smoke from parents or family members who smoke.

Cough Medicines

There are medicines to help you stop coughing (antitussives) and others to help you cough more effectively (protussives). Some medicines are available without prescription, while others must be prescribed by a physician. No cough medicine should be taken for long periods of time (3 weeks or more) without a medical examination. You could be taking the wrong medicine without realizing it, or you could be inadvertently using cough medicine to cover up a serious problem such as asthma or lung cancer.

For tobacco smokers, the most effective way to stop coughing is to stop smoking.

Don't Spread Infection

Remember that coughing spreads disease by dispersing germs through the air and on skin.

- You should always cover your mouth and nose while coughing.

- If you cough into your hands or blow your nose, wash your hands immediately to remove germs deposited on the skin.

- If you have been covering your mouth while coughing, do not handle or prepare food until you have washed your hands.

Chapter 11

Croup

Croup is an infection that commonly occurs in children aged six months to three years in the late fall and winter. There are different viruses that can cause croup and they include the parainfluenza virus, RSV, and more rarely the influenza virus or adenovirus. While these viruses will usually just cause cold symptoms in older children and adults, in younger children they can cause inflammation and infection in the lower throat, including the windpipe (trachea) and voice box (larynx). This causes swelling and building up of mucus and other secretions that can cause narrowing of these air passages. It is this narrowing that causes the distinctive cough, which sounds like a barking seal. Your child may also make another noise, called stridor, which is a loud, high pitched sound that your child may make when breathing in and is often confused with 'wheezing' by many parents.

The barking cough of croup most commonly begins in the middle of the night, and most children had been fine earlier in the night when they went to bed. Your child may have had cold symptoms for a few days already and then wakes up with a loud, dry, barking cough.

While there is no cure for croup, some steps you can take to improve your child's breathing include increasing the moisture or humidity of the air he is breathing. This can be done by taking your child

"Croup," © 2000 Keep Kids Healthy, LLC., available online at http://www.keepkidshealthy.com/welcome/infectionsguide/croup.html, last updated August 2000; reprinted with permission. This document was written by Vincent Iannelli, M.D., F.A.A.P., President, Keep Kids Healthy, LLC. For additional information, visit www.keepkidshealthy.com.

into the bathroom, closing all of the doors and windows and turning on all of the hot water. This will fill the room with steam and warm moisture and may help loosen the mucus and soothe the inflammation in his throat. Be sure to stay with your child and keep him away from direct contact with the hot water. This treatment may take up to 15–20 minutes to become effective. Keep in mind that it will not make the cough go away, it should, however, help him to breath better.

Another way to improve your child's breathing is to take him outside, where the air will be cooler and probably more humid than the dry air inside the house. A cool mist humidifier may also help.

While no medications are used for mild symptoms of croup, if your child is having a moderate or severe attack, your physician may prescribe a steroid medication to help decrease the inflammation in your child's lower throat. Another medicine called racemic epinephrine may also be given as a breathing treatment in a hospital setting if needed.

The first night of symptoms of croup are usually the worse, and while your child may be totally fine during the next day, symptoms may return the next night (but usually they are not as bad). Symptoms usually last about 5–6 days, but the first few nights are usually the worst.

Since there are different viruses that can cause croup, it is possible to get it more than once.

You should seek help from your physician if your child isn't improving with these measures or if he is having a lot of trouble breathing. Some signs that your child is having difficulty breathing include a fast breathing rate, flaring of his nostrils, retracting (where you can see the muscles moving in and out between his ribs and at the base of his neck), being lethargic or inconsolable, making the harsh stridor noise when he is breathing in, or if he is turning blue. You should seek emergency care for any of these signs.

Chapter 12

Influenza

Colds and Flu: Identify the Enemy

Flu is like the cold in many ways—most basically, they're both respiratory infections caused by viruses. If a cold is misdiagnosed as flu, there's no problem. At worst, a cold can occasionally lead to secondary bacterial infections of the middle ear or sinuses, which can be treated with antibiotics. But if the flu is misdiagnosed as a bad cold, potentially life-threatening flu complications like pneumonia may be overlooked.

Some of the symptoms of a cold and flu are similar, but the two diseases can usually be distinguished.

Colds

Typically, colds begin slowly, two to three days after infection with the virus. The first symptoms are usually a scratchy, sore throat, followed by sneezing and a runny nose. Temperature is usually normal or only slightly elevated. A mild cough can develop several days later.

This chapter contains text from "Colds and Flu: Time Only Sure Cure," by Tamar Nordenberg, *FDA Consumer*, Food and Drug Administration (FDA) Pub. No. 99-1264, http://www.fda.gov/fdac/features/896_flu.html, May 1999, and "Influenza in the Child Care Setting," Centers for Disease Control and Prevention (CDC), January 1997. Reviewed in July 2002 by Dr. David A. Cooke, MD, Diplomate, American Board of Internal Medicine.

Symptoms tend to be worse in infants and young children, who sometimes run temperatures of up to 102° Fahrenheit (39° Celsius). Cold symptoms usually last from two days to a week.

Flu

Signs of the flu include sudden onset with a headache, dry cough, and chills. The symptoms quickly become more severe than those of a cold. The flu sufferer often experiences a "knocked-off-your-feet" feeling, with muscle aches in the back and legs. Fever of up to 104 degrees Fahrenheit (40 degrees Celsius) is common. The fever typically begins to subside on the second or third day, and then respiratory symptoms like nasal congestion and sore throat appear. Fatigue and weakness may continue for days or even weeks.

"The lethargy, achiness and fever are side effects of the body doing its job of trying to fight off the infection," according to Dominick Iacuzio, Ph.D., influenza program officer with the National Institutes of Health (NIH).

Other Illnesses

Influenza rarely causes stomach upset. What is popularly called "stomach flu"—with symptoms like nausea, diarrhea and vomiting—is technically another malady: gastroenteritis.

Cold and flu-like symptoms can sometimes mimic more serious illnesses like strep throat, measles, and chickenpox. Allergies, too, can resemble colds with their runny noses, sneezing, and general miserable feeling.

If symptoms persist, become severe or localized in the throat, stomach or lungs, or if other symptoms such as vomiting and behavioral changes occur, consult your physician. "With the typical symptoms, it's not necessary to contact your physician immediately," Iacuzio says.

The Treatment Arsenal

There is no proven cure for colds or flu but time. However, over-the-counter medications are available to relieve the symptoms.

"OTC cough-cold products can make you more comfortable while you suffer," says Debbie Lumpkins, a scientist with the Food and Drug Administration's division of over-the-counter drug products. "They are intended to treat the symptoms of minor conditions, not to treat the underlying illness."

Don't bother taking antibiotics to treat your flu or cold; antibiotics do not kill viruses, and they should be used only for bacterial complications such as sinus or ear infections. Overuse of antibiotics has become a very serious problem, leading to a resistance in disease-causing bacteria that may render antibiotics ineffective for certain conditions.

Children and teenagers with symptoms of flu or chickenpox should not take aspirin or products containing aspirin or other salicylates. Use of these products in young flu and chickenpox sufferers has been associated with Reye syndrome, a rare condition that can be fatal. Because cold symptoms can be similar to those of the flu, it's best not to give aspirin to people under 20 with these types of symptoms.

The active ingredients Food and Drug Administration (FDA) considers safe and effective for relieving certain symptoms of colds or flu fall into the following categories:

- Nasal decongestants open up the nasal passages. They can be applied topically, in the form of sprays or drops, or taken orally. But using sprays or drops longer than three days may cause nasal congestion to worsen.

- Antitussives, also known as cough suppressants, can quiet coughs due to minor throat irritations. They include drugs taken orally, as well as topical medications like throat lozenges and ointments to be rubbed on the chest or used in a vaporizer.

- Expectorants, taken orally, help loosen mucus and make coughs more productive.

Until recently, another category of over-the-counter (OTC) drugs called "antihistamines" was approved only for use by sufferers of hay fever and some other allergies. In October, clemastine fumarate, the active ingredient in products such as Tavist-1 and Tavist-D, was approved to treat cold symptoms. The effectiveness of other OTC antihistamines for this use is still being studied.

Most nonprescription cough-cold remedies contain a combination of ingredients to attack multiple symptoms. These combination products often contain antipyretics to reduce fever and analgesics to relieve minor aches, pains and headaches.

Users of OTC medicines should carefully follow the labeling instructions and warnings. Under a new FDA rule, all OTC products will soon have labels with a standardized format and simplified language to help consumers understand the information.

The Flu Fighters

Flu typically affects 20 to 50 percent of the U.S. population each winter. It's a highly contagious disease, spreading mostly by direct person-to-person contact. "With the flu, coughing—even more than sneezing—is the most effective method of transmission," Iacuzio says.

The flu virus can linger in the air for as long as three hours. In close quarters, conditions are ripe for the spread of the virus. That explains why the highest incidence of the flu is in 5- to 14-year-olds, who spend much of their time in school, in close contact with their classmates. The most serious complications occur in older adults, however.

Years ago, there were no practical tools to protect people from flu. In 1918–1919, a global flu epidemic, or pandemic, struck half the world's population and claimed the lives of 20 million. Still today, 10,000 to 20,000 Americans—almost all of them elderly, newborns, or chronically ill—die each year from flu complications, usually pneumonia.

The challenge for scientists trying to protect us from the disease is that influenza viruses can change themselves, or mutate, to become different viruses. Scientists have classified flu viruses as types A, B and C. Type A is the most common and leads to the most serious epidemics. Type B can cause epidemics, but usually produces a milder disease than type A. Type C viruses have never been associated with a large epidemic.

Vaccine a Powerful Weapon

The most important tool for fighting the ever-changing flu virus is immunization by a killed virus vaccine licensed by FDA. The vaccine is made from highly purified, egg-grown viruses that have been made noninfectious.

Vaccination is available to anyone who wants to reduce their chances of getting the flu. Studies have shown the vaccine's effectiveness rate to be 70 to 90 percent in healthy young adults. In the elderly and in people with certain chronic illnesses, the vaccine sometimes doesn't prevent illness altogether, but it does reduce its severity and the risk of complications.

The government's Advisory Committee on Immunization Practices strongly recommends vaccination for the following high-risk groups:

- people aged 65 or older

- residents of nursing homes and other facilities that provide care for chronically ill persons

- people over the age of 6 months, including pregnant women, who have certain underlying medical conditions that required hospitalization or regular doctors' visits during the preceding year. These conditions include:

  - asthma, anemia, metabolic disease such as diabetes, or heart, lung or kidney disease

  - impaired immune system due to Human Immunodeficiency Virus (HIV) infection, treatment with drugs such as long-term steroids, or cancer treatment with radiation or chemotherapy

- children and teenagers (6 months to 18 years) who must take aspirin regularly and, therefore, may be at risk of developing Reye syndrome if they get the flu.

The Flu Vaccine

To reduce the risk of transmitting flu to high-risk persons—and to protect themselves from infection—the advisory committee recommends flu shots for people with regular close contact with high-risk groups. Such people include health-care workers, nursing home personnel, and home-care providers. Police, firefighters, and other community service providers may also find vaccination useful.

Because it takes the immune system about six to eight weeks to respond to vaccination, the best time to get the flu vaccine is mid-October to mid-November, before the December-to-March U.S. flu season hits.

The vaccine's most common side effect is soreness at the vaccination site for up to two days. Some people may experience post-shot fever, malaise, sore muscles, and other symptoms resembling the flu that can last for one to two days. Actually, the flu vaccine can't cause flu because it contains only inactivated viruses.

The vaccine should be repeated annually, since the immunity is believed to last only about a year, and because the vaccine's composition changes each year based on the flu strains scientists expect to be most common.

To decide which strains of influenza virus should be incorporated into the vaccine for the coming flu season, FDA's Vaccines and Related Biologicals Advisory Committee meets in late January each year to consider reports from national and international surveillance systems. A World Health Organization panel meets in Geneva in mid-February to make final recommendations for the next season's flu vaccine. The strains are labeled by their type (A, B, or C) and the place where the strain was isolated.

"In the not-too-distant future," says Iacuzio, "consumers may have alternatives to the flu shot, including different delivery methods like nasal drops or a spray." Major pharmaceutical companies, in cooperation with scientists representing the National Institutes of Health (NIH), the Food and Drug Administration's (FDA) Center for Biologics Evaluation and Research, and academia, are making significant strides, also, toward an even more protective vaccine.

Some people—but not many—should avoid the flu shot. People allergic to eggs and people with certain other allergies and medical problems like bronchitis or pneumonia should consult a doctor before getting a flu shot. And those with a high fever should not receive the vaccine until they feel better.

Pregnant women who have a high-risk condition should be immunized regardless of the stage of pregnancy; healthy pregnant women may also want to consult their health-care providers about being vaccinated.

In the rare cases when the vaccine is not advisable, two prescription drugs are available for prevention of type A influenza: Symmetrel (amantadine), approved by FDA in 1976, and Flumadine (rimantadine), approved by FDA in 1993. Either drug also can be used to reduce symptoms and shorten the illness if administered within 48 hours after symptoms appear.

First Do No Harm

If, despite precautions, you do get a cold or flu, besides taking an OTC medication if needed and as directed, drink fluids and get plenty of bed rest. "Your body is trying to attack the virus," Iacuzio says. "Give in, and give your body a chance to fight off the infection. It takes energy to do that."

Many people are convinced that vitamin C can prevent colds or relieve symptoms. There is no conclusive evidence of this, but the vitamin may reduce the severity or duration of symptoms, according to the National Institute of Allergy and Infectious Diseases. But taking vitamin C in large amounts over long periods can be harmful, sometimes causing diarrhea and distorting common medical tests of the urine and blood.

Another proposed therapy, interferon-alpha nasal spray, can prevent infection and illness but causes unacceptable side effects like nosebleeds, according to the Institute.

Many patients have their own, unproven theories about what works. "As long as it's not harmful, why not try it?" says Iacuzio. "But be skeptical of something that hasn't been clinically proven in a well-designed, placebo-controlled study." So what about chicken soup? It may soothe a sore throat, unstuff clogged passageways, and hydrate a thirsty body. At the very least, according to Iacuzio, "It's good TLC. Psychologically, that's important when you're sick."

Influenza in the Child Care Setting

Children who are in frequent contact, at home or in the child care setting, with people who are in any of the above high-risk categories should be vaccinated against influenza.

If a child or staff person in a child care setting develops a fever (100° F or higher under the arm, 101° F orally, or 102° F rectally) AND chills, cough, sore throat, headache, or muscle aches, he or she should be sent home.

During an epidemic of influenza you should:

- Closely observe all children for symptoms and refer anyone developing symptoms to his or her physician.

- Make sure all children and adults follow good handwashing and hygiene practices, including use and proper disposal of paper tissues.

- Make sure all children and adults follow good handwashing and hygiene practices, including use and proper disposal of paper tissues.

- In large child care facilities, follow appropriate group separation practices.

- Closely observe all children for symptoms and refer anyone developing symptoms to his or her physician.

- Notify parents.

Chapter 13

Pneumonia

Signs and Symptoms

Pneumonia is a general term that refers to an infection of the lungs, which can be caused by a variety of microorganisms, including viruses, bacteria, and parasites.

Often pneumonia begins after an upper respiratory tract infection (an infection of the nose and throat). When this happens, symptoms of pneumonia begin after 2 or 3 days of a cold or sore throat.

Symptoms of pneumonia vary, depending on the age of the child and the cause of the pneumonia. Some common symptoms include:

- fever
- chills
- cough
- unusually rapid breathing
- breathing with grunting or wheezing sounds
- labored breathing that makes a child's rib muscles retract (when muscles under the rib cage or between ribs draw inward with each breath)

- vomiting
- chest pain
- abdominal pain
- decreased activity
- loss of appetite (in older children) or poor feeding (in infants)
- in extreme cases, bluish or gray color of the lips and fingernails

Sometimes a child's only symptom is rapid breathing. Sometimes when the pneumonia is in the lower part of the lungs near the abdomen, there may be no breathing problems at all, but there may be fever and abdominal pain or vomiting.

When pneumonia is caused by bacteria, an infected child usually becomes sick relatively quickly and experiences the sudden onset of high fever and unusually rapid breathing. When pneumonia is caused by viruses, symptoms tend to appear more gradually and are often less severe than in bacterial pneumonia. Wheezing may be more common in viral pneumonia.

Some types of pneumonia cause symptoms that give important clues about which germ is causing the illness. For example, in older children and adolescents, pneumonia due to *Mycoplasma* (also called walking pneumonia) is notorious for causing a sore throat and headache in addition to the usual symptoms of pneumonia.

In infants, pneumonia due to *Chlamydia* may cause conjunctivitis (redness of the eyes) with only mild illness and no fever. When pneumonia is due to pertussis (whooping cough), the child may have long coughing spells, turn blue from lack of air, or make a classic "whoop" sound when trying to take a breath.

Description

Pneumonia is a lung infection that can be caused by different types of germs, including bacteria, viruses, fungi, and parasites. Although different types of pneumonia tend to affect children in different age groups, pneumonia is most commonly caused by viruses. Some viruses that cause pneumonia are adenoviruses, rhinovirus, influenza virus (flu), respiratory syncytial virus (RSV), and parainfluenza virus (the virus that causes croup).

Incubation

The incubation period for pneumonia varies, depending on the type of virus or bacteria causing the infection. Some common incubation periods are: respiratory syncytial virus, 4 to 6 days; influenza, 18 to 72 hours.

Duration

With treatment, most types of bacterial pneumonia can be cured within 1 to 2 weeks. Viral pneumonia may last longer. Mycoplasmal pneumonia may take 4 to 6 weeks to resolve completely.

Contagiousness

The viruses and bacteria that cause pneumonia are contagious and are usually found in fluid from the mouth or nose of an infected person. Illness can spread when an infected person coughs or sneezes on a person, by sharing drinking glasses and eating utensils, and when a person touches the used tissues or handkerchiefs of an infected person.

Prevention

There are vaccines to prevent infections by viruses or bacteria that cause some types of pneumonia.

Children usually receive routine immunizations against *Haemophilus influenzae* and pertussis (whooping cough) beginning at 2 months of age. (The pertussis immunization is the "P" part of the routine DTaP injection.) Vaccines are now also given against the pneumococcus organism (PCV), a common cause of bacterial pneumonia.

Children with chronic illnesses, who are at special risk for other types of pneumonia, may receive additional vaccines or protective immune medication. The flu vaccine is recommended for children with chronic illnesses such as chronic heart or lung disorders or asthma.

Because they are at higher risk for serious complications, infants who were born prematurely may be given treatments that temporarily protect against RSV, which can lead to pneumonia in younger children.

Doctors may give prophylactic (disease-preventing) antibiotics to prevent pneumonia in children who have been exposed to someone with certain types of pneumonia, such as pertussis. Children with HIV infection may also receive prophylactic antibiotics to prevent pneumonia caused by *Pneumocystis carinii*.

Antiviral medication is now available, too, and can be used to prevent some types of viral pneumonia or to make symptoms less severe.

In addition, regular tuberculosis screening is performed yearly in some high-risk areas because early detection will prevent active tuberculosis infection including pneumonia.

In general, pneumonia is not contagious, but the upper respiratory viruses that lead to it are, so it is best to keep your child away from anyone who has an upper respiratory tract infection. If someone in your home has a respiratory infection or throat infection, keep his or her drinking glass and eating utensils separate from those of other family members, and wash your hands frequently, especially if you are handling used tissues or dirty handkerchiefs.

When to Call Your Child's Doctor

Call your child's doctor immediately if your child has any of the signs and symptoms of pneumonia, but especially if your child is having trouble breathing or is breathing abnormally fast, if your child has a bluish or gray color to her fingernails or lips, or if your child has a fever of 102 degrees Fahrenheit (38.9 degrees Celsius) or above 100.4 degrees Fahrenheit (38 degrees Celsius) in infants under 6 months of age.

Professional Treatment

Doctors usually make the diagnosis of pneumonia after a physical examination of your child. The doctor may possibly use a chest X-ray, blood tests, and (sometimes) bacterial cultures of mucus produced by coughing when making a diagnosis.

In most cases, pneumonia can be treated with oral antibiotics given to your child at home. The type of antibiotic used depends on the type of pneumonia.

Children may be hospitalized for treatment if their pneumonia is caused by pertussis or other bacterial pneumonia that are causing high fevers and respiratory distress. If supplemental oxygen is needed or if they have lung infections that may have spread into the bloodstream, they may also be hospitalized.

Children may be also be hospitalized if they have chronic illnesses that affect the immune system, if they are vomiting so much that they cannot take medicine by mouth, or if they have recurrent episodes of pneumonia.

Home Treatment

If your child's doctor has prescribed antibiotics for your child's bacterial pneumonia, give the medicine on schedule for as long as the doctor directs. This will help your child recover faster and will decrease the chance that infection will spread to other household members.

Don't force your child to eat if she's not feeling well, but encourage your child to drink fluids, especially if she has a fever. Ask your child's doctor before you use a medicine to treat your child's cough because cough suppressants stop the lungs from clearing mucus, which may not be helpful in some types of pneumonia.

If your child has chest pain, try a heating pad or warm compress on the chest area. Take your child's temperature at least once each morning and each evening, and call your child's doctor if it goes above 102 degrees Fahrenheit (38.9 degrees Celsius) or above 100.4 degrees Fahrenheit (38 degrees Celsius) in infants under 6 months of age.

Check your child's lips and fingernails to make sure that they are rosy and pink, not bluish or gray, which is a sign that your child's lungs are not getting enough oxygen.

Chapter 14

Tuberculosis (TB)

Tuberculosis in the Child Care Setting

Tuberculosis (TB) is a disease caused by bacteria called *Mycobacterium tuberculosis*. These germs can be spread from one person to others. These germs can be spread through the air when a person with TB disease coughs, sneezes, yells, or sings. Children, although they may be infectious, usually are not as likely as adults to transmit TB to others. (TB is not spread by objects such as clothes, toys, dishes, walls, floors, and furniture.) When a person is sick from the TB germ, the person has TB disease. TB can be serious for anyone, but is especially dangerous for children younger than 5 years old and for any persons who have weak immune systems, such as those with HIV (human immunodeficiency virus) infection or AIDS (acquired immune deficiency syndrome).

You should know the difference between the two stages of TB:

1. TB infection is just having the TB germ in the body without being sick, and

2. Active TB or TB disease is having the germ and also being sick from it, with the symptoms of active TB (see description of symptoms below).

This chapter contains text from "Tuberculosis (TB) in the Child Care Setting," Centers for Disease Control and Prevention (CDC), January 1997, updated in July 2002 by Dr. David A. Cooke, MD, Diplomate, American Board of Internal Medicine, and "Tuberculosis," National Institute of Allergy and Infectious Diseases (NIAID), National Institutes of Health (NIH), http://www.niaid.nih.gov/factsheets/tb.htm, March 2002.

When a child has TB infection, it means that the child was infected by an adult with active TB—often a person in the home. Most persons who have TB infection do not know it because it does not make them sick. A person with only TB infection cannot spread TB to others and does not pose an immediate danger to the public. TB infection is diagnosed only by the TB skin test. This safe, simple test is given at most local health departments. A small injection is made under the skin, usually on the forearm. In persons who are infected with the TB germ, the skin test causes a firm swelling in the skin where the test was given. After 1 or 2 days, a health care provider reads the results of the TB skin test.

A TB-infected person can take 9 to 12 months of medicine, usually isoniazid, to get rid of the TB germs and to prevent active TB (the illness with symptoms). This preventive treatment is most important for TB-infected children younger than 5 years old, persons infected with the TB germ within the past 2 years, and TB-infected persons who have a weak immune system (especially HIV infection or AIDS) because these persons are more likely to get active TB after infection.

Active TB (when infection develops into a disease with symptoms) is preventable and curable. Active TB can attack any part of the body, but it usually affects the lungs. Persons with active TB in the lungs may spread TB germs through the air by coughing, sneezing, or yelling. People who share this air have a chance of breathing in the germs and getting the infection in their lungs, too.

Persons with active TB have symptoms such as a cough that won't go away, a cough that brings up blood, a fever lasting longer than 2 weeks, night sweats, feeling very tired, or losing a noticeable amount of weight. The TB skin test cannot show active TB—active TB must be diagnosed by a physician, based on a physical exam, a chest x-ray, and laboratory tests. The treatment for active TB usually involves taking at least 3 different drugs and lasts for at least 6 months and usually cures the TB. The law states that doctors must report active TB to the local health department.

In child care settings, TB has been spread from adults to children, although the spread of TB in such settings is rare. In family home child care settings, TB infection has been passed from sick adults living in the home to children, even thought the sick adults may not have been taking care of the children directly. As noted before, a person with only TB infection cannot infect another person. Only a person with active TB can infect another person. Also, children younger than 5 years old who have active TB usually cannot infect other persons. The spread of TB from child to child in a child care setting has not been reported. Still, children under 5 years old who have active TB should not attend child care until they have been given permission. Usually, they may return to child care as soon as they are feeling well and on medication, but this should be decided by the local health department. Well children should not be kept out of child care [or school] if they only have a positive skin test result.

In the United States, TB is more common in some populations, for example immigrants coming from Asia, Africa, and Latin America, and medically underserved minority populations. However, overall, TB infection in children younger than 5 years old is rare. Therefore, TB skin testing of all children in child care centers is not useful. However, a local health department may decide to test children who have more risk for infection. Some programs (e.g., Head Start) and some states require children to have a TB skin test before they can attend. A child who has a positive skin test result should be seen by a doctor to check for active TB and to start medicine that will prevent TB disease, if appropriate. A child should not be kept out of child care [or school] only because of a positive TB skin test result.

Persons who are beginning work as a child care provider should have a TB skin test to check for infection with TB bacteria. Child care providers who come from a community with high rates of TB may want to take preventive medicine so they will not develop active TB. Local health department TB control programs can help with these activities.

Tuberculosis: Questions and Answers about the Disease

Many people think tuberculosis (TB) is a disease of the past. But, TB is still a leading killer of young adults worldwide. Some 2 billion people—one-third of the world's population—are infected with the TB bacterium, *M. tuberculosis*. TB is a chronic bacterial infection. It is spread through the air and usually infects the lungs, although other organs are sometimes involved. Most persons that are infected with *M. tuberculosis* harbor the bacterium without symptoms but many develop active TB disease. Each year, 8 million people worldwide develop active TB and 3 million die.

How do people catch TB?

TB is primarily an airborne disease. The disease is spread from person to person in tiny microscopic droplets when a TB sufferer coughs, sneezes, speaks, sings, or laughs. Only people with active disease are contagious.

It usually takes lengthy contact with someone with active TB before a person can become infected. On average, people have a 50 percent chance of becoming infected with *M. tuberculosis* if they spend eight hours a day for six months or 24 hours a day for two months working or living with someone with active TB. However, people with TB who have been treated with appropriate drugs for at least two weeks are no longer contagious and do not spread the germ to others.

Adequate ventilation is the most important measure to prevent the transmission of TB.

What happens when someone gets infected with M. tuberculosis?

Between two to eight weeks after being infected with *M. tuberculosis*, a person's immune system responds to the TB germ by walling off infected cells. From then on the body maintains a standoff with the infection, sometimes for years. Most people undergo complete healing of their initial infection, and the bacteria eventually die off. A positive TB skin test, and old scars on a chest x-ray, may provide the only evidence of the infection.

If, however, the body's resistance is low because of aging, infections such as HIV, malnutrition, or other reasons, the bacteria may break out of hiding and cause active TB.

What is active disease?

One in ten people that are infected with *M. tuberculosis* may develop active TB at some time in their lives. The risk of developing active disease is greatest in the first year after infection, but active disease often does not occur until many years later.

Early symptoms of active TB can include weight loss, fever, night sweats, and loss of appetite, or they may be vague and go unnoticed by the affected individual. One in three patients with TB will die within weeks to months if the disease is not treated. For the rest, their disease either goes into remission (halts) or becomes chronic and more debilitating with cough, chest pain, and bloody sputum.

Symptoms of TB involving areas other than the lungs vary, depending upon the organ affected.

How is TB diagnosed?

Doctors can identify most people infected with *M. tuberculosis* with a skin test. They will inject a substance under the skin of the forearm. If a red welt forms around the injection site within 72 hours, the person may have been infected. This doesn't necessarily mean he or she has active disease. Most people with previous exposure to *M. tuberculosis* will test positive on the tuberculin test, as will some people exposed to bacteria that are related to the TB germ.

If a person has an obvious reaction to the skin test, other methods can help to show if the individual has active TB. In making a diagnosis, doctors rely on symptoms and other physical signs, a person's history of exposure to TB, and x-rays that may show evidence of *M. tuberculosis* infection.

The doctor also will take sputum and other samples, to see if the TB bacteria will grow in the lab. If bacteria are growing, this positive culture confirms the diagnosis of TB. Because *M. tuberculosis* grows very slowly, it can take four weeks to confirm the diagnosis. An additional two to three weeks usually are needed to determine which antibiotics the bacteria are susceptible to.

Can TB be cured?

With appropriate antibiotic treatment, TB can be cured in more than nine out of ten patients.

Successful treatment of TB depends on close cooperation between the patient and doctor and other health care workers. Treatment usually combines several different antibiotic drugs which are given for at least six months, sometimes for as long as 12 months.

Patients must take their medicine on time every day for the 6 to 12 months. Some TB patients stop taking their prescribed medicines because they may feel better after only a couple of weeks of treatment. Another reason they may stop taking their medicine is because TB drugs can have unpleasant side effects.

Why is it so important to finish all of the TB medicine?

If patients don't take all their medicine the way their doctor tells them, they can become sick again and spread TB to their friends and family. Additionally, when patients do not take all the drugs the doctor has prescribed or skip times when they are supposed to take them, the TB bacteria learn to outwit the TB antibiotics, and soon those medications no longer work against the disease. If this happens, the person now has resistant TB infection. Some patients have disease that is resistant to two or more drugs. This is called multidrug-resistant TB or MDR-TB because the TB germ, *M. tuberculosis* resists eradication with more than one drug. This form of TB is much more difficult to cure.

107

Can MDR-TB be treated?

Treatment for MDR-TB often requires the use of special TB drugs, all of which can produce serious side effects. To cure MDR-TB, patients may have to take several antibiotics, at least three to which the bacteria still respond, every day for up to two years. However, even with this treatment, between four and six out of ten patients with MDR-TB will die, which is the same as for patients with normal TB who do not receive treatment.

How is TB prevented?

TB is largely a preventable disease. In the United States, doctors try to identify persons infected with *M. tuberculosis* as early as possible, before they have developed active TB. They will give a drug called isoniazid (INH) to prevent the active disease. This drug is given every day for 6 to 12 months. INH can cause hepatitis in a small percentage of patients, especially those older than 35 years. A nurse may watch the patients take their medicine to make sure all pills are taken.

Hospitals and clinics can take precautions to prevent the spread of TB. Precautions include using ultraviolet light to sterilize the air, special filters, and special respirators and masks. Until they can no longer spread the TB germs, TB patients in hospitals should be isolated in special rooms with controlled ventilation and airflow.

Is there a vaccine for TB?

In those parts of the world where the disease is common, the World Health Organization (WHO) recommends that infants receive a vaccine called BCG (bacille Calmette-Guérin) made from a live weakened bacterium related to *M. tuberculosis*. BCG vaccine prevents *M. tuberculosis* from spreading within the body, thus preventing TB from developing.

However, the vaccine has its drawbacks. It does not protect adults very well against TB. In addition, BCG interferes with the TB skin test, showing a positive skin test reaction in people who have received BCG vaccine. In countries where BCG vaccine is used, the ability of the skin test to identify persons that are infected with *M. tuberculosis* is limited. Because of these limitations, more effective vaccines are needed and BCG is not recommended for general use in the United States.

Part Three

Ailments of the
Head, Throat, and Mouth

Chapter 15

Ear Infections

What Is Otitis Media?

Otitis media is an ear infection. Three out of four children experience otitis media by the time they are 3 years old. In fact, ear infections are the most common illnesses in babies and young children.

Are There Different Types of Otitis Media?

Yes. There are two main types. The first type is called acute otitis media (AOM). This means that parts of the ear are infected and swollen. It also means that fluid and mucus are trapped inside the ear. AOM can be painful.

The second type is called otitis media with effusion (fluid), or OME. This means fluid and mucus stay trapped in the ear after the infection is over. OME makes it harder for the ear to fight new infections. This fluid can also affect your child's hearing.

How Does Otitis Media Happen?

Otitis media usually happens when viruses and/or bacteria get inside the ear and cause an infection. It often happens as a result of

Excerpted from "Otitis Media: Facts for Parents," National Institute on Deafness and Other Communication Disorders (NIDCD), NIH Pub. No. 00-4216, July 2001; available online at http://www.nidcd.nih.gov/health/parents/otitismedia.htm.

another illness, such as a cold. If your child gets sick, it might affect his or her ears.

It is harder for children to fight illness than it is for adults, so children develop ear infections more often. Some researchers believe that other factors, such as being around cigarette smoke, can contribute to ear infections.

What's Happening inside the Ear When My Child Has an Ear Infection?

When the ears are infected the eustachian tubes become inflamed and swollen. The adenoids can also become infected.

The eustachian tubes are inside the ear. They keep air pressure stable in the ear. These tubes also help supply the ears with fresh air. Swollen and inflamed eustachian tubes often get clogged with fluid and mucus from a cold. If the fluids plug the openings of the eustachian tubes, air and fluid get trapped inside the ear. These tubes are smaller and straighter in children than they are in adults. This makes it harder for fluid to drain out of the ear and is one reason that children get more ear infections than adults. The infections are usually painful.

Adenoids are located in the throat, near the eustachian tubes. Adenoids are clumps of cells that fight infections. Adenoids can become infected and swollen. They can also block the openings of the eustachian tubes, trapping air and fluid. Just like the eustachian tubes, the adenoids are different in children than in adults. In children, the adenoids are larger, so they can more easily block the opening of the eustachian tube.

Can Otitis Media Affect My Child's Hearing?

Yes. An ear infection can cause temporary hearing problems. Temporary speech and language problems can happen, too. If left untreated, these problems can become more serious.

An ear infection affects important parts in the ear that help us hear. Sounds around us are collected by the outer ear. Then sound travels to the middle ear, which has three tiny bones and is filled with air. After that, sound moves on to the inner ear. The inner ear is where sounds are turned into electrical signals and sent to the brain. An ear infection affects the whole ear, but especially the middle and inner ear. Hearing is affected because sound cannot get through an ear that is filled with fluid.

How Do I Know if My Child Has Otitis Media?

It is not always easy to know if your child has an ear infection. Sometimes you have to watch carefully. Your child may get an ear infection before he or she has learned how to talk. If your child is not old enough to say, "My ear hurts," you need to look for other signals that there is a problem.

Here are a few signs your child might show you if he or she has otitis media:

- Does she tug or pull at her ears?
- Does he cry more than usual?
- Do you see fluid draining out of her ears?
- Does he have trouble sleeping?
- Can she keep her balance?
- Does he have trouble hearing?
- Does she seem not to respond to quiet sounds?

A child with an ear infection may show you any of these signs. If you see any of them, call a doctor.

What Will a Doctor Do?

Your doctor will examine your child's ear. The doctor can tell you for sure if your child has an ear infection. The doctor may also give your child medicine. Medicines called antibiotics are sometimes given for ear infections. It is important to know how they work. Antibiotics only work against organisms called bacteria, which can cause illness. Antibiotics are not effective against viruses, such as those associated with a cold. In order to be effective, antibiotics must be taken until they are finished. A few days after the medicine starts working, your child may stop pulling on his or her ear and appear to be feeling better. This does not mean the infection is gone. The medicine must still be taken. If not, the bacteria can come back. You need to follow the doctor's directions exactly.

Your doctor may also give your child pain relievers, such as acetaminophen. Medicines such as antihistamines and decongestants do not help in the prevention or treatment of otitis media.

How Can I Be Sure I Am Giving the Medicine Correctly?

If your doctor gives you a prescription for medicine for your child, make sure you understand the directions completely before you leave his or her office. Here are a few suggestions about giving medicine to your child.

Read. Make sure the pharmacy has given you printed information about the medicine and clear instructions about how to give it to your child. Read the information that comes with the medicine. If you have any problems understanding the information, ask the pharmacist, your doctor, or a nurse. You should know the answers to the following questions:

- Does the medicine need to be refrigerated?
- How many times a day will I be giving my child this medicine?
- How many days will my child take this medicine?
- Should it be given with food or without food?

Plan. Sometimes it is hard to remember when you have given your child a dose of medicine. Before you give the first dose, make a written plan or chart to cover all of the days of the medication. Some children may require 10 to 14 days of treatment.

Put your chart on the refrigerator so you can check off the doses at every meal. Be sure to measure carefully. Use a measuring spoon or special medicine-measuring cup if one comes with the medicine. Do not use spoons that come with tableware sets because they are not always a standard size.

Follow through. Be sure to give all of the medicine to your child. Make sure it is given at the right times. If your doctor asks you to bring your child back for a recheck, do it on schedule. Your doctor wants to know if the ears are clear of fluid and if the infection has stopped. Write down and ask the doctor any questions you have before you leave his or her office.

Will My Child Need Surgery?

Some children with otitis media need surgery. The most common surgical treatment involves having small tubes placed inside the ear. This surgery is called a myringotomy. It is recommended when fluids from an ear infection stay in the ear for several months. At that stage, fluid may cause hearing loss and speech problems. A doctor called an otolaryngologist (ear, nose, and throat surgeon) will help you through this process if your child needs an operation. The operation will require anesthesia.

In a myringotomy, a surgeon makes a small opening in the ear drum. Then a tube is placed in the opening. The tube works to relieve pressure in the clogged ear so that the child can hear again. Fluid cannot build up in the ear if the tube is venting it with fresh air.

After a few months, the tubes will fall out on their own. In rare cases, a child may need to have a myringotomy more than once.

Another kind of surgery removes the adenoids. This is called an adenoidectomy. Removing the adenoids has been shown to help some children with otitis media who are between the ages of 4 and 8. We know less about whether this can help children under age 4.

What about Children in Daycare, Pre-School, or School?

Even before your child has an ear infection or needs to take medicine, ask the daycare program or school about their medication policy. Sometimes you will need a note from your doctor for the staff at the school. The note can tell the people at your child's school how and when to give your child medicine if it is needed during school hours. Some schools will not give children medicine. If this is the case at your child's school, ask your doctor how to schedule your child's medicine.

What Else Can I Do for My Child?

The best thing you can do is to pay attention to your child. Know the warning signs of ear infections, and be on the lookout if your child gets a cold. If you think your child has an ear infection, call the doctor.

Do not smoke around your child. Smoke is not good for the delicate parts inside your child's ear.

Chapter 16

Labyrinthitis

What Is Labyrinthitis?

Labyrinthitis is an ear disorder involving inflammation of the canals of the inner ear (semicircular canals, labyrinth), resulting in dizziness.

Causes, Incidence, and Risk Factors

The cause of labyrinthitis is unknown but since it commonly occurs following otitis media or an upper respiratory infection (URI), it is thought to be a consequence of viral or bacterial infection. It may also follow allergy, cholesteatoma, or ingestion of toxic drugs.

The semicircular canals of the inner ear (labyrinth) become inflamed. This disrupts their function, including the regulation of balance. Risk factors include recent viral illness, respiratory infection, or ear infection; use of prescription or nonprescription drugs (especially aspirin); stress; fatigue; and a history of allergy, smoking, or alcohol consumption.

Prevention

Prompt treatment of respiratory infections and ear infections may help prevent labyrinthitis.

Symptoms

- dizziness
- abnormal sensation of movement (vertigo)
  - may be accompanied by nausea and vomiting
  - may be severe
  - may be continuous for up to a week at a time
  - severe episodes may be followed by transient episodes for several weeks
- loss of balance, especially falling toward the affected side
- hearing loss in the affected ear (especially with bacterial labyrinthitis)
- ringing or other noises in the ears (tinnitus)
- involuntary eye movements

Signs and Tests

An ear examination may not reveal any changes. Differentiation from other causes of dizziness or vertigo may include:

- head computed tomography (CT) scan or magnetic resonance imaging (MRI) scan
- hearing testing (audiology/audiometry)
- caloric stimulation (tests reflexes of the eye)
- electronystagmography
- electroencephalogram (EEG), evoked auditory potential studies

Treatment

Labyrinthitis usually runs its course over a few weeks. However, symptoms may need treatment. Medications that may reduce symptoms include antihistamines, anticholinergics, sedative-hypnotics, antiemetics (antinausea medications), and benzodiazepines. To prevent worsening of symptoms during episodes of labyrinthitis, keep still, rest during attacks, and gradually resume activity. Avoid sudden position changes. Do not try to read during attacks, and avoid bright lights.

Assistance with walking may be needed during attacks. Avoid hazardous activities such as driving, operating heavy machinery, and climbing, until 1 week after symptoms disappear.

Expectations (Prognosis)

Recovery is usually spontaneous and hearing usually returns to normal.

Complications

- injury to self or others during attacks of vertigo
- permanent hearing loss in the affected ear (rare)
- spread of inflammation to other ear areas or to the brain (rare)

Calling Your Health Care Provider

Call your health care provider if dizziness, vertigo, loss of balance, or other symptoms of labyrinthitis are present. Also call if hearing loss occurs.

Urgent or emergency symptoms include convulsions, fainting, persistent vomiting, or vertigo accompanied by fever over 101 degrees Fahrenheit.

Chapter 17

Sore Throats

What Causes a Sore Throat?

Sore throat is a symptom of many medical disorders. Infections cause the majority of sore throats and are contagious. Infections are caused either by viruses such as the flu, the common cold, mononucleosis, or by bacteria such as strep, mycoplasma, or haemophilus.

While bacteria respond to antibiotic treatment, viruses do not.

Viruses. Most viral sore throats accompany flu or colds along with a stuffy, runny nose, sneezing, and generalized aches and pains. These viruses are highly contagious and spread quickly, especially in winter. The body builds antibodies that destroy the virus, a process that takes about a week.

Sore throats accompany other viral infections such as measles, chicken pox, whooping cough, and croup. Canker sores and fever blisters in the throat also can be very painful.

One viral infection takes much longer than a week to be cured: infectious mononucleosis, or mono. This virus lodges in the lymph system, causing massive enlargement of the tonsils, with white patches on their surface and swollen glands in the neck, armpits, and groin. It creates a severely sore throat and, sometimes, serious breathing difficulties. It can affect the liver, leading to jaundice—yellow skin and eyes. It also causes extreme fatigue that can last six weeks or more.

Mono, a severe illness in teenagers but less severe in children, can he transmitted by saliva. So it has been nicknamed the kissing disease, but it can also be transmitted from mouth-to-hand to hand-to-mouth or by sharing of towels and eating utensils.

Bacteria. Strep throat is an infection caused by a particular strain of streptococcus bacteria. This infection can also damage the heart valves (rheumatic fever) and kidneys (nephritis), cause scarlet fever, tonsillitis, pneumonia, sinusitis, and ear infections.

Because of these possible complications, a strep throat should be treated with an antibiotic. Strep is not always easy to detect by examination, and a throat culture may be needed. These tests, when positive, persuade the physician to prescribe antibiotics. However, strep tests might not detect other bacteria that also can cause severe sore throats that deserve antibiotic treatment. For example, severe and chronic cases of tonsillitis or tonsillar abscess may be culture negative. Similarly, negative cultures are seen with diphtheria, and infections from oral sexual contacts will escape detection by strep culture tests.

Tonsillitis is an infection of the lumpy tissues on each side of the back of the throat. In the first two to three years of childhood, these tissues catch infections, sampling the child's environment to help develop his immunities (antibodies). Healthy tonsils do not remain infected. Frequent sore throats from tonsillitis suggest the infection is not fully eliminated between episodes. A medical study has shown that children who suffer from frequent episodes of tonsillitis (such as three to four times each year for several years) were healthier after their tonsils were surgically removed.

Infections in the nose and sinuses also can cause sore throats, because mucus from the nose drains down into the throat and carries the infection with it.

The most dangerous throat infection is epiglottitis, caused by bacteria that infect a portion of the larynx (voice box) and cause swelling that closes the airway. This infection is an emergency condition that requires prompt medical attention. Suspect it when swallowing is extremely painful (causing drooling), when speech is muffled, and when breathing becomes difficult. A strep test may miss this infection.

Allergy. The same pollens and molds that irritate the nose when they are inhaled also may irritate the throat. Cat and dog dander and house dust are common causes of sore throats for people with allergies to them.

Irritation. During the cold winter months, dry heat may create a recurring, mild sore throat with a parched feeling, especially in the mornings. This often responds to humidification of bedroom air and increased liquid intake. Patients with a chronic stuffy nose, causing mouth breathing, also suffer with a dry throat. They need examination and treatment of the nose.

Pollutants and chemicals in the air can irritate the nose and throat, but the most common air pollutant is tobacco smoke. Other irritants include smokeless tobacco, alcoholic beverages, and spicy foods.

A person who strains his or her voice (yelling at a sports event, for example) gets a sore throat not only from muscle strain but also from the rough treatment of his or her throat membranes.

Reflux. An occasional cause of morning sore throat is regurgitation of stomach acids up into the back of the throat. To avoid reflux, tilt your bedframe so that the head is elevated four- to six-inches higher than the foot of the bed. You might find antacids helpful. You should also avoid eating within three hours of bedtime, and eliminate caffeine and alcohol. If these tips fail, see your doctor.

Tumors. Tumors of the throat, tongue, and larynx (voice box) are usually (but not always) associated with long-time use of tobacco and alcohol. Sore throat and difficulty swallowing, sometimes with pain radiating to the ear, may be symptoms of such a tumor. More often the sore throat is so mild or so chronic that it is hardly noticed. Other important symptoms include hoarseness, a lump in the neck, unexplained weight loss, and/or spitting up blood in the saliva or phlegm.

When Should I See a Doctor?

Whenever a sore throat is severe, persists longer than the usual five- to seven-day duration of a cold or flu, and is not associated with an avoidable allergy or irritation, you should seek medical attention. The following signs and symptoms should alert you to see your physician:

- Severe and prolonged sore throat.
- Difficulty breathing.
- Difficulty swallowing.

- Difficulty opening the mouth.
- Joint pain.
- Earache.
- Rash.
- Fever (over 101° F).
- Blood in saliva or phlegm.
- Frequently recurring sore throat.
- Lump in neck.
- Hoarseness lasting over two weeks.

When Should I Take Antibiotics?

Antibiotics are drugs that kill or impair bacteria. Penicillin or erythromycin (well-known antibiotics) are prescribed when the physician suspects streptococcal or another bacterial infection that responds to them. However, a number of bacterial throat infections require other antibiotics instead. Antibiotics do not cure viral infections, but viruses do lower the patient's resistance to bacterial infections. When such a combined infection occurs, antibiotics may be recommended. When an antibiotic is prescribed, it should be taken as the physician directs for the full course (usually 10 days). Otherwise the infection will probably be suppressed rather than eliminated, and it can return. Some children will experience recurrent infection despite antibiotic treatment. When some of these are strep infections or are severe, your child may require a tonsillectomy.

Should Other Family Members Be Treated or Cultured?

When a strep test is positive, many experts recommend treatment or culturing of other family members. Practice good sanitary habits; avoid close physical contact; and avoid sharing of napkins, towels, and utensils with the infected person. Hand washing makes good sense.

What If My Throat Culture Is Negative?

A strep culture tests only for the presence of streptococcal infections. Many other infections, both bacterial and viral, will yield negative cultures and sometimes so does a streptococcal infection. Therefore, when your culture is negative, your physician will base his/her decision for treatment on the severity of your symptoms and the appearance of your throat on examination.

How Can I Treat My Sore Throat?

A mild sore throat associated with cold or flu symptoms can be made more comfortable with the following remedies:

- Increase your liquid intake.
- Warm tea with honey is a favorite home remedy.
- Use a steamer or humidifier in your bedroom.
- Gargle with warm salt water several times daily: ¼ tsp. salt to ½ cup water.
- Take over-the-counter pain relievers such as acetaminophen or ibuprofen.

Chapter 18

Tonsils and Adenoids

Chapter Contents

Section 18.1

Tonsils and Tonsillectomy

"Tonsils and Tonsillectomy: Frequently Asked Questions (FAQs)," by Michael Poole, MD, Department of Pediatric Otolaryngology–Head and Neck Surgery, © 2001 Texas Pediatric Surgical Associates (www.pedisurg.com); reprinted with permission. Available online at http://www.pedisurg.com/PtEducENT/tonsils.htm.

What are tonsils?

The tonsils are two clumps of tissue, on either side of the throat, embedded in a pocket at the side of the palate (roof of the mouth). The lower edge of each tonsil is beside the tongue, way in the back of the throat.

What function do they serve? Aren't they important?

The tonsils are mostly composed of lymphoid tissue, which is found throughout the gastrointestinal tract and on the base of the tongue. Lymphoid tissue is composed of lymphocytes, which are mostly involved in antibody production. Since we generally consider antibody production to be a good thing, many studies have been performed to try to clarify the importance of the tonsils. There seems to be no adverse effect on the immune status or health of patients who have had them removed. Any noticeable effect has generally been positive. It appears that the tonsils were not "designed" to effectively handle the multitude of viral infections that occur in children in an urban population. Rather, the immune system, including the tonsils and adenoids, developed during a era where the child was rarely exposed to a large number of other people and the germs they carried. It may also be that these organs are relatively more important in dealing with certain types of infections, such as worms or other parasites, that are relatively uncommon in today's society. It is clear that in many cases, the tonsils become "dysfunctional" and are more of a liability than an asset.

Why are the tonsils removed?

There are a number of well-established valid reasons for removal. Some patients will have more the one reason. The most common are listed below.

- **Blockage of the throat; they are too big:** This is now the most common reason for removal. The tonsils can be large enough to impede breathing, swallowing, or clear speech production. The blockage of breathing can range from simple "mouth breathing" to severe snoring, or sleep apnea (blockage of breathing at night). The health risks of this can be slight to life-threatening. Not all tonsils that appear to be large are actually causing obstruction. A history and an examination by a skilled practitioner is usually sufficient for the diagnosis.

- **Chronic and recurrent tonsillitis; sore throats:** This used to be the most common reason for removal and remains so in some parts of the world. Some patients will have frequent severe bouts of tonsillitis. Other patients have a pattern of low-grade, constant, or very frequent sore throats. Unrelenting strep (Group A streptococcus) infection or colonization is still encountered, despite antibiotics.

- **White debris in the tonsils; "chronic cryptic tonsillitis":** The tonsils contain many pits and pockets called crypts. These, in some patients tend to become impacted with white foul-smelling (especially to the owner) debris that is composed of bacteria and dead cells. It may cause a low grade intermittent sore throat. Antibiotics are only transiently helpful. Some patients will use various mechanical picks and swabs to attempt removal. The only consistent cure is a tonsillectomy, although the problem often is minor enough that no therapy is necessary.

- **Unusual enlargement or appearance:** Like any other tissue, the tonsils can be the site of benign or malignant tumors. An unusual or markedly enlarged tonsil is sometimes seen in this situation. Lymphoma is the most common tumor of the tonsil in children. In adults, lymphoma or carcinoma can be seen.

Will he/she outgrow the problem?

In general, yes. We rarely see patients over 40 years old with significant enlargement or infections of the tonsils. However, we have also seen 35-year-old patients in severe heart failure due to sleep apnea and severely enlarged tonsils about to undergo a heart transplant, and their doctor had said they did not need the tonsils out because they would outgrow the problem. (A tonsillectomy would have prevented the heart failure and years of sleep deprivation.) In short, the potential gain of a tonsillectomy (or any other procedure) has to be weighed against the likelihood of resolution, the risks of the procedure, the discomfort, and the expense. For many patients, tonsillectomy is still an appropriate decision.

Should the adenoids be removed also?

At least in young children, enlargement or infection frequently affects the adenoids as well as the tonsils, so they are often removed together. Compared to a tonsillectomy, an adenoidectomy is less traumatic and painful.

How are tonsils removed?

There are many techniques used for tonsillectomy. General anesthesia is usually employed; but it is possible to perform tonsillectomy with sedation and local anesthesia. In the United States, some degree of electrocautery assisted dissection is most commonly employed, because of the ability to rapidly stop bleeding. Some surgeons use very little cautery with more bleeding, but with less burned tissue. Use of lasers has been studied and considered by most surgeons. We feel that laser use is primarily a marketing gimmick at this point, since it offers no apparent advantage over certain cautery techniques, and has some very real hazards and extra costs.

What are the complications of tonsillectomy?

Most surgical procedures share the general risks of anesthesia, bleeding, and infection. The anesthetic risk is, in general, proportional to the health of the patient; and serious problems should be very rare. Bleeding is most commonly encountered in a delayed fashion—five to ten days after surgery—when an eschar (scab) comes off. Postoperative bleeding is more likely in teenagers and adults, as opposed to younger children (who have smaller vessels). The area where the tonsils were removed (the tonsillar fossae) always becomes colonized with high numbers of bacteria and often causes a low-grade fever. Serious infections are very rare. If tonsils are very large, speech may be different post-operatively (often temporarily high-pitched and "whiney").

Most often the post-op speech is actually more normal. Remember, very rarely, someone can die from complications of tonsillectomy (or any other surgery); so no surgical procedure should be undertaken lightly.

Is hospitalization necessary?

Not usually. Nine out of ten patients do well enough to go home. We will admit anyone who doesn't meet standard discharge criteria: significant breathing problems, no oral intake, severe nausea/vomiting, or serious co-existing illnesses. An occasional patient goes home, but comes back to the hospital, because of poor liquid consumption or bleeding.

Note

The information above, although based on a thorough knowledge and careful review of current medical literature, is the opinion of the doctors at Texas Pediatric Surgical Associates and is presented to inform you about surgical conditions. It is not meant to contradict any information you may receive from your personal physician and should not be used to make decisions about surgical treatment. If you have any questions about the information above or your child's care, please contact our doctors at any time by calling (713) 704-5869.

Section 18.2

Adenoids and Adenoidectomy

"Adenoids and Adenoidectomy," by Michael Poole, MD, Department of Pediatric Otolaryngology–Head and Neck Surgery, © 2001 Texas Pediatric Surgical Associates (www.pedisurg.com); reprinted with permission. Available online at http://www.pedisurg.com/PtEducENT/adenoids.htm.

What are adenoids?

The adenoids are a single clump of tissue in the back of the nose (nasopharynx). They are located (in the adult) on the back wall of the throat (pharynx), about one inch above the uvula (the little teardrop shaped piece of tissue that hangs down in the middle of the soft palate).

What function do they serve? Aren't they important?

The adenoids are mostly composed of lymphoid tissue, which is found throughout the gastrointestinal tract and on the base of the tongue. Lymphoid tissue is composed of lymphocytes, which are mostly involved in antibody production. To date, there seems to be no adverse effect on the immune status or health of patients who have had them removed. Any noticeable effect has generally been positive. It appears that the adenoids were not designed to effectively handle the multitude of viral infections that occur in children in an urban population. Rather, the immune system, including the tonsils and adenoids, developed during a era where the child was rarely exposed to a large number of other people and the germs they carried. It may also be that these organs are relatively more important in dealing with certain types of infections, such as worms or other parasites, that are relatively uncommon in today's society. It is clear that in many cases, the adenoids become dysfunctional and are more of a liability than an asset.

Why are the adenoids removed?

There are a number of well-established, valid reasons for removal (called an adenoidectomy). Some patients will have more than one reason. The most common are listed below.

- **Blockage of the back of the nose; they are too big:** This is now one of the more common reasons for removal. The adenoids may be large enough to cause mouth breathing, snoring, or even sleep apnea (blockage of breathing during sleep). This degree of enlargement may be associated with chronic fluid or infection in ears. Inability to breathe through the nose causes a reduction in smell (and therefore taste). This is most commonly seen in pre-school children but can exist as early as several months of age.

- **Chronic and recurrent fluid or infections of the ears:** The adenoids may be enlarged or chronically infected to the extent that they cause ear problems, either recurrent infections or chronic fluid. The infection or blockage may affect eustachian tube function. An adenoidectomy is often recommended for children who continue to have ear problems after the first set of tubes. We will occasionally recommend an adenoidectomy with the first set of tubes if some of the other problems exist.

- **Chronic or recurrent sinus infections, or rhinosinusitis:** Similar to the problem with the middle ear, enlarged or infected adenoids may cause accumulation of nasal secretions or recurrent sinus infections. Many surgeons feel that an adenoidectomy is the most appropriate surgical procedure for young children with severe sinus problems.

Should the tonsils be removed also?

In general, only if they are enlarged, or otherwise have been causing problems themselves. The tonsils rarely, if ever, are associated with ear disease. However, if we are removing adenoids because they are enlarged or obstructed, we tend to be relatively aggressive with borderline enlarged tonsils. Too often, several months later, when we left such tonsils, they became enough of a problem to warrant removal.

Will the child outgrow the problem?

In general, yes, the adenoids usually shrink (regress) in the second decade of life. However, years of any of the problems above may be too high of a price to pay for waiting. In particular, blockage and sleep apnea may result in permanent adverse changes in facial or dental development, in addition to the adverse effects on growth and learning caused by chronic poor sleeping.

How are adenoids removed?

General anesthesia is the norm. Most often, with the assistance of a small mirror, adenoid tissue is shaved or curetted from the back of the nose. Occasionally, some other devices or electrocautery is used. With the advent of special cautery devices, we almost always completely dry the surgical site before the patient wakes up, eliminating the low-grade bleeding that used to be associated with adenoidectomies. The procedure typically takes 5–15 minutes to complete.

What are the complications of adenoidectomy?

Complications are rare, and usually minor. Anesthetic risk is usually related to the health of the patient. Serious anesthetic complications can occur, but are very unusual. Bleeding is rare; we have had no serious bleeding in over 3000 patients, and only a few minor bleeding episodes. The adenoid bed usually becomes superficially infected, and can cause 7–10 days of bad breath, but serious infections are very rare. If adenoids are routinely removed in all children, without careful consideration and examination, a few children will have velopharyngeal insufficiency, meaning that sounds or liquids can escape up the back of the nose, affecting speech and/or swallowing. We have never encountered that complication, but it has been reported by other surgeons. In other words, some children should not undergo adenoidectomy—because of their special anatomy.

What should we expect post-operatively?

Adenoidectomy typically is much less painful than a tonsillectomy. Most children need no pain medications. A few benefit from acetaminophen (Tylenol). Bad breath is common for 7–10 days. A few children will complain of a stiff or sore neck (from irritation of the neck muscles underneath the adenoid bed). We do not limit activity (playing or swimming) although some surgeons do so. The patient may consume a normal diet. We usually see patients 2–4 weeks post-operatively—to ensure normal function and healing.

Note

The information above, although based on a thorough knowledge and careful review of current medical literature, is the opinion of the doctors at Texas Pediatric Surgical Associates and is presented to inform you about surgical conditions. It is not meant to contradict any information you may receive from your personal physician and should not be used to make decisions about surgical treatment. If you have any questions about the information above or your child's care, please contact our doctors at any time by calling (713) 704-5869.

Chapter 19

Sinusitis in Children

Chapter Contents

Section 19.1

What Is Sinusitis?

Excerpted from: "Sinusitis," Office of Communications and Public Liaison, National Institute of Allergy and Infectious Diseases (NIAID), National Institutes of Health (NIH), U.S. Department of Health and Human Services, http://www.niaid.nih.gov/factsheets/sinusitis.htm, April 2002.

Sinusitis simply means the sinuses are infected or inflamed, but this gives little indication of the misery and pain this condition can cause. Health care experts usually divide sinusitis cases into:

- Acute, which lasts for 3 weeks or less

- Chronic, which usually lasts for 3 to 8 weeks but can continue for months or even years

- Recurrent, which is several acute attacks within a year

Sinuses are hollow air spaces in the human body. When people say, "I'm having a sinus attack," they usually are referring to symptoms in one or more of four pairs of cavities, or sinuses, known as paranasal sinuses. These cavities, located within the skull or bones of the head surrounding the nose, include the:

- Frontal sinuses over the eyes in the brow area

- Maxillary sinuses inside each cheekbone

- Ethmoid sinuses just behind the bridge of the nose and between the eyes

- Sphenoid sinuses behind the ethmoids in the upper region of the nose and behind the eyes

Each sinus has an opening into the nose for the free exchange of air and mucus, and each is joined with the nasal passages by a continuous mucous membrane lining. Therefore, anything that causes a swelling in the nose—an infection, an allergic reaction, or an immune reaction—also can affect the sinuses. Air trapped within a blocked sinus, along with pus or other secretions, may cause pressure on the sinus wall. The result is the sometimes intense pain of a sinus attack. Similarly, when air is prevented from entering a paranasal sinus by a swollen membrane at the opening, a vacuum can be created that also causes pain.

Acute Sinusitis

Most cases of acute sinusitis start with a common cold, which is caused by a virus. These viral colds do not cause symptoms of sinusitis, but they do inflame the sinuses. Both the cold and the sinus inflammation usually go away without treatment in two weeks. The inflammation, however, might explain why having a cold increases your likelihood of developing acute sinusitis. For example, your nose reacts to an invasion by viruses that cause infections (such as the common cold or flu) by producing mucus and sending white blood cells to the lining of the nose, which congest and swell the nasal passages.

When this swelling involves the adjacent mucous membranes of your sinuses, air and mucus are trapped behind the narrowed openings of the sinuses. When your sinus openings become too narrow, mucus cannot drain properly. This increase in mucus sets up prime conditions for bacteria to multiply.

Most healthy people harbor bacteria, such as *Streptococcus pneumoniae* and *Haemophilus influenzae*, in their upper respiratory tracts with no problems until the body's defenses are weakened or drainage from the sinuses is blocked by a cold or other viral infection. Thus, bacteria that may have been living harmlessly in your nose or throat can multiply and invade your sinuses, causing an acute sinus infection.

Sometimes, fungal infections can cause acute sinusitis. Although fungi are abundant in the environment, they usually are harmless to healthy people, indicating that the human body has a natural resistance to them. Fungi, such as *Aspergillus*, can cause serious illness in people whose immune systems are not functioning properly. Some people with fungal sinusitis have an allergic-type reaction to the fungi.

Chronic inflammation of the nasal passages also can lead to sinusitis. If you have allergic rhinitis or hay fever, you can develop episodes of acute sinusitis. Vasomotor rhinitis, caused by humidity, cold air, alcohol, perfumes, and other environmental conditions, also may be complicated by sinus infections.

Acute sinusitis is much more common in some people than in the general population. For example, sinusitis occurs more often in people who have reduced immune function (such as those with immune deficiency diseases or HIV infection) and with abnormality of mucus secretion or mucus movement (such as those with cystic fibrosis).

Chronic Sinusitis

If you have asthma, an allergic disease, you may have frequent episodes of chronic sinusitis.

If you are allergic to airborne allergens, such as dust, mold, and pollen, which trigger allergic rhinitis, you may develop chronic sinusitis. In addition, people who are allergic to fungi can develop a condition called allergic fungal sinusitis.

If you are subject to getting chronic sinusitis, damp weather, especially in northern temperate climates, or pollutants in the air and in buildings also can affect you.

Like acute sinusitis, you might develop chronic sinusitis if you have an immune deficiency disease or an abnormality in the way mucus moves through and from your respiratory system. In addition, if you have severe asthma, nasal polyps (small growths in the nose), or a severe asthmatic response to aspirin and aspirin-like medicines such as ibuprofen, you might have chronic sinusitis often.

Section 19.2

Pediatric Sinusitis

Your child's sinuses are not fully developed until age 20. Although small, the maxillary (behind the cheek) and ethmoid (between the eyes) sinuses are present at birth. Unlike in adults, pediatric sinusitis is difficult to diagnose because symptoms can be subtle and the causes complex.

How Do I Know When My Child Has Sinusitis?

The following symptoms may indicate a sinus infection in your child:

- a "cold" lasting more than 10 to 14 days, sometimes with a low-grade fever

- thick yellow-green nasal drainage

- post-nasal drip, sometimes leading to or exhibited as sore throat, cough, bad breath, nausea and/or vomiting

- headache, usually in children age six or older

- irritability or fatigue

- swelling around the eyes

Young children have immature immune systems and are more prone to infections of the nose, sinus, and ears, especially in the first several years of life. These are most frequently caused by viral infections (colds), and they may be aggravated by allergies. However, when your child remains ill beyond the usual week to ten days, a serious sinus infection is likely.

You can reduce the risk of sinus infections for your child by reducing exposure to known environmental allergies and pollutants such

141

as tobacco smoke, reducing his/her time at day care, and treating stomach acid reflux disease.

How Will the Doctor Treat Sinusitis?

Acute sinusitis: Most children respond very well to antibiotic therapy. Nasal decongestants or topical nasal sprays may also be prescribed for short-term relief of stuffiness. Nasal saline (saltwater) drops or gentle spray can be helpful in thinning secretions and improving mucous membrane function.

If your child has acute sinusitis, symptoms should improve within the first few days. Even if your child improves dramatically within the first week of treatment, it is important that you continue therapy until all the antibiotics have been taken. Your doctor may decide to treat your child with additional medicines if he/she has allergies or other conditions that make the sinus infection worse.

Chronic sinusitis: If your child suffers from one or more symptoms of sinusitis for at least twelve weeks, he or she may have chronic sinusitis. Chronic sinusitis or recurrent episodes of acute sinusitis numbering more than four to six per year, are indications that you should seek consultation with an ear, nose, and throat (ENT) specialist. The ENT may recommend medical or surgical treatment of the sinuses.

Diagnosis of Sinusitis

If your child sees an ENT specialist, the doctor will examine his/her ears, nose, and throat. A thorough history and examination usually leads to the correct diagnosis. Occasionally, special instruments will be used to look into the nose during the office visit. An x-ray called a CT scan may help to determine how your child's sinuses are formed, where the blockage has occurred, and the reliability of a sinusitis diagnosis.

When Is Surgery Necessary?

Surgery is considered for the small percentage of children with severe or persistent sinusitis symptoms despite medical therapy. Using an instrument called an endoscope, the ENT surgeon opens the natural drainage pathways of your child's sinuses and makes the narrow passages wider. This also allows for culturing so that antibiotics can be directed specifically against your child's sinus infection. Opening up the sinuses and allowing air to circulate usually results in a reduction in the number and severity of sinus infections.

Also, your doctor may advise removing adenoid tissue from behind the nose as part of the treatment for sinusitis. Although the adenoid tissue does not directly block the sinuses, infection of the adenoid tissue, called adenoiditis, or obstruction of the back of the nose, can cause many of the symptoms that are similar to sinusitis, namely, runny nose, stuffy nose, post-nasal drip, bad breath, cough, and headache.

Summary

Sinusitis in children is different than sinusitis in adults. Children more often demonstrate a cough, bad breath, crankiness, low energy, and swelling around the eyes along with a thick yellow-green nasal or post-nasal drip. Once the diagnosis of sinusitis has been made, children are successfully treated with antibiotic therapy in most cases. If medical therapy fails, surgical therapy can be used as a safe and effective method of treating sinus disease in children.

Chapter 20

Headaches in Children

- Headaches can be a common problem in children.

- Somewhere between 4% and 10% of children have migraine headaches.

- Many adults with headaches started having their headaches as children, with 20% reporting the onset before age 10.

- Most headaches in children are benign—meaning they are not symptoms of some serious disorder or disease.

- Migraine headaches often run in families, so information on other family member's headaches are important.

- Headache may interfere with participation in activities and school and can be a significant health problem.

Aren't Headaches Just Headaches?

Headaches can be divided into two categories, primary or secondary. Primary refers to headaches that occur on their own and not as the result of some other health problem. Primary headaches include migraine, migraine with aura, tension-type headache, and cluster headache. Secondary refers to headaches that result from some cause or condition, such as a head injury or concussion, blood vessel problems, medication side effects, infections in the head or elsewhere in the body, sinus disease, or tumors. There are many different causes for secondary headaches, ranging from rare, serious diseases to easily treated conditions. Sometimes headaches occur almost every day and are called chronic daily headaches.

You should consult your family doctor if headaches are frequent or severe or include unusual symptoms. Your physician may ask you to describe features of your headaches (for example, the location of the pain, pain severity, and any other symptoms associated with the headache attack). To rule out the possibility of secondary headache, the physician may decide to order special tests, including a CT (Computed Tomography) scan or an MRI (Magnetic Resonance Imaging). Worrisome symptoms that should be brought to your doctor's attention include:

- Headaches that wake a child from sleep.

- Early morning vomiting without nausea (upset stomach).

- Worsening or more frequent headaches.

- Personality changes.

- Complaints that "this is the worst headache I've ever had!"

- The headache is different than previous headaches.

- Headaches with fever or a stiff neck.

- Headaches that follow an injury.

What Is a Tension-Type Headache?

This type of headache has also been called a tension headache, muscle contraction headache, stress-related headache, and ordinary headache. These headaches can be either episodic or chronic and may include tightness in the muscles of the head or neck.

A tension-type headache can last from 30 minutes to several days. Chronic tension headaches may persist for many months. The pain usually occurs on both sides of the head, is steady and nonthrobbing. Some people say "it feels like a band tightening around my head." The pain is usually mild to moderate in severity. Most of the time the headache does not affect the person's activity level.

Tension-type headaches are usually not associated with other symptoms, such as nausea or vomiting. Some people may experience sensitivity to light or sound with the headache, but not both. Muscle tightness may be noticed by some patients but doesn't always have to occur.

What Is a Migraine Headache?

Migraine headaches are recurrent headaches that occur at intervals of days, weeks, or months. There may or may not be a pattern to the attacks—for example, teenage girls may tend to have attacks at a particular point in their monthly menstrual cycle.

Migraines generally have some of the following symptoms and characteristics:

- Untreated, they can last from 2 to 48 hours in children. Sleep or medical treatment can reduce this time period.

- Headache starts on one side of the head. This may vary from headache to headache and in children, they may start in the front or in both temples.

- Throbbing or pounding pain during the headache.

- Pain is rated as moderate to severe.

- Pain gets worse with exertion. The pain may be so severe that it is difficult or almost impossible to continue with normal daily activities.

- Nausea, vomiting, and/or stomach pain commonly occur with the attacks.

- Light and/or sound sensitivity is also common.

- Pain may be relieved with rest or sleep.

- Other members of the family have had migraines or sick headaches.

- Warnings called auras may start before the headache. These auras can include blurry vision, flashing lights, colored spots, strange tastes, or weird sensations and usually precede the headache by 5 to 60 minutes.

What Are Chronic Daily Headaches?

In adults, headaches that occur at least 15 days per month for at least 3 months have been called chronic daily headaches. In children there is not yet a clear definition.

Some chronic daily headaches may have started as migraine and build to a daily frequency. These are sometimes called transformed migraines. Tension-type headaches that increase to near-daily frequency are known as chronic tension-type headaches. Chronic headaches can result from taking some types of medication—for example, acetaminophen (Tylenol), ibuprofen (Motrin), caffeine, and some prescription medications—almost every day. These are called drug rebound headaches. These headaches either return shortly after taking the medication, or the medication stops working. The most effective way to make these headaches better is to stop taking pain medicines altogether for a few weeks. After that time, use of pain-relievers is limited to no more that 2 to 3 times per week.

Some people with chronic daily headaches are low in certain vitamins and minerals. It is important to eat balanced meals. Many children and adolescents may need to take a daily multivitamin. Your doctor or nurse practitioner may talk to you about getting blood tests to see if you need more vitamins or minerals.

What Causes Headaches?

There are different theories about the cause of migraine headaches. Often several family members are affected, suggesting genetic factors are partly responsible. Some individuals may become hypersensitive to triggers in their environment, such as flickering lights, changing weather patterns, or strong odors. The true cause may be a combination of factors. Some of the possible causes include:

- Blood vessel changes. Blood vessels in the head may first tighten and then expand during a migraine attack, changes that may explain the aura before and the throbbing pain during the migraine. Some migraine medication and other treatments may work by counteracting or blocking these changes in the blood vessels.

- Brain and nervous system changes. Imaging studies have identified an area in the brainstem at the back of the head that is activated during a migraine attack. A spreading wave of decreased activation occurs in the brain at the onset of an attack, which may account for the blurred vision or numbness that some people experience in the migraine aura.

- Serotonin system abnormalities. Serotonin is a natural chemical in the brain that has an important function in transmission of signals from one brain cell to another. Some migraine medication and other treatments affect serotonin action in the brain and can stop a migraine.

What Can I Do to Prevent Headaches?

Taking good care of yourself can decrease the frequency and severity of headaches:

1. Make sure you drink enough fluids. Children and adolescents need from 4 to 8 glasses of fluid a day. Caffeine should be avoided. Sports drinks may also help during a headache as well as during exercise by keeping sugar and sodium levels normal.

2. Make sure you get plenty of regular sleep at night (but don't oversleep). Fatigue and over exertion are two factors that can trigger headaches. Most children and adolescents need to sleep 8 to 10 hours each night and keep a regular sleep schedule to help prevent headaches.

3. Be sure that you eat balanced meals at regular hours. Do not skip meals.

4. Try to avoid foods that seem to trigger headaches. Remember that everyone is different, so your triggers may be different from someone else's.

5. Plan and schedule your activities sensibly. Try to avoid overcrowded schedules or stressful and potentially upsetting situations.

Also, if your doctor prescribed daily medication to reduce headache frequency (called preventive or prophylactic medication), remember to take it every day, whether you're having headaches or not.

What Do I Do If I Get a Headache?

Keep a record of your headaches. Write down everything that might relate to your headache (foods, odors, situations), how long it lasted, and how much pain the headache caused.

Take pain medication for your headache as soon as you feel pain. You may be taking over-the-counter medication or prescription medication when you get a headache. Follow your doctor's instructions in using your medication and treatment plan.

You need to be able to treat your headaches at school. This means that your school nurse needs to know your treatment plan. It is important that you discuss this with your doctor, so that all of the forms and permission are completed for treating your headaches at school without having to go home. You may even need to educate your teachers about headaches and migraines.

Remember that using pain-relievers (analgesics) every day can cause an increase in your headaches. Drinking more fluids (especially sports drinks) during a headache may also be very important to help it to go away faster.

Chapter 21

Periodontal (Gum) Disease

What Is Gum Disease?

Gum disease or periodontal disease or gingivitis as it is also called is the number one cause of tooth loss today. The reason you lose teeth from gum disease is because this disease attacks the gums as well as the bones, which are the foundation in which your teeth rest. As the bone literally dissolves away from around your teeth, your teeth become loose and eventually fall out.

Anyone at any age is susceptible to gum disease. Gum disease is caused by plaque. If the plaque is not removed on a daily basis it will form calculus, which is the breeding ground for the germs which cause gum disease. Bleeding gums are the first sign that there may be a problem with the gums. Puffy, tender red gums are also a sign that there is an infection present. Bleeding gums, however, are not always present even in severe cases of gum disease.

Routine and regular visits to the dentist are the best way of catching gum disease in its early stages before too much damage has been caused. Gum disease will not go away by itself or with improved home care. The only way of removing plaque deep under the gums is with professional cleanings. Once you have had a gum problem you will always be susceptible to recurring problems, so be sure to see your dentist on a regular basis—every three to four months, unless he or she recommends otherwise.

Excerpted from "Periodontal Disease," Smiles4ever.com, http://www. smiles4ever. com/perio-news.htm, 2001. This information is reprinted with permission of Richard M. Weledniger, DDS, PC. For more information, visit www.smiles4ever.com. © 2001.

Signs of Periodontal Disease

If you notice any of the following signs, please call and make an appointment with your child's dentist immediately

- gums that bleed when you brush the teeth
- red, swollen, puffy or tender gums
- gums that have pulled away from the teeth
- bad breath, that just does not want to go away
- exudate or pus that is between teeth
- a loose or several loose teeth [excluding baby teeth]
- a change in the way your teeth come together when you close your mouth

What Is Root Planing?

Normal tooth cleanings remove plaque and calculus deposits from above the gum line. When these deposits extend below the gum line, root planing is necessary.

Root planing is performed with the same tools as normal cleanings, but the procedure is more aggressive. Often it is necessary to numb the affected area before the procedure. Once the accumulated plaque and calculus have been removed, the gums will heal, tightening around the teeth.

Depending upon the extent of disease found in the examination, root planing may be done over several office visits. In this way, your dentist can assess the progress of treatment, and alter tactics if necessary.

Simply stated, root planing may be considered as an extension of a "routine cleaning." A "routine cleaning" is intended to clean hardened deposits that form above the gums. Over time, these deposits often form below the gums, on the roots. It is at this point that we recommend a more therapeutic procedure, called root planing.

What Does It Accomplish?

During this procedure the root surfaces are literally planed. This accomplishes several things:

- removes hard deposits and the bacteria they harbor
- creates a smooth root surface that is easier to keep clean
- reduces infection because the bacteria will not re-attach to the smooth surface as readily

Chapter 22

Canker Sores and Cold Sores

Questions and Answers about Canker Sores

What are canker sores?

They're small, painful, crater-like nuisances that sprout on the tongue or on the inside of the cheeks. The sores are usually white, gray, or yellowish with a red rim and last up to two weeks. (Some people confuse them with cold sores, which form blisters instead of craters and usually show up on or around the lips.) Canker sores are most common in teenagers and women, but they can strike children as young as two.

What causes canker sores?

These simple sores are a real mystery. Nobody knows why they erupt, but several factors seem to set the stage for their arrival, including emotional stress, irritation from sour or spicy foods, or injury to the mouth's lining from toothbrushing, biting, hot liquids, or rough foods such as corn chips. If your child frequently gets sores, he may have a more deep-rooted problem such as a food allergy or a deficiency of vitamin B_{12}, folic acid, or iron.

This chapter includes "Canker Sores (Children)" and "Cold Sores," both by Chris Woolston, M.S., reviewed by Karen Buchi, M.D., associate professor of pediatrics, University of Utah School of Medicine, Salt Lake City, Utah. © 1999 Consumer Health Interactive, updated September 2001; reprinted with permission.

Unlike cold sores, canker sores aren't caused by a virus or any other type of germ, and they can't spread from one person to another. So don't turn down a goodnight kiss just because your child has a canker sore. (Remember, the kiss supply will run awfully low in a few years.)

How can I treat them?

Once canker sores appear, there's no way to speed their healing. But you can take some steps to make the sores less painful and annoying. Have your child avoid spicy, sour, or rough-edged foods like corn chips that can irritate the sores. If he's old enough, have him rinse his mouth several times each day with a cup of warm water mixed with half a teaspoon of salt (don't let him swallow). For younger children, apply a paste of baking soda and water directly on the sore after meals. You can also ease the pain with an over-the-counter salve, Zilactin, which contains tannic acid that will numb the sore; it stings terribly for a few minutes, though, so it's not a realistic option for young children. Ibuprofen or acetaminophen will also lessen pain from the sores. (Don't use aspirin in anyone under 20; it may cause Reye syndrome, a rare but potentially life-threatening illness.) With luck, you might be able to coax your child into eating a dish of cold ice cream to numb the spot.

When should I call the doctor?

Schedule an appointment with your pediatrician if the sores last more than two weeks, the pain becomes severe, or your child has trouble swallowing. Consult the doctor as well if the sores continually crop up.

How can I prevent my child from getting canker sores?

Buy your child a soft-bristled toothbrush, and make sure he uses it at least twice each day. Give him toothpaste that doesn't contain sodium lauryl sulfate, a detergent that seems to promote the sores. Biotene Dry Mouth Toothpaste and Rembrandt Natural Toothpaste are two of the brands that don't contain the ingredient.

If your child is allergic to certain foods, make sure he avoids them. If canker sores are a chronic problem, your pediatrician may recommend a daily multivitamin to help boost your child's immune system.

Questions and Answers about Cold Sores

What are cold sores?

Cold sores, also known as fever blisters, are small red blisters that crop up near the lips or on them. More rarely, they sprout on the roof of the mouth. (Some people confuse them with canker sores, which are painful crater-like sores that appear on the tongue or on the inside of the cheeks.) Despite their name, cold sores actually have nothing to do with colds; they're caused by the herpes simplex virus type 1 (HSV-1), a close relative of the virus that causes genital herpes.

How do you get cold sores?

Most children pick up the virus by sharing food with or kissing someone who has a cold sore. They can also get the infection from someone who doesn't have a visible sore but has the virus in his or her saliva. Once you contract the virus, it stays in your body for good, hiding in nerve cells near your ear. In some people, the virus lies dormant and never causes harm. In others, it periodically wakes up and triggers cold sores. Nobody knows what stirs the virus into action, but stress, fever, colds, and sunburn seem to encourage outbreaks.

What are the symptoms?

Children don't develop cold sores immediately after the first time they catch the virus. Instead, your child may have swollen gums and a sore feeling in the mouth. A few days later, you may see a cluster of small blisters that turn into a shallow, painful sore, possibly accompanied by fever and swollen lymph glands in the neck. In a few days the sore will crust over and slowly disappear. The whole flare-up lasts about seven to ten days.

What's the best way to treat cold sores?

Cold sores will go away on their own, but there are some things you can do to help your child feel better in the meantime.

- To ease the pain, apply ice to the sore or give your child a mild pain reliever, such as ibuprofen or acetaminophen. (Never give aspirin to children or teenagers; it may trigger Reye syndrome, a rare but potentially life-threatening illness.)

- Have your child avoid salty, spicy, and sour foods, which irritate the raw nerves in the sore.

- Dab on a water-based zinc ointment. It helps dry out the sore so it can heal faster, and the zinc may also aid the immune system.

To keep your child from infecting other parts of his body or giving the virus to someone else, encourage him to wash his hands regularly and keep him from picking at his sores.

One last caution: Urge your child to avoid touching his eyes when he has a cold sore. HSV-1 can cause ocular herpes, a serious eye infection. If your child develops a painful sore on his eyelid or the surface of his eye, schedule a prompt appointment with his pediatrician: Your child may need antiviral drugs to keep the infection from scarring his cornea. In rare cases, ocular herpes can weaken vision and even cause blindness.

Also, any kind of herpes virus is dangerous to newborns. If you have a newborn, keep any of your children who have a cold sore away from him until it's healed.

How can I prevent cold sores?

The first thing you can do is try to keep your child free of the virus that causes cold sores, which may be difficult, given how contagious HSV-1 is. Remember, one peck with an infected lip is all it takes to pass on the virus. If you have sores and your child doesn't, cut out kissing until you've healed.

If you are the parent of a newborn and have a cold sore, you don't need to separate yourself from your new baby. Do wash your hands frequently, though, and avoid kissing your baby until the cold sore goes away. You may consider wearing a surgical mask to cover the sore as well. Infectious disease experts do recommend that women with herpes sores on their breasts refrain from breast feeding until the sores are healed.

If your child already has the virus, the best thing you can do is keep his immune system strong by making sure he gets a healthful diet, plenty of sleep, and regular exercise. Giving your child a daily multivitamin may also help boost his immune system.

You should protect your child from the sun as well. If he ventures outside on a sunny day, slather him with sunscreen and put on a lip balm that contains sunblock.

Resources and References

"Fever Blisters and Canker Sores," U.S. Department of Health and Human Services, Public Health Service, National Institutes of Health. NIH Publication No. 87-247.

Health Magazine, The Self-Care Advisor: The Essential Home Health Guide for You and Your Family, Time Life, 2000, p. 78–80.

Robert H. Pantell M.D., James F. Fries M.D., Donald M. Vickery M.D., *Taking Care of Your Child: A Parent's Illustrated Guide to Complete Medical Care*. Perseus Books Publishing, L.L.C.: 1999.

—by Chris Woolston, M.S.
—Consumer Health Interactive

About the Author

Chris Woolston is a health and medical writer with a master's degree in biology. He is a contributing editor at Consumer Health Interactive, and was the staff writer at *Hippocrates*, a magazine for physicians. He has also covered science issues for Time, Inc., Health, WebMD, and the *Chronicle of Higher Education*. His reporting on occupational health earned him an award from the northern California Society of Professional Journalists.

Part Four

Digestive and Genitourinary Diseases and Disorders

Chapter 23

Vomiting and Diarrhea in Children

Vomiting

Why does vomiting occur?

- Vomiting is common. Often it is caused by stomach upset from a virus. An infection, pain, excitement, or other problems can also cause it.

- Vomiting that lasts for more than 6 hours should be considered serious. Call your child's doctor.

- Vomiting can cause drying out or dehydration, which can be very serious. Dehydration happens when your child loses too much liquid. You can prevent dehydration by increasing the amount of liquid your child drinks.

Signs of Dehydration

Call your child's doctor immediately if your child shows any of these signs. Do not wait for the later signs of dehydration.

- Child has not urinated in 6 hours.

This chapter includes excerpts from "Vomiting," © 1998 Cincinnati Children's Hospital Medical Center (www.cincinnatichildrens.org); reprinted with permission. The section "Acute Diarrhea" is excerpted from "Childhood Diarrhea: Messages for Parents," Centers for Disease Control and Prevention (CDC), August 2000; "Chronic Diarrhea" is excerpted from a fact sheet produced by CDC's Division of Parasitic Diseases, August 1999.

- Child is less active than normal or is unusually sleepy.
- Child's urine is dark yellow and may smell strong like ammonia.
- Child's mouth is dry and sticky.

Later signs of dehydration include:

- Child's eyes are sunken.
- Child has no energy and is difficult to wake up.
- Child has a fever.

Call Your Child's Doctor

- If your child shows any signs of dehydration.
- If your child has green or bloody vomit.
- If your child experiences severe stomach pain.

Liquids to Give Your Children

- Gatorade® (Check with your child's doctor about other sports drinks. They may not be right for your child.)
- Caffeine-free tea
- Popsicles
- Broth

How to Give Liquids to Children

Give liquids in small amounts and frequently. For example, give 1 or 2 ounces every half hour. If your child takes this well, increase the amount a little every half hour. If your child vomits, decrease the amount of liquid for the next feeding and then try to slowly increase the amount again with every feeding after that.

Slowly advance the diet to a regular diet. Greasy foods and foods high in sugar should be added slowly because they may increase vomiting.

Foods to start with:

- Rice
- Plain crackers
- Chicken
- Noodles

- Potatoes
- Bananas
- Applesauce

Foods to avoid until the vomiting improves:

- Fruit juice
- Kool-Aid®
- Fried foods
- Dairy products

Warning: Do not use any medication for your child unless your child's doctor tells you to give it to your child. Medications that are good for adults or older children can be dangerous for babies or small children.

Acute Diarrhea

Diarrhea is the passage of loose or watery stools that may contain blood, pus, or mucus. Children with diarrhea often have additional symptoms including nausea, vomiting, stomach aches, headache, and fever.

Diarrhea can impact the ability of the body to process and absorb necessary water, salts and nutrition and can lead to dehydration, shock and even death.

What causes acute diarrhea?

Mild, acute diarrhea can be caused by a number of conditions, including:

- a change in dietary habits, such as eating rich or different foods
- food allergies
- taking medicines such as antibiotics

Serious, acute diarrhea can be caused by a variety of viruses, bacteria, and parasites including:

- rotavirus
- *E. coli* O157:H7
- *Salmonella*

- certain respiratory infections

Most episodes of serious, acute diarrhea in children are caused by viruses. Diarrheal illness can be seasonal or may occur in outbreaks where many people are affected.

How do you treat diarrhea?

Dehydration is the biggest threat from diarrheal diseases in children. Illnesses that cause diarrhea or vomiting can lead to dehydration if the child loses more body fluids and salts (electrolytes) than he/she takes in. To prevent dehydration, your child may require special fluids.

- The best fluid to give children with diarrhea is an oral rehydration solution such as Ceralyte, Pedialyte or Oralyte. These solutions can be purchased in nearly all drug stores and grocery stores. Parents should keep two bottles or packages of these solutions on hand in case your child gets diarrhea. Follow the instructions on the solution according to your child's age.

- Sports drinks do not replace the fluid losses correctly and should not be used for the treatment of diarrheal illness.

- Children who are breastfeeding, taking formula, or eating solids should continue to follow their usual diet.

The best chance to prevent dehydration, hospitalization or death from diarrheal diseases is by making sure children receive enough fluids, and by seeking medical care when diarrhea is severe or you are concerned about dehydration. It is vital to replace fluids properly. Your health care provider can help you decide what is right for your child.

When should you call a doctor if your child has diarrhea?

Contact your health care provider if diarrhea is accompanied by the following (particularly if your child is less than 6 months of age):

- High fever (temperature over 101.5° F, measured orally)

- Blood in stools

- Prolonged vomiting that prevents keeping liquids down (which can lead to dehydration)

- Signs of dehydration, including:
  - Decrease in urination
  - Sunken eyes
  - No tears when child cries
  - Extreme thirst
  - Unusual drowsiness or fussiness
  - Dry, sticky mouth

Are antibiotics needed to treat diarrheal diseases?

Do not be surprised if your doctor does not prescribe an antibiotic to treat a diarrheal illness. Many diarrheal illnesses are caused by viruses and will improve in two or three days without antibiotics. In fact, antibiotics have no effect on viruses, and using an antibiotic to treat a virus infection could cause harm and will do the child no good. Antibiotics are often not needed to treat mild bacterial infections.

How are diarrheal illnesses spread?

Children and adults can become infected by coming in direct contact with the feces of an infected child and then passing the infection to the mouth (fecal-oral transmission). Often, another child or adult touches a surface that has been contaminated, touches his or her mouth and then ingests the germs. A child with a diarrheal illness may be contagious before the onset of diarrhea and for a few days after the diarrhea has ended. Germs that cause diarrhea can also be spread by contaminated food.

How do you prevent spreading diarrheal illnesses?

Careful and frequent handwashing can prevent the spread of infection to other people.

- Adults should wash their hands after using the toilet, helping a child use the toilet, and diapering a child and before preparing, serving, or eating food.
- Children should wash their hands after using the toilet, after having their diapers changed (an adult should wash infant's or small child's hands), and before eating snacks or meals.
- Disinfect toys, bathrooms, and food preparation surfaces frequently, especially if a sick child has been in the home.

- Use diapers with waterproof outer covers that can contain liquid stool or urine, or use plastic pants

- Make sure that children wear clothes over diapers.

Chronic Diarrhea

What is chronic diarrhea?

Diarrhea that lasts for more than two weeks is considered persistent or chronic. In an otherwise healthy person, chronic diarrhea may be a nuisance, or, for someone who has a weak immune system, a life-threatening illness.

What causes chronic diarrhea?

There are many causes of chronic diarrhea; these may be different for children and adults. Causes of chronic diarrhea can be grouped into two categories: diarrhea caused by an infection and diarrhea not caused by an infection. Sometimes, the cause of chronic diarrhea remains unknown.

Diarrhea caused by an infection may result from:

- parasites, such as *Cryptosporidium parvum, Cyclospora cayetanensis, Entamoeba histolytica, Giardia lamblia,* microsporidia.

- bacteria, such as *Campylobacter, Clostridium difficile, Escherichia coli, Listeria monocytogenes, Salmonella enteritidis, Shigella.*

- viral infections, such as HIV, rotavirus, Norwalk agent

Diarrhea not caused by an infection may result from:

- antibiotics
- high blood pressure medications
- cancer drugs
- Crohn disease
- colitis
- diabetes, thyroid, and other endocrine diseases
- food additives (sorbitol, fructose, and others)
- food allergies

- previous surgery or radiation of the abdomen or gastrointestinal tract
- tumors
- reduced blood flow to the intestine
- heredity—certain diseases occur more often in related family members
- travel

How is chronic diarrhea diagnosed?

Diagnosis may be difficult and requires that your health care provider take a careful history and perform a physical exam. The types of tests that your health care provider orders will be based on your symptoms and history. Tests may include blood or stool tests; stool cultures may be used to test for bacteria. To detect parasites, the Centers for Disease Control and Prevention (CDC) recommends that three or more stool samples be examined. Special stains may be required to look for some parasites. If these initial tests do not reveal the cause of your diarrhea, additional tests may include radiographs (x-rays) and endoscopy. Endoscopy is a procedure in which a tube is inserted into the mouth or rectum so that the doctor, usually a gastroenterologist, can look at the intestine from the inside.

Who is at risk for chronic diarrhea?

Persons with severely weakened immune systems, such as those with HIV/AIDS, those taking certain types of chemotherapy, or persons who have recently received an organ transplant are at risk. So are travelers to developing countries where the water and food supply may be contaminated.

How is chronic diarrhea treated?

The key to treating chronic diarrhea is to determine its cause.

- Diarrhea caused by an infection can often be treated with antibiotics. However, the correct diagnosis must be made so the proper medication can be prescribed.
- Diarrhea not caused by an infection is more difficult to diagnose and treat. Long-term medication or surgery may be required. Specific treatment for chronic diarrhea not caused by an infection should be discussed with your health care provider.

For diarrhea whose cause has not been determined, follow these important treatment guidelines to relieve symptoms:

- Prevent dehydration. Serious health problems can occur if you don't maintain your body's proper fluid levels. Diarrhea may become worse and hospitalization may be required if dehydration occurs. Many oral rehydration solutions such as Pedialyte and Oralyte are available at drug stores. Ask your pharmacist or health care provider for the product best for you.

- Do not drink beverages containing caffeine, such as tea, coffee, and soft drinks.

- Do not drink alcohol; it causes dehydration.

- Do not rely on sports drinks and broths alone to maintain adequate fluid balance. They should not be used to prevent severe dehydration.

- Maintain well-balanced nutrition. Doing so may help you recover more quickly.

How is chronic diarrhea spread?

Chronic diarrhea caused by an infection can be spread by drinking water or eating food contaminated with stool. Close contact with a person who has diarrhea may also spread infection. This occurs when a person accidentally puts something that is contaminated with stool in or around his or her mouth. In general, chronic diarrhea not caused by an infection is not spread to other people.

How can chronic diarrhea be prevented?

- Drink clean or purified water.
- Use proper food handling techniques.
- Maintain proper hand-washing habits.

Chapter 24

Bacterial Foodborne Illnesses

Chapter Contents

Section 24.1

Escherichia Coli *O157:H7*

Excerpted from *"Escherichia Coli* O157:H7," Division of Bacterial and Mycotic Diseases, Centers for Disease Control and Prevention, June 2001.

Questions and Answers about E. Coli

What is Escherichia coli *O157:H7?*

E. coli O157:H7 is one of hundreds of strains of the bacterium *Escherichia coli*. Although most strains are harmless and live in the intestines of healthy humans and animals, this strain produces a powerful toxin and can cause severe illness. *E. coli* O157:H7 was first recognized as a cause of illness in 1982 during an outbreak of severe bloody diarrhea; the outbreak was traced to contaminated hamburgers. Since then, most infections have come from eating undercooked ground beef. The combination of letters and numbers in the name of the bacterium refers to the specific markers found on its surface and distinguishes it from other types of *E. coli*.

How is E. coli *O157:H7 spread?*

The organism can be found on a small number of cattle farms and can live in the intestines of healthy cattle. Meat can become contaminated during slaughter, and organisms can be thoroughly mixed into beef when it is ground. Bacteria present on the cow's udders or on equipment may get into raw milk.

Eating meat, especially ground beef, that has not been cooked sufficiently to kill *E. coli* O157:H7 can cause infection. Contaminated meat looks and smells normal. Although the number of organisms required to cause disease is not known, it is suspected to be very small.

Among other known sources of infection are consumption of sprouts, lettuce, salami, unpasteurized milk and juice, and swimming in or drinking sewage-contaminated water.

Bacteria in diarrheal stools of infected persons can be passed from one person to another if hygiene or handwashing habits are inadequate. This is particularly likely among toddlers who are not toilet trained. Family members and playmates of these children are at high risk of becoming infected. Young children typically shed the organism in their feces for a week or two after their illness resolves. Older children rarely carry the organism without symptoms.

What illness does E. coli O157:H7 cause?

E. coli O157:H7 infection often causes severe bloody diarrhea and abdominal cramps; sometimes the infection causes nonbloody diarrhea or no symptoms. Usually little or no fever is present, and the illness resolves in 5 to 10 days.

In some persons, particularly children under 5 years of age and the elderly, the infection can also cause a complication called hemolytic uremic syndrome, in which the red blood cells are destroyed and the kidneys fail. About 2%–7% of infections lead to this complication. In the United States, hemolytic uremic syndrome is the principal cause of acute kidney failure in children, and most cases of hemolytic uremic syndrome are caused by *E. coli* O157:H7.

How is E. coli O157:H7 infection diagnosed?

Infection with *E. coli* O157:H7 is diagnosed by detecting the bacterium in the stool. Most laboratories that culture stool do not test for *E. coli* O157:H7, so it is important to request that the stool specimen be tested on sorbitol-MacConkey (SMAC) agar for this organism. All persons who suddenly have diarrhea with blood should get their stool tested for *E. coli* O157:H7.

How is the illness treated?

Most persons recover without antibiotics or other specific treatment in 5–10 days. There is no evidence that antibiotics improve the course of disease, and it is thought that treatment with some antibiotics may precipitate kidney complications. Antidiarrheal agents, such as loperamide (Imodium), should also be avoided.

Hemolytic uremic syndrome is a life-threatening condition usually treated in an intensive care unit. Blood transfusions and kidney dialysis are often required. With intensive care, the death rate for hemolytic uremic syndrome is 3%–5%.

What are the long-term consequences of infection?

Persons who only have diarrhea usually recover completely.

About one-third of persons with hemolytic uremic syndrome have abnormal kidney function many years later, and a few require long-term dialysis. Another 8% of persons with hemolytic uremic syndrome have other lifelong complications, such as high blood pressure, seizures, blindness, paralysis, and the effects of having part of their bowel removed.

What can you do to prevent E. coli O157:H7 infection?

- Cook all ground beef and hamburger thoroughly. Ground beef should be cooked until a thermometer inserted into several parts of the patty, including the thickest part, reads at least 160° F.

- If you are served an undercooked hamburger or other ground beef product in a restaurant, send it back for further cooking. You may want to ask for a new bun and a clean plate, too.

- In your kitchen, keep raw meat separate from ready-to-eat foods. Wash hands, counters, and utensils with hot soapy water after they touch raw meat. Never place cooked hamburgers or ground beef on the unwashed plate that held raw patties. Wash meat thermometers in between tests of patties that require further cooking.

- Drink only pasteurized milk, juice, or cider.

- Wash fruits and vegetables thoroughly, especially those that will not be cooked. Children under 5 years of age, immunocompromised persons, and the elderly should avoid eating alfalfa sprouts until their safety can be assured. Methods to decontaminate alfalfa seeds and sprouts are being investigated.

- Drink municipal water that has been treated with chlorine or other effective disinfectants.

- Avoid swallowing lake or pool water while swimming.

- Make sure that persons with diarrhea, especially children, wash their hands carefully with soap after bowel movements to reduce the risk of spreading infection, and that persons wash hands after changing soiled diapers. Anyone with a diarrheal illness should avoid swimming in public pools or lakes, sharing baths with others, and preparing food for others.

For More Information

An estimated 73,000 cases of *Escherichia coli* O157:H7 infection and 61 deaths occur in the United States each year. Most illness has been associated with eating undercooked, contaminated ground beef. Person-to-person contact in families and child care centers is also an important mode of transmission.

For more information about reducing your risk of foodborne illness, visit the U.S. Department of Agriculture's Food Safety and Inspection Service website at http://www.fsis.usda.gov or the Partnership for Food Safety Education at www.fightbac.org.

Section 24.2

Salmonellosis

This section contains text from "Salmonellosis: Frequently Asked Questions," http://www.cdc.gov/ncidod/dbmd/diseaseinfo/salmonellosis_g.htm, reviewed June 2001, and "*Salmonella* Infections in the Child Care Setting," January 1997, updated in June, 2002 by Dr. David A. Cooke, MD, Diplomate, American Board of Internal Medicine. Both documents are from the Centers for Disease Control and Prevention (CDC).

Salmonellosis: Frequently Asked Questions

What is salmonellosis?

Salmonellosis is an infection with a bacteria called *Salmonella*. Most persons infected with *Salmonella* develop diarrhea, fever, and abdominal cramps 12 to 72 hours after infection. The illness usually lasts 4 to 7 days, and most persons recover without treatment. However, in some persons the diarrhea may be so severe that the patient needs to be hospitalized. In these patients, the *Salmonella* infection may spread from the intestines to the blood stream, and then to other body sites and can cause death unless the person is treated promptly with antibiotics. The elderly, infants, and those with impaired immune systems are more likely to have a severe illness.

How can **Salmonella** *infections be diagnosed?*

Many different kinds of illnesses can cause diarrhea, fever, or abdominal cramps. Determining that *Salmonella* is the cause of the illness depends on laboratory tests that identify *Salmonella* in the stools of an infected person. These tests are sometimes not performed unless the laboratory is instructed specifically to look for the organism. Once *Salmonella* has been identified, further testing can determine its specific type, and which antibiotics could be used to treat it.

How can Salmonella *infections be treated?*

Salmonella infections usually resolve in 5–7 days and often do not require treatment unless the patient becomes severely dehydrated or the infection spreads from the intestines. Persons with severe diarrhea may require rehydration, often with intravenous fluids. Antibiotics are not usually necessary unless the infection spreads from the intestines, then it can be treated with ampicillin, gentamicin, trimethoprim/sulfamethoxazole, or ciprofloxacin. Unfortunately, some *Salmonella* bacteria have become resistant to antibiotics, largely as a result of the use of antibiotics to promote the growth of feed animals.

Are there long-term consequences to a Salmonella *infection?*

Persons with diarrhea usually recover completely, although it may be several months before their bowel habits are entirely normal. A small number of persons who are infected with *Salmonella*, will go on to develop pains in their joints, irritation of the eyes, and painful urination. This is called Reiter's syndrome. It can last for months or years, and can lead to chronic arthritis which is difficult to treat. Antibiotic treatment does not make a difference in whether or not the person later develops arthritis.

How do people catch Salmonella?

Salmonella live in the intestinal tracts of humans and other animals, including birds. *Salmonella* are usually transmitted to humans by eating foods contaminated with animal feces. Contaminated foods usually look and smell normal. Contaminated foods are often of animal origin, such as beef, poultry, milk, or eggs, but all foods, including vegetables may become contaminated. Many raw foods of animal origin are frequently contaminated, but fortunately, thorough cooking kills *Salmonella*. Food may also become contaminated by the unwashed hands of an infected food handler, who forgot to wash his or her hands with soap after using the bathroom.

Salmonella may also be found in the feces of some pets, especially those with diarrhea, and people can become infected if they do not wash their hands after contact with these feces. Reptiles are particularly likely to harbor *Salmonella* and people should always wash their hands immediately after handling a reptile, even if the reptile is healthy. Adults should also be careful that children wash their hands after handling a reptile.

What can a person do to prevent this illness?

There is no vaccine to prevent salmonellosis. Since foods of animal origin may be contaminated with *Salmonella*, people should not eat raw or undercooked eggs, poultry, or meat. Raw eggs may be unrecognized in some foods such as homemade hollandaise sauce, caesar and other salad dressings, tiramisu, homemade ice cream, homemade mayonnaise, cookie dough, and frostings. Poultry and meat, including hamburgers, should be well-cooked, not pink in the middle. Persons also should not consume raw or unpasteurized milk or other dairy products. Produce should be thoroughly washed before consuming.

Cross-contamination of foods should be avoided. Uncooked meats should be keep separate from produce, cooked foods, and ready-to-eat foods. Hands, cutting boards, counters, knives, and other utensils should be washed thoroughly after handling uncooked foods. Hands should be washed before handling any food, and between handling different food items.

People who have salmonellosis should not prepare food or pour water for others until they have been shown to no longer be carrying the *Salmonella* bacterium.

People should wash their hands after contact with animal feces. Since reptiles are particularly likely to have *Salmonella*, everyone should immediately wash their hands after handling reptiles. Reptiles (including turtles) are not appropriate pets for small children and should not be in the same house as an infant.

How common is salmonellosis?

Every year, approximately 40,000 cases of salmonellosis are reported in the United States. Because many milder cases are not diagnosed or reported, the actual number of infections may be twenty or more times greater. Salmonellosis is more common in the summer than winter.

Children are the most likely to get salmonellosis. Young children, the elderly, and the immunocompromised are the most likely to have severe infections. It is estimated that approximately 1,000 persons die each year with acute salmonellosis.

What can I do to prevent salmonellosis?

- Cook poultry, ground beef, and eggs thoroughly before eating. Do not eat or drink foods containing raw eggs, or raw unpasteurized milk.

- If you are served undercooked meat, poultry, or eggs in a restaurant, don't hesitate to send it back to the kitchen for further cooking.

- Wash hands, kitchen work surfaces, and utensils with soap and water immediately after they have been in contact with raw meat or poultry.

- Be particularly careful with foods prepared for infants, the elderly, and the immunocompromised.

- Wash hands with soap after handling reptiles or birds, or after contact with pet feces.

- Avoid direct or even indirect contact between reptiles (turtles, iguanas, other lizards, snakes) and infants or immunocompromised persons.

- Don't work with raw poultry or meat and an infant (e.g., feed, change diaper) at the same time.

- Mother's milk is the safest food for young infants. Breast-feeding prevents salmonellosis and many other health problems.

Salmonella *Infections in the Child Care Setting*

Salmonella is present in the feces of ill and recently recovered persons and infections may be spread from person to person. However, outbreaks in child care settings are rare and most persons are believed to have acquired their infections from contaminated food.

While child care providers are most likely to encounter this condition as a result of infection outside their facility, they need to be aware of good hygiene and food handling practices to prevent foodborne illness from occurring within their facility. Additionally, providers may reduce the likelihood of *Salmonella* infection by making sure that children wash their hands after handling animals and cleaning their cages or pens. Because of the risk of *Salmonella* infection, turtles, lizards, and other reptiles should not be kept as pets in child care centers.

Limit the serving of snacks and treats prepared outside the facility and served for special occasions to those from commercial sources. Home-prepared snacks may be not only prepared under less than optimal circumstances but may be transported and stored under conditions that will allow bacteria to grow. Avoid food containing raw eggs, including homemade ice cream made with raw eggs. Make sure that lunches brought from home are refrigerated when necessary. These include meals containing raw vegetables as well as those with meats. Dairy products and liquid formula should also be kept refrigerated in order to limit the growth of bacteria, including *Salmonella*. In most states, laws require that you notify your state or local health department if you become aware that a child or staff person in your facility is infected with *Salmonella*. In addition to helping ensure that infected persons receive proper treatment, it will help prevent further spread of the infection.

Section 24.3

Shigellosis

"Shigellosis in the Child Care Setting," Centers for Disease Control and Prevention (CDC), January 1997. Reviewed in July 2002 by Dr. David A. Cooke, MD, Diplomate, American Board of Internal Medicine.

Shigellosis is a diarrheal illness caused by the *Shigella* group of bacteria. Infection is spread by the fecal-oral route. Only a few bacteria are needed to cause an infection and, unlike many of the diarrheal agents in child care settings, *Shigella* may spread through groups of children who are toilet trained as well as through groups of children who are in diapers.

Depending on the infectious dose, infection with *Shigella* may be very mild, or it may result in severe bloody diarrhea, fever, cramping, nausea, and vomiting. Numerous outbreaks have been reported from child care settings. Children may spread infections acquired in child care facilities to their parents and siblings and whole families may be ill within a matter of days. Deaths have been reported from this illness and it is one of the more serious infections providers are likely to encounter in the child care setting.

If you suspect a case of shigellosis in your child care facility: Contact your state or local health department. Prompt intervention may help prevent the spread of shigellosis to others and your health department should be in a position to give assistance and advice. Exclude the ill child and any children who subsequently develop diarrhea from child care until they no longer have diarrhea and have been shown to be free of the *Shigella* bacteria. In many areas, public health regulations require proof that an infected person is no longer excreting *Shigella* bacteria before they can return to their normal activities. Your health department should be able to tell you when infected persons can return to child care.

Make sure all children and adults use careful handwashing and that staff are practicing good diapering practices. Make sure procedures for cleaning and disinfecting toys are being followed; that toys are being cleaned and disinfected between use by children who are likely to put them in their mouths, especially in groups where there have been ill children. Notify parents of children in the involved classroom of the illness, ask that they have any child with diarrhea, vomiting, or severe cramping evaluated by a physician and that they inform you of diarrheal illness in their child and family. Explain to them the value of handwashing with soap and running water in stopping the spread of infection in the home. In the event of an outbreak, your health department may recommend a more extensive notification of parents.

Section 24.4

Staphylococcus Aureus

"Staphylococcus Aureus: A Most Common Cause," by Nancy Stehulak, © 1998 Ohio State University Extension Department of Family and Consumer Sciences; reprinted with permission. Available online at http://ohioline.osu.edu/hyg-fact/5000/5564.html.

Questions and Answers about Staphylococcus Aureus

What is Staphylococcus aureus?

Staphylococcus aureus is the most common cause of foodborne illness. Commonly called staph, this bacterium produces a poison/toxin that causes the illness.

Symptoms of staphylococcal food poisoning are usually rapid and in many cases serious, depending on individual response to the toxin, the amount of contaminated food eaten, the amount of toxin in the food ingested, and the general health of the victim. The most common symptoms are nausea, vomiting, abdominal cramping, and prostration. Some individuals may not always demonstrate all the symptoms associated with the illness. In more severe cases, headache, muscle cramping, and changes in blood pressure and pulse rate may occur. Recovery generally takes two days. It is not unusual for complete recovery to take three days and sometimes longer.

Foods that are frequently a problem with staphylococcal food poisoning include meat and meat products; poultry and egg products; salads such as egg, tuna, chicken, potato, and macaroni; bakery products such as cream-filled pastries, cream pies, and chocolate eclairs; sandwich fillings; and milk and dairy products. Foods that require considerable handling during preparation and that are kept at slightly elevated temperatures after preparation are frequently involved in staphylococcal food poisoning.

Staph may also be present in raw milk and raw milk products. Staph can cause mastitis in dairy cows, and other infections in meat animals. In this way, such meat sources may cause staph outbreaks in people.

Where do staphylococci come from?

Staphylococci exist in air, dust, sewage, water, milk, and food or on food equipment, environmental surfaces, humans, and animals. Humans and animals are the primary methods of transport. Staphylococci are present in the nasal passages and throats and on the hair and skin of 50 percent or more of healthy individuals. This incidence is even higher for those who associate with or who come in contact with sick individuals and hospital environments. Although food handlers are usually the main source of food contamination in food poisoning outbreaks, equipment and environmental surfaces can also be sources of contamination with staph. People can contract the illness by eating food that is contaminated with any one of many strains of staph, usually because the food has not been kept hot enough or cold enough. Staph bacteria grow and reproduce at temperatures from 50° F to 120° F, with the most rapid growth occurring near body temperature (about 98° F).

The toxin produced by staph bacteria is very heat-stable—it is not easily destroyed by heat at normal cooking temperatures. The bacteria themselves may be killed, but the toxin remains. Careful handling of food that is prepared ahead is important. This is especially important of foods left over after one meal and planned to be used again at a later meal. Quick cooling and refrigeration, or holding at or above 140° F, can help ensure that the toxin has no chance to be formed.

How is staph treated or prevented?

It is hard to determine how often staph food poisoning has occurred because many persons do not report it or it is confused with flu symptoms. Death from staphylococcal food poisoning is rare, although such cases have occurred among the elderly, in infants, and ill persons. The objective of treatment is to replace fluids, salt, and minerals that are lost by vomiting or diarrhea.

To prevent spreading staph, wash hands thoroughly before and after all food preparation. Any food service worker who has skin infections should not be handling food. Food preparation equipment must be thoroughly washed before it is used. Refrigerate meats and leftovers promptly. Keep hot foods hot (over 140° F) and cold foods cold (below 40° F).

A Case in Point

In one example, 1,364 children became ill out of a total of 5,824 who had eaten lunch served at 16 elementary schools in Texas. The lunches were prepared in a central kitchen and transported to the schools by truck. Studies revealed that 95% of the children who became ill had eaten a chicken salad. The afternoon of the day preceding the lunch, frozen chickens were boiled for three hours. After cooking, the chickens were deboned, cooled to room temperature with a fan, ground into small pieces, placed into 12-inch deep aluminum pans and stored overnight in a walk-in refrigerator at 42°–45° F.

The following morning, the remaining ingredients of the salad were added and the mixture was blended with an electric mixer. The food was placed in thermal containers and transported to the various schools at 9:30 a.m. to 10:30 a.m., where it was kept at room temperature until served between 11:30 a.m. and noon. Upon examination of the chicken salad, large numbers of *S. aureus* were found.

Contamination of the chicken probably occurred when it was deboned. The chicken was not cooled rapidly enough because it was stored in 12-inch deep layers. Growth of the *Staphylococcus* probably occurred also during the period when the food was kept in the warm classrooms. Prevention of this incident would have entailed screening the individuals who deboned the chicken for carriers of *Staphylococcus*, more rapid cooling of the chicken, and adequate refrigeration of the salad from the time of preparation until it was eaten.

Section 24.5

Yersinia Enterocolitica

From "*Yersinia Enterocolitica*," Centers for Disease Control and Prevention (CDC), Division of Bacterial and Mycotic Diseases (DBMD), http://www.cdc.gov/ncidod/dbmd/diseaseinfo/yersinia_g.htm, March 29, 2000.

Questions and Answers about Yersinia Enterocolitica

What is yersiniosis?

Yersiniosis is an infectious disease caused by a bacterium of the genus *Yersinia*. In the United States, most human illness is caused by one species, *Y. enterocolitica*. Infection with *Y. enterocolitica* can cause a variety of symptoms depending on the age of the person infected. Infection with *Y. enterocolitica* occurs most often in young children. Common symptoms in children are fever, abdominal pain, and diarrhea, which is often bloody. Symptoms typically develop 4 to 7 days after exposure and may last 1 to 3 weeks or longer. In older children and adults, right-sided abdominal pain and fever may be the predominant symptoms, and may be confused with appendicitis. In a small proportion of cases, complications such as skin rash, joint pains, or spread of bacteria to the bloodstream can occur.

How do people get infected with Y. enterocolitica?

Infection is most often acquired by eating contaminated food, especially raw or undercooked pork products. The preparation of raw pork intestines (chitterlings) may be particularly risky. Infants can be infected if their caretakers handle raw chitterlings and then do not adequately clean their hands before handling the infant or the infant's toys, bottles, or pacifiers. Drinking contaminated unpasteurized milk or untreated water can also transmit the infection. Occasionally *Y. enterocolitica* infection occurs after contact with infected animals. On rare occasions, it can be transmitted as a result of the bacterium passing from the stools or soiled fingers of one person to the mouth of another person. This may happen when basic hygiene and handwashing habits are inadequate. Rarely, the organism is transmitted through contaminated blood during a transfusion.

Y. enterocolitica is a relatively infrequent cause of diarrhea and abdominal pain. Based on data from the Foodborne Diseases Active Surveillance Network (FoodNet), which measures the burden and sources of specific diseases over time, approximately one culture-confirmed *Y. enterocolitica* infection per 100,000 persons occurs each year. Children are infected more often than adults, and the infection is more common in the winter.

How can **Y. enterocolitica** *infections be diagnosed?*

Y. enterocolitica infections are generally diagnosed by detecting the organism in the stools. Many laboratories do not routinely test for *Y. enterocolitica*, so it is important to notify laboratory personnel when infection with this bacterium is suspected so that special tests can be done. The organism can also be recovered from other sites, including the throat, lymph nodes, joint fluid, urine, bile, and blood.

How can **Y. enterocolitica** *infections be treated?*

Uncomplicated cases of diarrhea due to *Y. enterocolitica* usually resolve on their own without antibiotic treatment. However, in more severe or complicated infections, antibiotics such as aminoglycosides, doxycycline, trimethoprim-sulfamethoxazole, or fluoroquinolones may be useful.

Most infections are uncomplicated and resolve completely. Occasionally, some persons develop joint pain, most commonly in the knees, ankles or wrists. These joint pains usually develop about one month after the initial episode of diarrhea and generally resolve after one to six months.

What can be done to prevent the infection?

1. Avoid eating raw or undercooked pork.

2. Consume only pasteurized milk or milk products.

3. Wash hands with soap and water before eating and preparing food, after contact with animals, and after handling raw meat.

4. After handling raw chitterlings, clean hands and fingernails scrupulously with soap and water before touching infants or

their toys, bottles, or pacifiers. Someone other than the foodhandler should care for children while chitterlings are being prepared.

5. Prevent cross-contamination in the kitchen:

    • Use separate cutting boards for meat and other foods.

    • Carefully clean all cutting boards, counter-tops, and utensils with soap and hot water after preparing raw meat.

6. Dispose of animal feces in a sanitary manner.

Chapter 25

Giardiasis:
A Foodborne Parasite

What is giardiasis?

Giardiasis is an illness caused by *Giardia lamblia*, a one-celled, microscopic parasite that lives in the intestines of people and animals. The parasite is passed in the bowel movement of an infected person or animal. During the past 15 years, *Giardia lamblia* has become recognized as one of the most common causes of waterborne disease in humans in the United States. This parasite is found in every region of the United States and throughout the world.

What are the symptoms of giardiasis?

Diarrhea, abdominal cramps, and nausea are the most common symptoms of giardiasis. These symptoms may lead to weight loss and dehydration. However, not everyone infected has symptoms.

How long after being infected do symptoms appear?

Symptoms usually appear 1–2 weeks after infection with the parasite.

How long do symptoms last?

In otherwise healthy persons, symptoms may last 4–6 weeks. Occasionally, symptoms last longer.

"Giardiasis," Division of Parasitic Diseases (DPD), Centers for Disease Control and Prevention (CDC), http://www.cdc.gov/ncidod/dpd/parasites/giardiasis/factsht_giardia.htm, reviewed May 2001.

How does someone get giardiasis?

You can become infected after accidentally ingesting (swallowing) the parasite. *Giardia* may be found in soil, food, water, or on surfaces.

- by swallowing water contaminated with *Giardia*. A person can swallow a *Giardia* cyst, the infectious stage of the parasite, by swallowing water from swimming pools, lakes, rivers, springs, ponds, or streams contaminated with sewage or feces from humans or animals.

- by eating uncooked food contaminated with *Giardia*. Thoroughly wash with safe water all vegetables and fruits you plan to eat raw.

- by accidentally swallowing the parasite picked up from surfaces (i.e., toys, bathroom fixtures, changing tables, diaper pails) contaminated with stool from an infected person. Hands become contaminated by not following good handwashing practices, particularly after using the toilet, changing diapers, and before eating.

Who is at risk?

Persons at increased risk for giardiasis include child care workers; diaper-aged children who attend day care centers; international travelers; hikers; campers; and others who drink untreated water from contaminated sources. Several community-wide outbreaks of giardiasis have been linked to drinking municipal water contaminated with *Giardia*. See your health care provider if you think you or your child may have giardiasis.

How is a Giardia *infection diagnosed?*

Your health care provider will likely ask you to submit stool samples to see if you have the parasite. Because *Giardia* can be difficult to diagnose, your health care provider may ask you to submit several stool specimens over several days.

What is the treatment for giardiasis?

Several prescription drugs are available to treat *Giardia*.

How can giardiasis be prevented?

- Wash hands with soap and water after using the toilet, changing diapers, and before handling food.

- Avoid drinking water or eating food that may be contaminated.

- Wash and peel all raw vegetables and fruits before eating.

- Avoid drinking water from lakes, rivers, springs, ponds, or streams unless it has been filtered and chemically treated.

- During community-wide outbreaks caused by contaminated drinking water, boil drinking water for 1 minute to kill the *Giardia* parasite and make the water safe to drink.

- When traveling in countries where the water supply may be unsafe, avoid drinking unboiled tap water and avoid uncooked foods washed with unboiled tap water. Bottled or canned carbonated beverages, seltzers, pasteurized fruit drinks, and steaming hot coffee and tea are safe to drink.

- If you work in a child care center where you change diapers, be sure to wash your hands thoroughly with soap and warm water after every diaper change, even if you wear gloves.

- If you or your child has *Giardia*, avoid swimming in pools for 2 weeks after the diarrhea or loose stools have cleared. *Giardia* cysts are fairly chlorine resistant and are passed in the stools of infected people for several weeks after they no longer have symptoms.

My water comes from a well. Should I have my well water tested?

Consider having your well water tested if you answer yes to the following questions:

- Are other members of your family or users of your well water ill? If yes, your well may be the source of infection.

- Is your well located at the bottom of a hill or is it considered shallow? If so, runoff from rain or flood water may be draining directly into your well causing contamination.

- Is your well in a rural area where animals graze? Well water can become fecally contaminated if animal waste seepage contaminates the ground water. This can occur if your well has cracked casings, is poorly constructed or is too shallow.

Tests specifically for *Giardia* are expensive, difficult, and usually require hundreds of gallons of water to be pumped through a filter. If you answered yes to the above questions, consider testing your well for fecal coliforms instead of *Giardia*. Although fecal coliform tests do not specifically test for *Giardia*, testing will show if your well has fecal contamination. If it does, the water may also be contaminated with *Giardia*, as well as other harmful bacteria and viruses. Look in your local telephone directory for a laboratory or cooperative extension that offers water testing.

My child was recently diagnosed as having giardiasis, but does not have any diarrhea. My health care provider says treatment is not necessary. Is this true?

In general, the answer supported by the American Academy of Pediatrics is that treatment is not necessary. However, there are a few exceptions. If your child does not have diarrhea, but is having nausea, or is fatigued, losing weight, or has a poor appetite, you and your health care provider may wish to consider treatment. If your child attends a day care center where an outbreak is continuing to occur despite efforts to control it, screening and treatment of children without obvious symptoms may be a good idea. The same is true if several family members are ill, or if a family member is pregnant and therefore not able to take the most effective anti-*Giardia* medications.

Chapter 26

Viral Digestive Illnesses

Chapter Contents

Section 26.1

Viral Gastroenteritis

From "Viral Gastroenteritis," National Centers for Infectious Diseases, Centers for Disease Control and Prevention (CDC), November 6, 2000. Available online at http://www.cdc.gov/ncidod/dvrd/gastro.htm.

What is viral gastroenteritis?

Gastroenteritis means inflammation of the stomach and small and large intestines. Viral gastroenteritis is an infection caused by a variety of viruses that results in vomiting or diarrhea. It is often called the stomach flu, although it is not caused by the influenza viruses.

Many different viruses can cause gastroenteritis, including rotaviruses, adenoviruses, caliciviruses, astroviruses, Norwalk virus, and a group of Norwalk-like viruses. Viral gastroenteritis is not caused by bacteria (such as *Salmonella* or *Escherichia coli*) or parasites (such as *Giardia*), or by medications or other medical conditions, although the symptoms may be similar. Your doctor can determine if the diarrhea is caused by a virus or by something else.

The main symptoms of viral gastroenteritis are watery diarrhea and vomiting. The affected person may also have headache, fever, and abdominal cramps ("stomach ache"). In general, the symptoms begin one to two days following infection with a virus that causes gastroenteritis and may last for one to ten days, depending on which virus causes the illness.

Is viral gastroenteritis a serious illness?

For most people, it is not. People who get viral gastroenteritis almost always recover completely without any long-term problems. Gastroenteritis is a serious illness, however, for persons who are unable to drink enough fluids to replace what they lose through vomiting or diarrhea. Infants, young children, and persons who are unable to care for themselves, such as the disabled or elderly, are at risk for dehydration from loss of fluids. Immune compromised persons are at risk for dehydration because they may get a more serious illness, with greater vomiting or diarrhea. They may need to be hospitalized for treatment to correct or prevent dehydration.

How are these viruses spread?

Viral gastroenteritis is contagious. The viruses that cause gastroenteritis are spread through close contact with infected persons (for example, by sharing food, water, or eating utensils). Individuals may also become infected by eating or drinking contaminated foods or beverages.

Food may be contaminated by food preparers or handlers who have viral gastroenteritis, especially if they do not wash their hands regularly after using the bathroom. Shellfish may be contaminated by sewage, and persons who eat raw or undercooked shellfish harvested from contaminated waters may get diarrhea. Drinking water can also be contaminated by sewage and be a source of spread of these viruses.

Viral gastroenteritis affects people in all parts of the world. Each virus has its own seasonal activity. For example, in the United States, rotavirus and astrovirus infections occur during the cooler months of the year (October to April), whereas adenovirus infections occur throughout the year. Viral gastroenteritis outbreaks can occur in institutional settings, such as schools, child care facilities, and nursing homes, and can occur in other group settings, such as banquet halls, cruise ships, dormitories, and campgrounds.

Who gets viral gastroenteritis?

Anyone can get it. Viral gastroenteritis occurs in people of all ages and backgrounds. However, some viruses tend to cause diarrheal disease primarily among people in specific age groups. Rotavirus infection is the most common cause of diarrhea in infants and young children under 5 years old. Adenoviruses and astroviruses cause diarrhea mostly in young children, but older children and adults can also be affected. Norwalk and Norwalk-like viruses are more likely to cause diarrhea in older children and adults.

How is viral gastroenteritis, diagnosed, treated, or prevented?

Generally, viral gastroenteritis is diagnosed by a physician on the basis of the symptoms and medical examination of the patient. Rotavirus infection can be diagnosed by laboratory testing of a stool specimen. Tests to detect other viruses that cause gastroenteritis are not in routine use.

The most important aspect of treating viral gastroenteritis in children and adults is to prevent severe loss of fluids (dehydration). This treatment should begin at home. Your physician may give you specific instructions about what kinds of fluid to give. Centers for Disease Control and Prevention (CDC) recommends that families with infants and young children keep a supply of oral rehydration solution (ORS) at home at all times and use the solution when diarrhea first occurs in the child. ORS is available at pharmacies without a prescription. Follow the written directions on the ORS package, and use clean or boiled water. Medications, including antibiotics (which have no effect on viruses) and other treatments, should be avoided unless specifically recommended by a physician.

Persons can reduce their chance of getting infected by frequent handwashing, prompt disinfection of contaminated surfaces with household chlorine bleach-based cleaners, and prompt washing of soiled articles of clothing. If food or water is thought to be contaminated, it should be avoided.

Section 26.2

Rotavirus

From "Rotavirus," National Center for Infectious Diseases, Centers for
Disease Control and Prevention, August 2001.

What is rotavirus?

Rotavirus is the most common cause of severe diarrhea among
children, resulting in the hospitalization of approximately 55,000
children each year in the United States and the death of over 600,000
children annually worldwide. The incubation period for rotavirus disease is approximately 2 days. The disease is characterized by vomiting and watery diarrhea for 3–8 days, and fever and abdominal pain
occur frequently. Immunity after infection is incomplete, but repeat
infections tend to be less severe than the original infection.

How is rotavirus spread?

The primary mode of transmission is fecal-oral. Because the virus
is stable in the environment, transmission can occur through ingestion of contaminated water or food and contact with contaminated
surfaces. In the United States and other countries with a temperate
climate, the disease has a winter seasonal pattern, with annual epidemics occurring from November to April. The highest rates of illness
occur among infants and young children, and most children in the
United States are infected by 2 years of age. Adults can also be infected, though disease tends to be mild.

How is rotavirus diagnosed and treated?

Diagnosis may be made by rapid antigen detection of rotavirus in
stool specimens. Strains may be further characterized by enzyme
immunoassay or reverse transcriptase polymerase chain reaction, but
such testing is not commonly done.

For persons with healthy immune systems, rotavirus gastroenteritis
is a self-limited illness, lasting for only a few days. Treatment is nonspecific and consists of oral rehydration therapy to prevent dehydration.

About one in 40 children with rotavirus gastroenteritis will require hospitalization for intravenous fluids.

Is there a vaccine against rotavirus?

In 1998, the U.S. Food and Drug Administration approved a live virus vaccine (Rotashield) for use in children. However, the Advisory Committee on Immunization Practices (ACIP) recommended that Rotashield no longer be recommended for infants in the United States because of data that indicated a strong association between Rotashield and intussusception (bowel obstruction) among some infants during the first 1–2 weeks following vaccination. More information about rotavirus vaccine is available from the National Immunization Program (www.cdc.gov/nip).

Chapter 27

Mushroom Poisoning in Children

Is it possible to tell if a wild mushroom is poisonous?

No. You can't tell for sure if a mushroom is poisonous by looking at it, unless you are an expert at identifying mushrooms. There are no tests to help you tell a poisonous mushroom from a nonpoisonous mushroom.

Does it help to see how the wild mushroom is growing?

Yes, a little. Mushrooms growing in the ground are more dangerous than mushrooms growing on living trees. Mushrooms on the ground in forests are usually more dangerous than mushrooms on lawns. The characteristics listed below often indicate danger:

- Warts or scales on the cap, or top, of the mushroom
- Gills (they look like thin, leaflike plates underneath the mushroom) on the underside of the mushroom cap
- Gills that are white or light-colored, not brown
- An upper ring around the upper part of the stem
- A lower ring around the lower part of the stem

- The base of the stem shaped a little like a bulb

What are the symptoms of mushroom poisoning?

Early symptoms of mushroom poisoning include feeling sick, stomach cramps, vomiting, and watery or bloody diarrhea. Symptoms may show up right after your child eats the mushroom, or may appear several hours later. If your child has any of these symptoms, call your doctor right away. Your child may need treatment.

What should be done if my child eats a wild mushroom?

Don't panic. There are thousands of kinds of mushrooms in North America. Only about 100 can hurt humans.

If your child has eaten a wild mushroom, you can take several simple steps. Collect the mushrooms your child was eating. A few should be carefully dug up so that even the underground parts can be saved for identification. The whole mushroom can then be shown to your child's doctor, which might help your doctor know whether the mushroom was poisonous or not. If you find more than one kind of mushroom around your child, collect all of the different kinds that your child might have eaten.

What should be done next?

Call your family doctor to see if your child can be seen right away. If your doctor can't see your child right away, call the emergency department at your local hospital. They will ask you questions about your child and tell you what to do. Bring the mushrooms you collected to the emergency room. You can also get help from your local poison control center. Look up this number in your telephone book. It's a good idea to keep this number by your telephone at all times.

Should syrup of ipecac be given to children who may have eaten wild mushrooms?

Check with your child's doctor, the local poison control center, or the hospital emergency room. If your child is alert and has not vomited, you might be told to give your child syrup of ipecac. First give your child several glasses of water or clear juice to drink. Then give the ipecac. Give 1 teaspoon to an infant, 1 tablespoon to children 1 to 12 years of age, and 2 tablespoons to children over 12 years of age. Your child should throw up everything in his or her stomach very soon after taking the ipecac. If he or she hasn't vomited within 20 minutes, give the same ipecac dose again.

What will happen in the emergency room?

If your child has thrown up, the worst is probably over. If he or she has not thrown up, your child may be given ipecac or activated charcoal in the emergency room. The physician will find a local mushroom expert to talk to. Your child's temperature, heart rate, and blood pressure will be checked. He or she will be watched closely for signs of mushroom poisoning. If your child has no symptoms of mushroom poisoning after the ipecac has worn off, and if the mushroom is identified as harmless, you and your child will probably be sent home. Your doctor will ask you to watch your child for any symptoms of mushroom poisoning for the next 24 hours.

Chapter 28

Stomach Ulcers in Children

What is a stomach ulcer?

A stomach ulcer (also called a peptic ulcer) is a small erosion (hole) in the gastrointestinal tract. The most common type, duodenal, occurs in the first 12 inches of small intestine beyond the stomach. Ulcers that form in the stomach are called gastric ulcers. An ulcer is not contagious or cancerous. Duodenal ulcers are almost always benign, while stomach ulcers may become malignant.

Stomach ulcer disease is common, affecting millions of Americans yearly. The size of a stomach ulcer can range between 1/8 of an inch to 3/4 of an inch.

Stomach ulcers may be a symptom of another disease or condition. Ulcers are often common in mastocytosis. Bleeding from stomach ulcers may cause iron deficiency anemia.

Can stomach ulcers occur in children?

Stomach ulcers do not occur only in adults. Children can also develop stomach ulcers.

What usually causes ulcers?

The direct cause of peptic ulcers is the destruction of the gastric or intestinal mucosal lining of the stomach by hydrochloric acid, an

From "Stomach Ulcers," and "Stomach Ulcers in Children," May 12, 2000, © 2000 Mamashealth.com™; reprinted with permission. More information from Mamashealth.com is available online at http://www.mamashealth.com.

acid normally present in the digestive juices of the stomach. Infection with the bacterium *Helicobacter pylori* is thought to play an important role in causing both gastric and duodenal ulcers. *H. pylori* may be transmitted from person to person through contaminated food and water. Antibiotics are the most effective treatment for *H. pylori* peptic ulcers.

Injury of the gastric mucosal lining, and weakening of the mucous defenses are also responsible for gastric ulcers. Excess secretion of hydrochloric acid, genetic predisposition, and psychological stress are important contributing factors in the formation and worsening of duodenal ulcers.

Another major cause of ulcers is the chronic use of anti-inflammatory medications, such as aspirin. Cigarette smoking is also an important cause of ulcer formation and ulcer treatment failure.

Why do children develop stomach ulcers?

Researchers are not sure of the exact reason children develop stomach ulcers. Unlike adults who develop stomach ulcers mostly as a result of a *H. pylori* infection, children do not usually develop stomach ulcers because of *H. pylori* infections. It is believed that many children develop gastric (stomach) ulcers as a result of medication.

What are the symptoms of stomach ulcers?

The major symptom of an ulcer is a burning or gnawing feeling in the stomach area that lasts between 30 minutes and 3 hours. This pain is often interpreted as heartburn, indigestion, or hunger. The pain usually occurs in the upper abdomen, but sometimes it may occur below the breastbone. In some individuals the pain occurs immediately after eating. In other individuals, the pain may not occur until hours after eating. The pain frequently awakens the person at night. Weeks of pain may be followed by weeks of not having pain. Pain can be relieved by drinking milk, eating, resting, or taking antacids.

Appetite and weight loss are other symptoms. Persons with duodenal ulcers may experience weight gain because the persons eats more to ease discomfort. Recurrent vomiting, blood in the stool, and anemia are other symptoms.

What does a stomach ulcer affect?

The main thing that a stomach ulcer affects is the nerves surrounding it. The nerves become agitated and cause a great amount of pain.

However, stomach ulcers can cause hemorrhages from the erosion of a major blood vessel; a tear in the wall of the stomach or intestine, with resultant peritonitis; or obstruction of the gastrointestinal tract because of spasm or swelling in the area of the ulcer.

What are the risk factors for developing an ulcer?

- Family history of ulcers
- Smoking
- Excess alcohol consumption
- Use of nonsteroidal anti-inflammatory medications (aspirin) or corticosteroids
- Zollinger-Ellison syndrome
- Improper diet; irregular or skipped meals
- Type O blood (for duodenal ulcers)

Stress does not cause an ulcer, but may be a contributing factor. Chronic disorders such as liver disease, emphysema, or rheumatoid arthritis may increase vulnerability to ulcers.

What should you do if your child has an ulcer?

If your child is diagnosed with an *H. pylori*-related ulcer, make sure that your child takes all of the antibiotics as directed by the doctor. Follow the instructions that the doctor has given you even if the symptoms have disappeared. If the symptoms are no longer present, it doesn't mean that the infection is gone.

If your child has a drug-related ulcer, his/her doctor will tell you to avoid the medications that caused the ulcer, including any medication containing ibuprofen or aspirin. Also, be sure to give your child the medication prescribed by the doctor.

Chapter 29

Pinworm Infection

What Is Pinworm Infection?

This infection is caused by a small, white intestinal worm called *Enterobius vermicularis* (EN-ter-O-be-us ver-MIK-u-lar-is). Pinworms are about the length of a staple and live in the rectum of humans. While an infected person sleeps, female pinworms leave the intestines through the anus and deposit eggs on the surrounding skin.

What Are the Symptoms of a Pinworm Infection?

Itching around the anus, disturbed sleep, and irritability are common symptoms. If the infection is heavy, symptoms may also include loss of appetite, restlessness, and difficulty sleeping. Symptoms are caused by the female pinworm laying her eggs. Most symptoms of pinworm infection are mild; many infected people have no symptoms.

Who Is at Risk for Pinworm Infection?

Pinworm is the most common worm infection in the United States. School-age children, followed by preschoolers, have the highest rates of infection. In some groups nearly 50% of children are infected. Infection often occurs in more than one family member. Adults are less

Excerpted from "Pinworm Infection," National Center for Infectious Diseases, Division of Parasitic Diseases (DPD), Centers for Disease Control and Prevention (CDC); reviewed August 15, 1999. Full text available online at http://www.cdc.gov/ncidod/dpd/parasites/pinworm/factsht_pinworm.htm.

likely to have pinworm infection, except mothers of infected children. Child care centers and other institutional settings often have cases of pinworm infection.

How Is Pinworm Infection Spread?

Pinworm eggs are infective within a few hours after being deposited on the skin. They can survive up to 2 weeks on clothing, bedding, or other objects. You or your children can become infected after accidentally ingesting (swallowing) infective pinworm eggs from contaminated surfaces or fingers.

How Is Pinworm Infection Diagnosed?

If pinworms are suspected, transparent adhesive tape (often called the "scotch tape test") or a pinworm paddle (supplied by your health care provider) are applied to the anal region. The eggs become glued to the sticky tape or paddle and are identified by examination under a microscope. Because bathing or having a bowel movement may remove eggs, the test should be done as soon as you wake up in the morning. You may have to provide several samples to your health care provider for examination. Since scratching of the anal area is common, samples taken from under the fingernails may also contain eggs. Eggs are rarely found during lab examinations of stool or urine. At night, the adult worms can sometimes be seen directly in bedclothes or around the anal area.

How Is Pinworm Infection Treated?

With either prescription or over-the-counter drugs. You should consult your health care provider before treating a suspected case of pinworm. Treatment involves a two-dose course. The second dose should be given 2 weeks after the first.

What If the Pinworm Infection Occurs Again?

The infected person should be treated with the same two-dose treatment. Close family contacts should also be treated. If the infection occurs again, you should search for the source of the infection. Playmates, schoolmates, close contacts outside the house, and household members should be considered. Each infected person should receive the usual two-dose treatment. In some cases it may be necessary to treat with more than two doses. One option is four to six treatments spaced 2 weeks apart.

How Can I Prevent the Spread of Infection and Reinfection?

- Bathe when you wake up to help reduce the egg contamination.

- Change and wash your underwear each day. Frequent changing of night clothes are recommended.

- Change underwear, night clothes, and sheets after each treatment. Because the eggs are sensitive to sunlight, open blinds or curtains in bedrooms during the day.

- Personal hygiene should include washing hands after going to the toilet, before eating, and after changing diapers.

- Trim fingernails short.

- Discourage nail-biting and scratching bare anal areas. These practices help reduce the risk of continuous self reinfection.

Cleaning and vacuuming the entire house or washing sheets every day are probably not necessary or effective. Screening for pinworm infection in schools or institutions is rarely recommended. Children may return to day care after the first treatment dose, after bathing, and after trimming and scrubbing nails.

Chapter 30

Bowel Problems in Children

Chapter Contents

Section 30.1

Constipation in Children

National Digestive Diseases Information Clearinghouse (NIDDK), NIH Pub. No. 02-4633, October 2001. Available online at http://www.niddk.nih. gov/health/digest/summary/conchild/index.htm.

Constipation means that bowel movements are hard and dry, difficult or painful to pass, and less frequent than usual. It is a common problem for children, but it is usually temporary and no cause for parents to be concerned.

When a child does not eat enough fiber, drink enough liquids, or get enough exercise, constipation is more likely to occur. It also happens when children ignore the urge to have a bowel movement, which they often do out of either embarrassment to use a public bathroom, fear or lack of confidence in the absence of a parent, or unwillingness to take a break from play. Sometimes constipation is caused by medicines or a disease.

Symptoms of constipation include:

- no bowel movement for several days or daily bowel movements that are hard and dry
- cramping abdominal pain
- nausea
- vomiting
- weight loss
- liquid or solid, clay-like stool in the child's underwear—a sign that stool is backed up in the rectum

Constipation can make a bowel movement painful, so the child may try to prevent having one. Clenching buttocks, rocking up and down on toes, and turning red in the face are signs of trying to hold in a bowel movement.

Treatment depends on the child's age and the severity of the problem. Often eating more fiber (fruits, vegetables, whole-grain cereal), drinking more liquids, and getting more exercise will solve the problem. Sometimes a child may need an enema to remove the stool or a laxative to soften it or prevent a future episode. However, laxatives can be dangerous to children and should be given only with a doctor's approval.

Although constipation is usually harmless, it can be a sign or cause of a more serious problem. A child should see a doctor if:

- Episodes of constipation last longer than 3 weeks.

- The child is unable to participate in normal activities.

- Small, painful tears appear in the skin around the anus.

- A small amount of the intestinal lining is pushed out of the anus (hemorrhoids).

- Normal pushing is not enough to expel stool.

- Liquid or soft stool leaks out of the anus.

Section 30.2

Soiling and Bowel Control

Reprinted with permission from "Problems with Soiling and Bowel Control," part of the American Academy of Child & Adolescent Psychiatry's *Facts for Families Series*. © 2000. For more information about issues related to child and adolescent psychiatry, or for information about how to get help in your area, visit the Referral Directory on the AACAP website at http://www.aacap.org/Referral Directory/index.htm.

Most children can control their bowels and are toilet trained by the time they are four years of age. Problems controlling bowel movements can cause soiling which leads to frustration and anger on part of the child, parents, teachers, and other people important in the child's life. In addition, social difficulties with this problem can be severe—the child is often made fun of by friends and avoided by adults. These problems can cause children to feel badly about themselves.

Some of the reasons for soiling are:

- problems during toilet training
- physical disabilities, which make it hard for the child to clean him/herself
- physical illnesses, for example Hirschsprung's Disease
- family or emotional problems

Soiling which is not caused by an illness or disability is called encopresis. Children with encopresis may have other problems, such as short attention span, low frustration tolerance, hyperactivity, and poor coordination. Occasionally, this problem with soiling starts with a stressful change in the child's life, such as the birth of a sibling, separation/divorce of parents, family problems, or a move to a new home. Encopresis is more common in boys than in girls.

Although most children with soiling do not have a physical condition, they should have a complete physical evaluation by a family physician or pediatrician. If no physical causes are found, or if problems continue after examination by a family physician, the next step is an evaluation by a child and adolescent psychiatrist. The child and adolescent psychiatrist will review the results of the physical evaluation and then decide whether emotional problems are contributing to the encopresis.

Child and adolescent psychiatrists treat encopresis with a combination of educational, psychological, and behavioral methods. Most children with encopresis can be helped, but progress can be slow and extended treatment may be necessary. Early treatment of a soiling or bowel control problem can help prevent and reduce social and emotional suffering and pain for the child and family.

Chapter 31

Urinary Incontinence in Children

In the United States, at least 13 million people have problems holding urine until they can get to a toilet. This loss of urinary control is called urinary incontinence or just incontinence. Although it affects many young people, it usually disappears naturally over time, which suggests that incontinence, for some people, may be a normal part of growing up. No matter when it happens or how often it happens, incontinence causes great distress. It may get in the way of a good night's sleep and is embarrassing when it happens during the day. That's why it is important to understand that occasional incontinence is a normal part of growing up and that treatment is available for most children who have difficulty controlling their bladders.

Incontinence happens less often after age 5: About 10 percent of 5-year-olds, 5 percent of 10-year-olds, and 1 percent of 18-year-olds experience episodes of incontinence. It is twice as common in boys as in girls.

How Does the Urinary System Work?

Urination, or voiding, is a complex activity. The bladder is a balloon-like muscle that lies in the lowest part of the abdomen. The bladder

Excerpted from "Urinary Incontinence in Children," The National Kidney and Urologic Diseases Information Clearinghouse (NKUDIC), National Institute of Diabetes and Digestive and Kidney Diseases (NIDDK), NIH Pub. No. 02-4095, May 2002; available online at http://www.niddk.nih.gov/health/urolog/pubs/uichild/uichild.htm.

stores urine, then releases it through the urethra, the canal that carries urine to the outside of the body. Controlling this activity involves nerves, muscles, the spinal cord, and the brain.

The bladder is made of two types of muscles: the detrusor, a muscular sac that stores urine and squeezes to empty, and the sphincter, a circular group of muscles at the bottom or neck of the bladder that automatically stay contracted to hold the urine in and automatically relax when the detrusor contracts to let the urine into the urethra. A third group of muscles below the bladder (pelvic floor muscles) can contract to keep urine back.

A baby's bladder fills to a set point, then automatically contracts and empties. As the child gets older, the nervous system develops. The child's brain begins to get messages from the filling bladder and begins to send messages to the bladder to keep it from automatically emptying until the child decides it is the time and place to void.

Failures in this control mechanism result in incontinence. Reasons for this failure range from the simple to the complex.

What Causes Nighttime Incontinence?

After age 5, wetting at night—often called bed-wetting or sleep-wetting—is more common than daytime wetting in boys. Experts do not know what causes nighttime incontinence. Young people who experience nighttime wetting tend to be physically and emotionally normal. Most cases probably result from a mix of factors including slower physical development, an overproduction of urine at night, a lack of ability to recognize bladder filling when asleep, and, in some cases, anxiety. For many, there is a strong family history of bed-wetting, suggesting an inherited factor.

Slower Physical Development

Between the ages of 5 and 10, incontinence may be the result of a small bladder capacity, long sleeping periods, and underdevelopment of the body's alarms that signal a full or emptying bladder. This form of incontinence will fade away as the bladder grows and the natural alarms become operational.

Excessive Output of Urine during Sleep

Normally, the body produces a hormone that can slow the making of urine. This hormone is called antidiuretic hormone, or ADH. The body normally produces more ADH at night so that the need to urinate is lower. If the body doesn't produce enough ADH at night, the making of urine may not be slowed down, leading to bladder overfilling. If a child does not sense the bladder filling and awaken to urinate, then wetting will occur.

Anxiety

Experts suggest that anxiety-causing events occurring in the lives of children ages 2 to 4 might lead to incontinence before the child achieves total bladder control. Anxiety experienced after age 4 might lead to wetting after the child has been dry for a period of 6 months or more. Such events include angry parents, unfamiliar social situations, and overwhelming family events such as the birth of a brother or sister.

Incontinence itself is an anxiety-causing event. Strong bladder contractions leading to leakage in the daytime can cause embarrassment and anxiety that lead to wetting at night.

Genetics

Certain inherited genes appear to contribute to incontinence. In 1995, Danish researchers announced they had found a site on human chromosome 13 that is responsible, at least in part, for nighttime wetting. If both parents were bed-wetters, a child has an 80 percent chance of being a bed-wetter also. Experts believe that other, undetermined genes also may be involved in incontinence.

Obstructive Sleep Apnea

Nighttime incontinence may be one sign of another condition called obstructive sleep apnea, in which the child's breathing is interrupted during sleep, often because of inflamed or enlarged tonsils or adenoids. Other symptoms of this condition include snoring, mouth breathing, frequent ear and sinus infections, sore throat, choking, and daytime drowsiness. In some cases, successful treatment of this breathing disorder may also resolve the associated nighttime incontinence.

Structural Problems

Finally, a small number of cases of incontinence are caused by physical problems in the urinary system in children. Rarely, a blocked bladder or urethra may cause the bladder to overfill and leak. Nerve damage associated with the birth defect spina bifida can cause incontinence.

In these cases, the incontinence can appear as a constant dribbling of urine.

What Causes Daytime Incontinence?

Daytime incontinence that is not associated with urinary infection or anatomic abnormalities is less common than nighttime incontinence and tends to disappear much earlier than the nighttime versions. One possible cause of daytime incontinence is an overactive bladder. Many children with daytime incontinence have abnormal voiding habits, the most common being infrequent voiding.

An Overactive Bladder

Muscles surrounding the urethra (the tube that takes urine away from the bladder) have the job of keeping the passage closed, preventing urine from passing out of the body. If the bladder contracts strongly and without warning, the muscles surrounding the urethra may not be able to keep urine from passing. This often happens as a consequence of urinary tract infection and is more common in girls.

Infrequent Voiding

Infrequent voiding refers to a child's voluntarily holding urine for prolonged intervals. For example, a child may not want to use the toilets at school or may not want to interrupt enjoyable activities, so he or she ignores the body's signal of a full bladder. In these cases, the bladder can overfill and leak urine. Additionally, these children often develop urinary tract infections (UTIs), leading to an irritable or overactive bladder.

Other Causes

Some of the same factors that contribute to nighttime incontinence may act together with infrequent voiding to produce daytime incontinence. These factors include:

- a small bladder capacity
- structural problems
- anxiety-causing events
- pressure from a hard bowel movement (constipation)
- drinks or foods that contain caffeine, which increases urine output and may also cause spasms of the bladder muscle, or other

ingredients to which the child may have an allergic reaction, such as chocolate or artificial coloring

Sometimes overly strenuous toilet training may make the child unable to relax the sphincter and the pelvic floor to completely empty the bladder. Retaining urine (incomplete emptying) sets the stage for urinary tract infections.

What Treats or Cures Incontinence?

Growth and Development

Most urinary incontinence fades away naturally. Here are examples of what can happen over time:

- bladder capacity increases
- natural body alarms become activated
- an overactive bladder settles down
- production of ADH becomes normal
- the child learns to respond to the body's signal that it is time to void
- stressful events or periods pass

Many children overcome incontinence naturally (without treatment) as they grow older. The number of cases of incontinence goes down by 15 percent for each year after the age of 5.

Medications

Nighttime incontinence may be treated by increasing ADH levels. The hormone can be boosted by a synthetic version known as desmopressin, or DDAVP, which recently became available in pill form. Patients can also spray a mist containing desmopressin into their nostrils. Desmopressin is approved for use by children.

Another medication, called imipramine, is also used to treat sleepwetting. It acts on both the brain and the urinary bladder. Unfortunately, total dryness with either of the medications available is achieved in only about 20 percent of patients.

If a young person experiences incontinence resulting from an overactive bladder, a doctor might prescribe a medicine that helps to calm the bladder muscle. This medicine controls muscle spasms and belongs to a class of medications called anticholinergics.

Bladder Training and Related Strategies

Bladder training consists of exercises for strengthening and coordinating muscles of the bladder and urethra, and may help the control of urination. These techniques teach the child to anticipate the need to urinate and prevent urination when away from a toilet. Techniques that may help nighttime incontinence include:

- determining bladder capacity
- stretching the bladder (delaying urinating)
- drinking less fluid before sleeping
- developing routines for waking up

Unfortunately, none of the above has demonstrated proven success. Techniques that may help daytime incontinence include:

- urinating on a schedule, such as every 2 hours (this is called timed voiding)
- avoiding caffeine or other foods or drinks that you suspect may contribute to your child's incontinence
- following suggestions for healthy urination, such as relaxing muscles and taking your time

Moisture Alarms

At night, moisture alarms can awaken a person when he or she begins to urinate. These devices include a water-sensitive pad worn in pajamas, a wire connecting to a battery-driven control, and an alarm that sounds when moisture is first detected. For the alarm to be effective, the child must awaken or be awakened as soon as the alarm goes off. This may require having another person sleep in the same room to awaken the bed-wetter.

Chapter 32

Urinary Tract Infections in Children

Introduction

Aside from unexpected wetting, the most common urinary problem among children is infections. An estimated three percent of girls and one percent of boys have had a urinary tract infection (UTI) by the age of 11. Some researchers believe these estimates are low because many cases of UTI go undetected. The symptoms are not always obvious to parents, and younger children are usually unable to describe how they feel. Recognizing and treating urinary tract infections is important. Untreated UTIs can lead to serious kidney problems that could threaten the life of your child.

How Does the Urinary Tract Normally Function?

The kidneys filter and remove waste and water from the blood to produce urine. They get rid of about 1½ to 2 quarts of urine per day in an adult and less in a child, depending on the child's age. The urine travels from the kidneys down two narrow tubes called the ureters. The urine is then stored in a balloon-like container called the bladder. In a child, the bladder can hold about 1 to 1½ ounces of urine for

Excerpted from "Urinary Tract Infections in Children," The National Kidney and Urologic Diseases Information Clearinghouse (NKUDIC), National Institute of Diabetes and Digestive and Kidney Diseases (NIDDK), NIH Pub. No. 97-4246, 1997, updated September 2000; available online at http://www.niddk.nih.gov/health/urolog/pubs/utichild/utichild.htm.

each year of the child's age. So, the bladder of a 4-year-old child may hold about 4 to 6 ounces (less than 1 cup); an 8-year-old can hold 8 to 12 ounces. When the bladder empties, urine flows out of the body through the urethra, a tube at the bottom of the bladder. The opening of the urethra is at the end of the penis in boys and in front of the vagina in girls.

How Does the Urinary Tract Become Infected?

Normal urine contains no bacteria (germs). Bacteria may, at times, get into the urinary tract (and the urine) from the skin around the rectum and genitals by traveling up the urethra into the bladder. When this happens, the bacteria can infect and inflame the bladder, resulting in swelling and pain in the lower abdomen and side. This is called "cystitis."

If the bacteria travel further up through the ureters to the kidneys, a kidney infection can develop. The infection is usually accompanied by pain and fever. Kidney infections are much more serious than bladder infections.

In some children a urinary tract infection may be a sign of an abnormal urinary tract that may be prone to repeated problems (See "What Abnormalities Lead to Urinary Problems?"). For this reason, when a child is found to have a urinary infection, additional tests are often recommended (See "What Tests May Be Needed After the Infection Is Gone?") In other cases, children develop urinary tract infections because they are prone to such infections the way, for example, other children are prone to getting coughs, colds, or ear infections. Or a child may happen to get an infection with a type of bacteria that has a special ability to cause urinary tract infections.

What Are the Signs of Urinary Tract Infection?

The lining of the bladder, urethra, ureters, and kidneys become irritated with a urinary tract infection, just like the inside of the nose or throat with a cold. If your child is an infant or is only a few years old, the signs of a urinary tract infection may not be clear, since children that young cannot tell you just how they feel. Your child may have a high fever, be irritable, or not eat.

On the other hand, sometimes a child may have only a low-grade fever, experience nausea and vomiting, or just not seem healthy. The diaper urine may have an unusual smell. If your child has a high temperature and appears sick for more than a day without signs of a runny nose or other obvious cause for discomfort, he or she may need to be checked for a bladder infection.

An older child with bladder irritation may complain of pain in the abdomen and pelvic area. Your child may urinate often. If the kidney is infected, your child may complain of pain under the side of the rib cage (the flank) or low back pain. Crying or complaining that it hurts to urinate and producing only a few drops of urine at a time are other signs of urinary tract infection. Your child may have difficulty controlling the urine and may leak urine into clothing or bed sheets. The urine may smell unusual or look cloudy.

How Do You Find out Whether Your Child Has a Urinary Tract Infection?

Only by consulting a health care provider can you find out for certain whether your child has a urinary tract infection.

Some of your child's urine will be collected and examined. The way urine is collected may depend on how old your child is. The health care provider may place a plastic collection bag over your child's genital area (sealed to the skin with an adhesive strip) if the child is not yet toilet trained. An older child may be asked to urinate into a container. The sample needs to come as directly into the container as possible to avoid picking up bacteria from the skin or rectal area. A doctor or nurse may need to pass a small tube into the urethra. Urine will drain directly from the bladder into a clean container through this tube (called a catheter). Sometimes the best way to get the urine is by placing a needle directly into the bladder through the skin of the lower abdomen. Getting urine through the tube or needle will make sure that the urine collected is pure.

Some of the urine will be examined under a microscope. If an infection is present, bacteria and sometimes pus will be in the urine. If the bacteria from the sample are hard to see at first, the health care provider may place the sample in a tube or dish with a substance that encourages any bacteria present to grow. Once the germs have multiplied, they can then be identified and tested to see which medications will provide the most effective treatment. The process of growing bacteria in the laboratory is known as performing a culture and often takes a day or more to complete.

The reliability of the culture depends on how long the urine stands before the culture is started. If you collect your child's urine at home, it should be refrigerated as soon as collected and the container should be transported in a plastic bag filled with ice.

How Are Urinary Tract Infections Treated?

Urinary tract infections are treated with antibiotics (infection-fighting drugs). After a urine sample is obtained, the health care provider may begin treatment with a drug that treats the bacteria most likely to be causing the infection. Once culture results are known, the health care provider may switch your child to another antibiotic, if necessary.

The way the antibiotic is given and the number of days that it must be taken depend in part on the type of infection and how severe it is. When a child is sick or not able to drink fluids, the antibiotic may need to be put directly into the bloodstream through a vein in the arm or hand. Otherwise, the medicine (liquid or pills) may be given by mouth or by shots. The medicine is given for at least 3 to 5 days and possibly for as long as several weeks. The daily treatment schedule recommended depends on the specific drug prescribed: The schedule may call for a single dose each day or up to four doses each day. In some cases, your child will need to take the medicine until further tests are finished.

After a few doses of the antibiotic, your child may appear much better, but often several days may pass before all symptoms are gone. In any case, your child should take the medicine for as long as the doctor says. Do not stop medications because the symptoms have gone away. Infections may return, and germs can resist future treatment if the drug is stopped too soon.

Children should drink fluids when they wish. Make sure your child drinks what he or she needs, but do not force your child to drink large amounts of fluid. The health care provider needs to know if the child is not interested in drinking.

What Tests May Be Needed after the Infection Is Gone?

Once the infection has cleared, additional tests may be recommended to check for abnormalities in the urinary tract. Repeated infections in abnormal urinary tracts may cause kidney damage. The kinds of tests ordered will depend on your child and the type of urinary infection. Because no single test can tell everything about the urinary tract that might be important to know, more than one of the following tests may be needed:

- Kidney and bladder ultrasound: A test that examines the kidney and bladder using sound waves. This test shows shadows of the kidney and bladder that may point out certain abnormalities; this test cannot reveal all important urinary abnormalities. It also cannot measure how well a kidney works.

- Voiding cystourethrogram (VCUG): A test that examines the urethra and bladder while the bladder fills and empties. A liquid that can be seen on x-rays is placed into the bladder through a catheter. The bladder is filled until the child urinates. This test can reveal abnormalities of the inside of the urethra and bladder. The test can also determine whether the flow of urine is normal when the bladder empties.

- Intravenous pyelogram: A test that examines the whole urinary tract. A liquid that can be seen on x-rays is injected into a vein. The substance travels into the kidneys and bladder, revealing possible obstructions.

- Nuclear scans: A number of tests using radioactive materials that are usually injected into a vein to show how well the kidneys work, the shape of the kidneys, and whether urine empties from the kidneys in a normal way. The many kinds of nuclear scans each give different information about the kidneys and bladder. Nuclear scans expose a child to no more radiation than he or she would receive from a conventional x-ray. At times, it can even be less.

What Abnormalities Lead to Urinary Problems?

Many children who get urinary tract infections have normal kidneys and bladders, but children who have an abnormality need to have it detected as early as possible in life to try to protect their kidneys against damage. Abnormalities that could occur include the following:

- Vesicoureteral reflux. Urine normally flows from the kidneys down the ureters to the bladder in one direction. With reflux, when the bladder fills, the urine may also flow backward from the bladder up the ureters to the kidneys. This abnormality is common in children with urinary infections.

- Urinary obstruction. Blockages to urinary flow may occur at many sites in the urinary tract. Blockages usually occur if the ureter or urethra is too narrow or a kidney stone at some point stops the urinary flow from leaving the body. Occasionally, the ureter may join the kidney or bladder at the wrong place, preventing urine from leaving the kidney in a normal way.

Do Urinary Tract Infections Have Long-Term Effects?

Young children are at the greatest risk for kidney damage from urinary tract infections, especially if they have some unknown urinary tract abnormality. Such damage includes kidney scars, poor kidney growth, poor kidney function, high blood pressure, and other problems. For this reason it is important that children with urinary tract infections receive prompt treatment and careful evaluation.

Points to Remember

- Urinary tract infections occur in about three percent of girls and one percent of boys by age 11.

- A urinary tract infection in a young child may be a sign of an abnormality in the urinary tract that could lead to repeated problems.

- Symptoms of a urinary infection range from slight burning with urination or unusual smelling urine to severe pain and high fever.

- Untreated urinary infections can lead to serious kidney damage.

- Talk to a doctor if you suspect your child has a urinary tract infection.

Chapter 33

Appendectomy

What Is an Appendectomy?

An appendectomy is surgery to remove the appendix. The appendix is a narrow sack that hangs down from the large bowel. The appendix may be removed during other surgeries, such as bowel surgery, or for appendicitis. Appendicitis is when the appendix becomes swollen and infected. If appendicitis is not treated in a day or two, the appendix may break open. When the appendix breaks, the infection spreads inside the belly. This is called peritonitis.

Signs and Symptoms of Appendicitis

- Vomiting
- Nausea
- Diarrhea
- Fever
- Constipation
- Irritable
- Lack of hunger
- Right lower belly pain
- Belly pain worse when the child moves or coughs

"Appendectomy: Health Facts," © 1998 Children's Hospital of the King's Daughters, Norfolk, VA. Reprinted with permission.

Having an Appendectomy

Before surgery, your child will have an IV started for fluids and medicines. Your child will go to sleep with a medicine called an anesthetic, so your child will not feel anything during surgery. After your child is asleep, the doctor will make a small cut on the right side of the belly. This small cut is called an incision or wound. The doctor will remove the appendix through this small opening. The surgery will take about an hour to an hour and a half.

What to Expect after Surgery

- Your child may be sleepy for the rest of the day.
- The stitches will be under the skin and will dissolve.
- Steri-Strips (small, white tape bandages) will be over the wound.
- The wound may have a drain or tube if your child has infection.
- There may be a small amount of bloody drainage from the wound.
- An IV will be needed for fluids and antibiotics.
- The doctor will order medicine for pain relief.
- Your child's temperature may be increased (101° to 102° F) for a few days.
- Your child may still feel sick and vomit after surgery if there is infection in the belly.

There may be a tube in the nose that goes into the stomach. This is to keep the stomach empty and will be removed before he/she starts eating and drinking. The doctor will tell you when your child may eat. Usually, this is not until a day or two after surgery.

Special Care

- Keep wound clean and dry for at least 48 hours after surgery. No tub baths or showers during this time.
- Steri-Strips should remain on at least 3 days. When they begin to peel off, that is okay.
- Your child's doctor will tell you when your child can return to school.

- Your child should not take gym class, play sports or climbing games or ride bikes until his/her doctor says it is okay (usually in 3 weeks).

- Call the doctor's office or clinic to schedule a check-up in 10 days to 2 weeks after surgery.

- Your child's doctor will send you home with a prescription for antibiotics.

When to Call Your Child's Doctor

- Your child's wound looks red or has white or yellow drainage, or the drainage has a foul odor.

- There is a lot of swelling or the wound is hot to touch or has a lump that you can feel.

- Your child's temperature is greater than 101.5° rectally or by mouth. Slight fevers are normal.

- You have any questions or concerns.

Chapter 34

Hernia

Chapter Contents

Section 34.1

Could That Lump Be a Hernia?

Excerpted from "Inguinal and Umbilical Hernias in Infancy and Child-hood," © 1999 British Hernia Centre (www.hernia.org); reprinted with permission. The full text of this document is available online at http://www.hernia.org/paeds.html.

Groin or Inguinal Hernias

A pediatric inguinal hernia can appear or occur at any age, but the peak incidence is during infancy and early childhood with 80 to 90% occurring in boys.

Some Statistics

About 3% to 5% of healthy, full-term babies may be born with an inguinal hernia and one third of hernias of infancy and childhood appear in the first 6 months of life. In premature infants the incidence of inguinal hernia is substantially increased, up to 30%. In just over 10% of cases, other members of the family have also had a hernia at birth or in infancy. Right side hernias are commoner than left.

The occurrence of an inguinal hernia in boys is related to the development and descent of the testes. The testes develop within the abdomen and at around the seventh month of pregnancy they descend into the scrotum. On their way through the abdominal wall, they pass through the inguinal canal. After they reach the scrotum, the opening behind should close. Failure to close adequately results in a hernia with an opening remaining in the abdominal wall at this point.

Symptoms

A hernia in an infant or a child will be seen as a bulge or a swelling in the groin. In boys the swelling might be seen in the scrotum.

In many cases the swelling may only be seen during crying or straining. This may lead parents to assume that the crying is because of the hernia, whereas it is more often the case that the hernia appears because the child is crying for some other reason.

Inguinal hernias in children are prone to get stuck, i.e. the lump does not go away when the child relaxes, and this is called incarceration. Because incarceration is quite common most experts advise that groin or inguinal hernias should be repaired as soon is practicable after they are discovered or diagnosed. However, an incarcerated or irreducible hernia (that does not reduce or go back in) should be seen by a doctor urgently. In an acute situation, the child or infant should be admitted to the hospital and given some pain relief and sedation. Initial attempts are made by the doctors to gently negotiate the hernia back inside.

If the hernia does not go back, or the child is ill, the irreducible hernia should be operated upon urgently as it may contain intestine that is in danger of strangulating. Strangulation is extremely serious and must be avoided at all costs. If the hernia does go back without any emergency operation it should still be repaired (operated on) at an early stage.

Umbilical Hernia

This is one of the most common pediatric surgical conditions affecting perhaps 1 in 5 (20%) of all children. Umbilical hernias are more common in premature babies and children with Down syndrome and there is a slight familial tendency.

They appear as a bulge at the umbilicus (the navel), which can vary in size from that of a pea up to the size of a small plum. They are not usually painful and are much more obvious when the baby or child cries or strains.

What Happens If They Are Not Treated? Do They Need an Operation?

There is a general agreement that most infantile umbilical hernias will eventually close spontaneously, though experts disagree over what period of time. Probably 80 to 90% of umbilical hernias will have closed by the time the child is 3, but the larger ones may be present up to 11 years before finally closing. The time taken to close probably depends on the size of the opening, with 95% of umbilical hernias less than 0.5 cm in diameter closing by the age of 2 years. Umbilical hernias present after puberty will probably not close spontaneously.

In the case of infantile umbilical hernias, problems, particularly strangulation—where a portion of intestine becomes trapped in the hernia, rarely occur, so that surgery is rarely required. However the presence of pain in the hernia, particularly if associated with vomiting or constipation, requires an urgent surgical opinion and possible operation.

Where to Get Treatment

Unlike in the case of adult hernias—which are very demanding in terms of achieving completely reliable repair and which benefit greatly from hernia specialization, pediatric hernias can be very successfully treated by any good pediatric surgeon.

Section 34.2

Information about Hydrocele and Hernia Surgery

Excerpted from "Information about Hydrocele and Hernia," by Christopher S. Cooper, MD, © 2000 University of Iowa Virtual Hospital; available online at http://www.vh.org/Patients/IHB/Uro/Peds/HydroceleHernia.html, reviewed May 2000. Copyright protected material used with permission of the author and the University of Iowa's Virtual Children's Hospital, www.vh.org/VCH.

What Is a Hydrocele or Hernia?

A hydrocele is a collection of fluid around the testicle. In children, this fluid comes down from the normal fluid that is present in the abdomen into a balloon-like structure around the testicle (called the *tunica vaginalis*). The neck of this balloon runs along the spermatic cord and opens into the abdomen. Normally, this neck closes off by itself within the first year of life. If it does not close off, it continues to let fluid come through and it may enlarge. If the opening becomes large enough a piece of the bowel may slip into it. This is called a hernia. If the bowel in a hernia becomes trapped it might swell and choke off its blood supply, which can be life-threatening.

Is Surgery Necessary?

Most infants with a hydrocele will have it go away as the opening closes off within the first year of life and require no surgery. If the hydrocele persists, it is unlikely to go away by itself and should be surgically corrected. If the hydrocele has a big enough opening to let fluid flow freely in and out (as noted by the swelling getting bigger and smaller) it is unlikely to close on its own and surgery is indicated. A hernia (when a piece of bowel extends through the opening) can be very dangerous and should always be surgically corrected.

What Is the Surgery Like?

The operation is performed by a small incision made in the groin. The abnormal opening is found and closed off and the fluid in the sac is drained. Almost all children will go home on the same day of surgery. There are no drains or stitches to be removed.

What Can I Expect Following Surgery?

Your child will go home on the day of surgery. The diet should start with liquids and then advance to soft food and solid food over the next 12 to 24 hours. Most children only require pain medication for 1 to 2 days after the operation. It is not unusual to see some swelling in the scrotum after surgery which will also go away over the next several weeks.

What Are Some of the Specific Complications Associated with Hydrocele/Hernia Surgery?

Wound infection or bleeding may occur with any operation, but are uncommon. Injury to the testicular blood vessels or vas deferens (the tube that carries sperm) may occur during a hydrocele or hernia operation. These structures are delicate and avoidance of injury requires delicacy and precision while performing the surgery. Rarely, a child may develop another hernia or hydrocele requiring a second operation.

Part Five

Skin and Scalp Ailments

Chapter 35

Taking Care of Children's Skin Problems

Children's skin problems span nearly two decades from birth through adolescence. Several common pediatric skin conditions include diaper dermatitis, atopic dermatitis, and warts.

What is diaper dermatitis?

Diaper dermatitis, or diaper rash as it is more commonly known, is not a diagnosis but rather a category of skin conditions affecting the diaper area. There are four types of diaper dermatitis, including:

- Irritant contact dermatitis
- Overgrowth of yeast (*Candida albicans*)
- Allergic contact dermatitis
- Inflammatory skin conditions such as seborrheic dermatitis

The most common type of diaper dermatitis is irritant contact dermatitis, associated with skin exposure to either urine or feces (or both) for a long period of time. Irritant contact dermatitis usually appears as bright red, sometimes slightly swollen, or even blister-like patches in the diaper area. Prolonged irritant contact dermatitis can increase the risk of infection in the affected area.

The primary treatment and prevention of irritant contact dermatitis includes barrier creams and ointments, most commonly containing zinc oxide. A mild topical steroid ointment or cream can also be very helpful in more quickly reducing the inflammation.

The next most common type of diaper dermatitis is the overgrowth of yeast, most commonly *Candida albicans*. The warm, moist, and often irritated environment of the diaper makes the skin more prone to an overgrowth of yeast. This condition generally develops on top of irritant contact dermatitis.

Usually, it appears as bright red papules (small, solid raised skin lesion or sore), patches, and sometimes pustules (pus-containing lesions) which are found on the skin and in its folds. There are also usually other similar patches that appear, which are not connected with the primary rash.

The condition can be treated with an over-the-counter topical antifungal cream such as Mycelex (clotrimazole), Nystatin (Mycostatin), or with a prescription medication. A barrier cream, often containing zinc oxide, is also recommended to treat and prevent this skin condition. If irritant contact dermatitis is also present, sometimes an additional mild topical steroid is prescribed. If this condition is only treated with topical steroids, the yeast will spread.

Rarely, allergic contact dermatitis will occur. This condition is usually associated with a component of the diaper itself. Symptoms of this condition include redness and swelling with itchiness which continues to recur in the same area such as the near the diaper's adhesive tape, or around the leg where there is elastic in the diaper.

Treatment of allergic contact dermatitis is very similar to the treatment of irritant contact dermatitis: barrier creams and ointments, most commonly containing zinc oxide, or mild topical steroid ointment if necessary.

To prevent allergic contact dermatitis, you need to identify the material that's causing the problem and then avoid it.

Seborrheic dermatitis, commonly known as cradle cap in infants and dandruff in older children and adults, can also be the cause of diaper dermatitis. Usually, this condition also affects other areas of the body such as the scalp, eyebrows, nasal folds, and sometimes the chest area. After seborrheic dermatitis is identified, the usual treatment is the careful use of mild topical steroid cream.

Topical steroids require very careful use, especially in the diaper area, to prevent skin atrophy (skin damage). Skin atrophy symptoms include shiny, thinned-looking skin, and sometimes striae (stretch marks). Skin atrophy can be avoided by: using low potency topical steroids, such as hydrocortisone 1–2%, and applying topical steroids sparingly to the affected areas only twice daily as needed for no longer than two weeks at a time.

What is atopic dermatitis?

Atopic dermatitis, or eczema, is a skin condition that can occur at any time in life, but usually first appears when children are infants and may not diminish until early adulthood. Over half of the infants with atopic dermatitis grow out of the condition by age 2, though flare-ups can occur throughout life.

Atopic dermatitis is a chronic condition, which means that it cannot be cured but it can be treated and controlled with proper guidance from a physician.

The condition is most common among families who have a history of allergies. Though food allergies may cause flare-ups, removing suspected foods (such as eggs, milk, fish, wheat and peanuts) from your child's diet is not likely to cure the problem. If you suspect that a food is worsening the rash, discuss this with your health care provider.

Atopic dermatitis can also get worse when the skin comes into contact with irritating substances such as harsh soaps and scratchy, tight fitting clothing. Scratching can also promote infections that require treatment.

Symptoms of atopic dermatitis in infants include:

• Red, very itchy dry patches of skin

• Rash on the cheeks that often begins at 2 to 6 months of age

• Rash oozes when scratched

• Symptoms can become worse if the child scratches the rash

Symptoms in adolescence and early adulthood include:

• Rash on creases of hands, elbows, wrists and knees and sometimes on the feet, ankles and neck

• Dry, scaly, brownish gray skin rash

• Thickened skin with markings

• Skin rash may bleed and crust after scratching

Treatment is aimed at reducing extreme itching and dry skin symptoms and may include topical corticosteroid creams and antihistamines.

Treatment will depend on the age of the child and the severity of the symptoms. Follow your health care provider's instructions for using the medications.

To help your child, you can also:

- Avoid long, hot baths, which can dry the skin. Instead use luke-warm water and give your child sponge baths.

- Apply lotion after bathing. This step will help trap moisture in the skin.

- Keep the room temperature as regular as possible. Changes in room temperature and humidity can dry the skin.

- Keep your child dressed in cotton. Wool, silk, and man-made fabrics such as polyester can irritate the skin.

- Use mild laundry soap and make sure that clothes are well rinsed.

- Watch for skin infections, which are more likely with dermatitis. Contact your health care provider if you notice an infection.

- Do not rub or scratch the rash.

- Use moisturizers often.

If atopic dermatitis is severe, systemic steroids can be safely used for a short time. If open wounds result from excessive itching, a topical antibiotic (Bactroban) may be used. Occasionally, a systemic antibiotic is necessary to treat infection. If these treatment methods are not effective, alternative therapy such as phototherapy (light therapy) may be prescribed for older children.

What are warts?

Warts commonly affect children of all ages. The types of warts include:

- Common warts are small, round, hard elevated lumps which often affect the fingers, hands and feet.

- Flat warts are slightly raised and have a flat top. They usually appear in groups and often affect the hands and face.

- Warts referred to as molluscum contagiosum which often affect the face

Common and flat warts are caused by the human papilloma virus (HPV), while molluscum contagiosum warts are caused by a pox virus. Warts usually spread through direct contact. It is also possible to pick up the virus in moist environments such as showers and locker rooms.

Unfortunately there are no antiviral treatments that actually target the virus itself. Instead, the treatment available is targeted against the skin in which the virus is living.

Over-the-counter treatments include liquid and film medications containing salicylic acid, which softens the abnormal skin cells and dissolves them. The film type of wart medications tend to work better because they have a higher percentage of salicylic acid (40%).

Over-the-counter wart treatments should be used as directed. First, soak the wart in warm water to help the medication penetrate the skin. Then gently rub off dead skin with a washcloth or pumice stone. Apply the medicine and cover with a bandage (replace the bandage if it gets wet). The medication stays on for 48 to 72 hours.

Repeat this process until there is a depression where the wart once was. The skin at the base of the wart will be pink and slightly tender. After the area heals, re-check it to see if the wart is still present or not. Repeat the treatment as necessary to remove the wart. This may take many weeks.

In the dermatologist's office, wart treatment will depend on the age of the child, the number and location of the warts, and the patient's and parent's decision.

Common and flat wart removal methods by the doctor include:

- Freezing the wart with liquid nitrogen (cryotherapy)

- Destroying the wart with chemicals (trichloroacetic acid or cantharidin preparations)

- Burning the wart off with electricity or a laser (such as a flash lamp or CO_2 lasers)

- Rarely, sensitization removal methods (dinitrochlorobenzene or DNCB) can be used, as well as locally injected chemotherapy

Oral cimetidine (Tagamet) may be prescribed along with one of the methods above. It has been shown to boost the immune system to better counter an immune response to the wart virus infection. Cimetidine, when used, is given at a higher dose than for stomach acid and should only be used for a trial two to three months.

Molluscum contagiosum treatment methods by the doctor include:

• Topical tretinoin (Retin-A)

• Destroying the wart with chemicals (trichloroacetic acid or cantharidin preparations)

• Freezing the wart with liquid nitrogen (cryotherapy)

• Scraping the wart off (curettage)

It is important to mention that these wart treatments often need to be repeated every three to four weeks until the wart is gone. Individual molluscum lesions can usually be cured in less treatments.

All of these treatment methods may cause scarring and/or blisters so it is important to practice good wound care throughout the healing process.

Certain precautions can be taken to reduce the chance of getting warts, including:

• Wearing rubber sandals or shoes in public shower areas or swimming pools

• Avoiding physical contact with those who have visible warts

• Practicing good hygiene

• Eating balanced meals high in vitamins A, C, and E to boost your immune system

Chapter 36

Bites, Scratches, and Stings

Chapter Contents

Section 36.1

Bites and Scratches

Animal bites and scratches, even minor ones, can become infected and spread bacteria to other parts of the body. Whether the animal is a family pet or a creature from the wild, scratches and bites can carry disease. For example, cat scratch disease, a bacterial infection, can be transmitted by a cat scratch (usually from a kitten) even if the site of the scratch doesn't look infected. In addition, certain animals can transmit rabies and tetanus. Human bites that break the skin are even more likely to become infected.

What to Do for a Bite or Scratch

- If the bite or scratch wound is bleeding, apply pressure to the area with a clean bandage or towel until the bleeding stops. If available, use clean latex or rubber gloves to protect yourself from exposure to blood.

- Clean the wound with soap and water, and hold it under running water for at least 5 minutes. Do not apply an antiseptic or anything else to the wound.

- Dry the wound and cover it with sterile gauze or a clean cloth.

- Phone your child's doctor. Your child may need antibiotics, a tetanus booster, or a rabies vaccination. A bite or scratch on a child's hand or face is particularly prone to infection and should be evaluated by your doctor.

- If possible, locate the animal that inflicted the wound. Some animals may have to be captured, confined, and observed for rabies. Do not try to capture the animal yourself. Look in your phone book for the number of an animal control office or animal warden in your area.

• Go to the nearest hospital emergency department if:

  • the wound won't stop bleeding after 10 minutes of direct pressure.

  • the wound is more than ½ inch long or appears to be deep.

  • the attacking animal was wild (not tame) or behaving strangely.

  • a body part is severed. Wrap the severed part in sterile gauze or a clean cloth and take it with you to the emergency department.

Reminder to pet owners: Make sure that your pets are properly immunized and licensed.

Section 36.2

Cat Scratch Disease

This information was provided by KidsHealth, one of the largest resources online for medically reviewed health information written for parents, kids, and teens. For more articles like this one, visit www.KidsHealth.org, or www.TeensHealth.org. © 2001 The Nemours Center for Children's Health Media, a division of The Nemours Foundation. Reprinted with permission.

Signs and Symptoms

Cat scratch disease is an infection that causes swelling of the lymph nodes (swollen glands) after an animal scratch—most often from a cat.

A blister or a small bump often develops 3 to 10 days after the scratch and may be mistaken for an insect bite. The blister or bump at the site of a cat scratch is called an inoculation lesion (injury site where germs enter the body), and it is most commonly found on the arms and hands, head, and scalp.

The first clue to diagnosing this illness is history of exposure to a cat or kitten. About 55% to 70% of people with the infection have a cat scratch somewhere on their bodies.

Usually within 2 weeks of a cat scratch, lymph nodes close to the area of the inoculation lesion will swell and become tender (lymph nodes are bean-shaped organs of the immune system that are often called glands).

These swollen lymph nodes or glands appear most often in the underarm area, neck, and above the collar bone. They range in size from about ½ inch to 2 inches (1 to 5 centimeters) in diameter and may be surrounded by a larger area of swelling under the skin. The swollen lymph nodes may also be painful or tender, and the skin over them may be red. Swollen lymph nodes may persist for months.

In most children and adolescents, swollen lymph nodes are the main symptom of the disease. About one third of people with cat scratch disease have other, more generalized symptoms. These include fever (usually less than 101° Fahrenheit or 38.3° Celsius), fatigue, loss of appetite, headache, and a generally ill feeling.

Cat scratch disease does not appear in its usual form in about 9% to 14% of cases. Instead, it may appear in a form called Parinaud Oculoglandular Syndrome, with the following symptoms: an inoculation site that looks like a small sore on the conjunctiva (membrane lining the eye surface) of one eye; swollen lymph nodes in the area around the ears; and (sometimes) redness of the involved eye. Other unusual forms of cat scratch disease include osteomyelitis (bone infection), pneumonia (lung infection), liver and spleen abscesses, and prolonged fevers without any other findings.

Very rarely, people with cat scratch disease have symptoms that may include seizures. These symptoms usually begin 1 to 6 weeks after swollen lymph nodes appear and are severe for 1 to 2 weeks. People usually recover slowly, but completely.

Description

Bartonella henselae is the bacterium that causes cat scratch disease. It is found in all parts of the world, and over 80% of cases affect people under age 21. Most cases occur in fall and winter. In the United States, about 22,000 cases occur annually. Worldwide, the disease affects nine out of every 100,000 persons each year, and multiple cases within families are common, especially among those who have the same cat.

A cat with *Bartonella henselae* infection does not look sick. Experts believe that up to 44% of cats have a *Bartonella henselae* infection at some time in their lives.

Incubation

It usually takes 3 to 10 days for a blister or small bump to appear at the site of a cat scratch. Lymph node swelling usually begins about 2 weeks after the cat scratch, with a range of 7 to 60 days.

Duration

Swollen lymph nodes usually disappear within 2 to 6 months in nearly all cases. Having one episode of cat scratch disease usually makes people immune for the rest of their lives.

Contagiousness

Cat scratch disease is not contagious from person to person. It is transmitted by the scratch of an infected animal, most often a kitten. Kittens or cats may carry this bacteria in their blood for months. Cats with this bacteria do not need to be put to sleep.

Prevention

Teaching children to avoid stray or unfamiliar cats can prevent cat scratch disease. If your child is scratched by a pet—even one of your own household pets—wash the injured area thoroughly with soap and water.

If you have a cat in your home, ask your veterinarian's advice about having the cat declawed. If you suspect that someone in your family has caught cat scratch disease from your family pet, you don't need to worry that the animal will need to be put to sleep. Talk with your veterinarian about the problem.

When to Call Your Child's Doctor

Call your child's doctor whenever your child has swollen and/or painful lymph nodes in any area of the body.

Professional Treatment

Diagnosis is usually based on the following (although not all of the following are necessary for diagnosis):

- your child's history of being exposed to cats or kittens
- a physical examination for signs of a cat scratch and swollen lymph nodes

- negative skin tests, blood tests, and cultures to rule out other causes of swollen lymph nodes

- a positive cat scratch blood test, available through your child's doctor or hospital

- a microscopic examination of a removed lymph node consistent with cat scratch disease

Rarely, a swollen lymph node becomes so large and painful that your child's doctor may recommend its removal. This is usually done in a very simple surgical procedure with a small incision.

Antibiotics are generally used to treat the disease, especially the unusual forms of cat scratch disease. If your child's doctor has prescribed antibiotics, give medication to your child on schedule for as many days as your child's doctor has advised. Use nonprescription medicines, like acetaminophen, to relieve pain of swollen lymph nodes and to lower fever.

In most cases, swollen lymph nodes usually subside within 2 to 4 months.

Home Treatment

A child with cat scratch disease doesn't need to be isolated from other family members. Bed rest is not necessary, but it may help a child with cat scratch disease who tires easily. If your child feels like playing, encourage quiet play, taking care to avoid injuring areas of swollen lymph nodes. For localized care of swollen lymph nodes, try moist compresses of salty water.

Section 36.3

Insect Stings

Part 1: An Introduction to Insect Bites and Stings

Insect bites and stings are very common in children, especially during the spring and summer months. Among the arthropods that often bite and sting are spiders, ticks, mites, mosquitoes, flies, fleas, ants, bees, and wasps.

While most insect bites only result in mild local reactions, they can cause more serious conditions, such as anaphylactic reactions and Lyme disease.

Knowing how to prevent and treat common insect bites and stings, and knowing when to not overreact, can help keep your kids safe and healthy.

Symptoms

The symptoms that can be caused by insect bites depend on the type of insect and how sensitive you are to it. Symptoms can vary from mild swelling, pain, itchiness, and redness to large blisters or life threatening anaphylactic reactions.

Reactions that stay localized to the sight of the bite or sting are usually not serious.

More serious signs and symptoms of anaphylaxis, a type of life threatening reaction, can include trouble swallowing, throat and chest tightness, low blood pressure (hypotension), diaphoresis (sweating), dizziness, weakness, itching, hives, wheezing, and difficulty breathing. These symptoms usually develop fairly quickly and usually within 30 minutes of being stung. You should seek immediate medical attention or activate your local emergency services if your child has these symptoms following an insect bite or sting.

Mosquito bites commonly cause itchy red bumps, which can vary in size from being very small to ½ inch. They usually also have a central raised area.

Fire ants are notorious for causing severe local reactions, including pustules or pimples and red, swollen, and extremely itchy areas, which may turn into blisters. They often bite multiple times, most commonly on the feet and legs. A large number of bites, more than 10–20, in a young infant can lead to serious reactions and may require medical attention.

Bees, wasps, yellow jackets, and hornets usually cause painful red bumps. Honey bees have a barbed stinger and usually leave it behind at the site of the sting. The stinger will usually appear as a black dot inside the bite if it has been left behind. More serious local reactions can cause swelling of an entire limb.

Unlike other bites, tick bites are painless and usually don't itch.

Bedbugs also usually cause painless bites, which then become itchy. Since bedbugs usually only come out to feed at night, and they feed infrequently (often just weekly), they can be hard to detect.

Chiggers or harvest mites also commonly bite children, especially in the southern United States, where they are found in grasses and bushes. Chigger bites usually occur on the legs and along the belt line and can appear as small red bumps and are extremely itchy. Chigger bites are often confused with chickenpox infections.

Flea bites also commonly affect children, causing multiple grouped red bumps with a central area of crusting.

Spider bites cause a lot of fear in parents, but rarely cause serious reactions in children. Only two spiders in the United States, the black widow spider and the brown recluse spider, usually cause poisoning. These spiders can be readily identified by their characteristic markings, including the red or orange hour glass shape on the abdomen of the black widow spider and the violin shaped markings on the back of the brown recluse. These bites are usually painless or cause mild irritation. More serious reactions usually occur quickly and within 3–12 hours and can include muscle pain, diaphoresis (sweating), nausea, vomiting, headache, and high blood pressure.

Papular Urticaria

Papular urticaria is a delayed hypersensitivity type reaction to many bites and stings. Children, usually between the ages of 2 and 7 years, with this condition will commonly develop multiple small, red itchy bumps in clusters on the upper arms, shoulders and other exposed areas. New crops of bumps commonly appear and each last about 2–10 days.

Part 2: Prevention of Insect Bites and Stings

To help prevent your child from getting bitten or stung by insects, you can:

- Make sure to keep as much of her skin covered with clothing as possible, including a long sleeve shirt, long pants, socks, and a hat.

- Wear light colored clothing, so as not to attract bugs.

- Avoid using any scented soaps or other products on your baby, since the fragrances can also attract insects.

- Use an insect repellent regularly. Commonly used insect repellents that can usually be safely used in children include those with less than 10% DEET (n,n-diethyl-m toluamide), or others with citronella or soybean oil.

- Apply insect repellents to clothing instead of to skin so that it won't be absorbed.

- Wash off insect repellents as soon as possible.

- Follow the instructions, including age restrictions on any insect repellent you are considering using.

- Avoid areas where insects nest.

- Do daily tick checks of your child's body when he has a possible exposure, especially when camping or hiking, so as to prevent tick borne diseases, such as Lyme disease.

- Remember that insect repellents do not protect against most stinging insects, including wasps, bees, and fire ants.

- Use window and door screens to prevent insects from getting inside your house.

Part 3: Treatment of Insect Bites and Stings

Most children with insect bites or stings only need symptomatic treatment for the symptoms of pain and itching.

Anaphylaxis

Some children who are allergic to the venom in the insect sting can develop more serious anaphylactic reactions.

Since this type of reaction is life-threatening, treatment should be started as soon as possible and you should activate your local emergency medical services. An injection of epinephrine is the main treatment for anaphylactic reactions. Children with a history of anaphylactic reactions should have an auto-injector of epinephrine available for immediate administration, but you should still call 911.

Since children do not always outgrow these types of reactions, an evaluation by a pediatric allergist can be helpful to confirm the allergy (skin and/or RAST [Radioallergosorbent] testing) and consider venom immunotherapy (allergy shots). These shots can protect your child from having future reactions to an insect bite or sting. Children usually begin with weekly shots of a gradually increasing strength of insect venom. This is followed by monthly maintenance shots so that the protection lasts.

Children with anaphylactic reactions should be given an emergency kit with an epinephrine auto-injector and they should wear an identification tag, such as a MedicAlert bracelet.

Bee Stings

Unlike other insects that sting, the honey bee leaves its stinger behind. Proper removal of this stinger following a honey bee sting can help prevent worsening symptoms. What you should not do includes pulling the stinger out with tweezers or pinching it out with your fingers, since this can inject more venom and cause a worsening reaction. Instead, use a credit card or dull blade to scrape it out.

Symptomatic Treatment

Most insect bites and stings only cause local reactions, including redness, swelling, pain, and itching. After you thoroughly wash the area with soap and water, other symptomatic treatments that may help your child feel better include applying:

- an ice pack or cool compress

- a meat tenderizer solution, which can be made by mixing one part meat tenderizer and 4 parts of water. This is especially helpful for painful stings from bee, wasp, or ant. For best effect, soak a cotton ball in the meat tenderizer solution and use it to rub the area of the bite for 15–20 minutes.

- a baking soda paste

- a topical steroid or other topical anti-itch cream, such as Calamine lotion, to the area

Other medications, including an oral antihistamine for itching, such as diphenhydramine (Benadryl), and/or pain medications, such as ibuprofen or acetaminophen, may also help. More extensive local reactions may sometimes require a short course of an oral steroid.

Antibiotics may be needed if the bite becomes infected.

Is It Infected?

Insect bites and stings are commonly misdiagnosed as an infection. Or if the initial bite or sting is identified, the resulting redness and swelling is confused as a secondary cellulitis. While both conditions can cause similar symptoms, the local reaction of a bite or sting usually begins quickly and generally within 6–24 hours of the bite. A secondary infection usually occurs after the first twenty four hours and can cause spreading redness, especially red streaks, and fever.

Chapter 37

Head Lice Infestation (Pediculosis)

Head Lice Infestation

What are head lice?

Also called *Pediculus humanus capitis*, head lice are parasitic insects found on the heads of people. Having head lice is very common; as many as 6–12 million people worldwide get head lice each year.

Who is at risk for getting head lice?

Anyone who comes in close contact with someone who already has head lice, contaminated clothing, and other belongings. Preschool and elementary-age children, 3–10, and their families are infested most often. Girls get head lice more often than boys, women more than men. In the United States, African-Americans rarely get head lice.

What do head lice look like?

There are three forms of lice: the nit, the nymph, and the adult.

This chapter contains text from "Head Lice Infestation," http://www.cdc.gov/ncidod/dpd/parasites/headlice/factsht_head_lice.htm, reviewed 2001, "Treating Head Lice," http://www.cdc.gov/ncidod/dpd/parasites/headlice/factsht_head_lice_treating.htm, reviewed 2001, and "Treating Head Lice with Malathion," http://www.cdc.gov/ncidod/dpd/parasites/headlice/factsht_malathion.htm, reviewed August 1999, Centers for Disease Control and Prevention (CDC), Division of Parasitic Diseases (DPD).

Nit. Nits are head lice eggs. They are hard to see and are often confused for dandruff or hair spray droplets. Nits are found firmly attached to the hair shaft. They are oval and usually yellow to white. Nits take about 1 week to hatch.

Nymph. The nit hatches into a baby louse called a nymph. It looks like an adult head louse, but is smaller. Nymphs mature into adults about 7 days after hatching. To live, the nymph must feed on blood.

Adult. The adult louse is about the size of a sesame seed, has 6 legs, and is tan to grayish-white. In persons with dark hair, the adult louse will look darker. Females lay nits; they are usually larger than males. Adult lice can live up to 30 days on a person's head. To live, adult lice need to feed on blood. If the louse falls off a person, it dies within 2 days.

Where are head lice most commonly found?

On the scalp behind the ears and near the neckline at the back of the neck. Head lice hold on to hair with hook-like claws found at the end of each of their six legs. Head lice are rarely found on the body, eyelashes, or eyebrows.

What are the signs and symptoms of head lice infestation?

- tickling feeling of something moving in the hair
- itching, caused by the allergic reaction to the bites
- irritability
- sores on the head caused by scratching. These sores can sometimes become infected.

How did my child get head lice?

- By contact with an already infested person. Contact is common during play at school and at home (slumber parties, sports activities, at camp, on a playground).
- By wearing infested clothing, such as hats, scarves, coats, sports uniforms, or hair ribbons.
- By using infested combs, brushes, or towels.

- By lying on a bed, couch, pillow, carpet, or stuffed animal that has recently been in contact with an infested person.

How is head lice infestation diagnosed?

By looking closely through the hair and scalp for nits, nymphs, or adults. Finding a nymph or adult may be difficult; there are usually few of them and they can move quickly from searching fingers. If crawling lice are not seen, finding nits within a 1/4 inch of the scalp confirms that a person is infested and should be treated. If you only find nits more than 1/4 inch from the scalp, the infestation is probably an old one and does not need to be treated. If you are not sure if a person has head lice, the diagnosis should be made by a health care provider, school nurse, or a professional from the local health department or agricultural extension service.

Treating Head Lice

How can I treat a head lice infestation?

By treating the person infested with head lice, other infested family members, and by cleaning the house.

Treat the infested person. Requires using an over-the-counter (OTC) or prescription medication. Follow these treatment steps:

1. Before applying treatment, remove all clothing.

2. Apply lice medicine, also called pediculicide, according to label instructions. If your child has extra long hair, you may need to use a second bottle. WARNING: Do not use a creme rinse or combination shampoo/conditioner before using lice medicine. Do not re-wash hair for 1–2 days after treatment.

3. Have the infested person put on clean clothing after treatment.

4. If a few live lice are still found 8–12 hours after treatment, but are moving more slowly than before, do not retreat. Comb dead and remaining live lice out of the hair. The medicine may take longer to kill lice.

5. If, after 8–12 hours of treatment, no dead lice are found and lice seem as active as before, the medicine may not be working. See your health care provider for a different medication; follow treatment directions.

6. Nit (head lice eggs) combs, often found in lice medicine packages, should be used to comb nits and lice from the hair shaft. Many flea combs made for cats and dogs are also effective.

7. After treatment, check hair and comb with a nit comb to remove nits and lice every 2–3 days. Continue to check for 2–3 weeks until you are sure all lice and nits are gone.

8. If using OTC pediculicides, retreat in 7–10 days. If using Malathion, retreat in 7–10 days only if crawling bugs are found.

Treat the household. Head lice do not survive long if they fall off a person. You do not need to spend a lot of time or money on house cleaning activities.

Follow these steps to help avoid re-infestation by lice that have recently fallen off the hair or crawled onto clothing or furniture.

1. To kill lice and nits, machine wash all washable clothing and bed linens that the infested person touched during the 2 days before treatment. Use the hot water (130° Fahrenheit) cycle. Dry laundry using high heat for at least 20 minutes.

2. Dry clean clothing that is not washable, (coats, hats, scarves, etc.) OR

3. Store all clothing, stuffed animals, comforters, etc., that cannot be washed or dry cleaned into a plastic bag; seal for 2 weeks.

4. Soak combs and brushes for 1 hour in rubbing alcohol, Lysol, or wash with soap and hot (130° Fahrenheit) water.

5. Vacuum the floor and furniture. Do not use fumigant sprays; they can be toxic if inhaled or absorbed through the skin.

Prevent reinfestation. Lice are most commonly spread directly by head-to-head contact and indirectly though contaminated clothing or belongings. Teach your child to avoid playtime and other activities that are likely to spread lice.

- Avoid head-to-head contact common during play at school and at home (slumber parties, sports activities, at camp, on a playground).

- Do not share clothing, such as hats, scarves, coats, sports uniforms, or hair ribbons.

- Do not share infested combs, brushes, or towels.

- Do not lie on beds, couches, pillows, carpets, or stuffed animals that have recently been in contact with an infested person.

My child has head lice. I don't. Should I treat myself to prevent being infested?

No, although anyone living with an infested person can get head lice. Check household contacts for lice and nits every 2–3 days. Treat only if crawling lice or nits (eggs) within a 1/4 inch of the scalp are found.

Should my pets be treated for head lice?

No. Head lice do not live on pets.

My child is under 2 years old and has been diagnosed with head lice. Can I treat him or her with prescription or OTC drugs?

For children under 2 years old, remove crawling bugs and nits by hand. If this does not work, ask your child's health care provider for treatment recommendations. The safety of head lice medications has not been tested in children 2 years of age and under.

What OTC medications are available to treat head lice?

Many head lice medications are available at your local drug store. Each OTC product contains one of the following active ingredients.

1. Pyrethrins: often combined with piperonyl butoxide. Brand name products include A-200, Pronto, R&C, Rid, Triple X. Pyrethrins are natural extracts from the chrysanthemum flower. Though safe and effective, pyrethrins only kill crawling lice, not unhatched nits. A second treatment is recommended in 7–10 days to kill any newly hatched lice. Treatment failures are common.

2. Permethrin. Brand name product: Nix. Permethrins are similar to natural pyrethrins. Permethrins are safe and effective and may continue to kill newly hatched eggs for several days after treatment. A second treatment may be necessary in 7–10

days to kill any newly hatched lice. Treatment failures are common.

What are the prescription drugs used to treat head lice?

1. Malathion (Ovide): Malathion has just been reapproved for the treatment of head lice infestations. Malathion treats both lice and head lice eggs. When used as directed, Malathion is very effective in treating lice. Few side-effects have been reported. Open sores from scratching may cause Malathion to sting the scalp.

2. Lindane (Kwell): Lindane is one of the most common products used to treat head lice. When used as directed, the drug is probably safe. Overuse, misuse, or accidentally swallowing Lindane can be toxic to the brain and other parts of the nervous system. Lindane should not be used if excessive scratching has caused open sores on the head.

Which head lice medicine is best for me?

If you aren't sure, ask your pharmacist or health care provider. When using the medicine, always follow the instructions provided.

When Treating Head Lice

1. Do not use extra amounts of the lice medication unless instructed. These drugs are insecticides and can be dangerous when misused or overused.

2. Do not treat the infested person more than 3 times with the same medication if it does not seem to work. See your health care provider for alternative medication.

3. Do not mix head lice drugs.

Should household sprays be used to kill adult lice?

No. Spraying the house is NOT recommended. Fumigants and room sprays can be toxic if inhaled or absorbed through the skin.

Should I have a pest control company spray my house?

No. Vacuuming floors and furniture is enough to treat the household.

Treating Head Lice with Malathion

Malathion (Ovide lotion) was re-approved Food and Drug Administration (FDA) as a prescription drug for the treatment of head lice infestation in the United States. Follow the directions below to treat a head lice-infestation in your home with Malathion.

Treat the person infested with head lice:

1. Before applying Malathion lotion, remove all clothing.

2. Apply Malathion according to label directions, to dry hair until the scalp and hair are wet and thoroughly coated. Leave the medication on the hair for 8–12 hours; allow the hair to dry naturally. Have the person put on clean clothing once medication has been applied. (Consider treating just before bedtime. Once Malathion has been applied to the hair and scalp, cover any pillow(s) with a towel to keep medication from staining the pillow.)

3. After 8–12 hours, thoroughly wash hair.

4. A nit (head lice egg) comb should be used to remove lice and nits from the hair. Many flea combs made for cats and dogs are also effective.

5. After treatment, check hair and comb with a nit comb to remove nits and lice every 2–3 days. Continue checking for 2–3 weeks until you are sure all lice and nits are gone.

6. If crawling bugs are found 7–10 days after treatment, retreat with the same or different louse medication.

After completing the steps above, follow instructions for "Treat the Household" and "Prevent Reinfestation" above.

What warnings and precautions are associated with Malathion?

1. Malathion may cause stinging, especially if the scalp has open sores from scratching.

2. Malathion is flammable. Keep medication out of the eyes and away from heat sources such as hair dryers, electric curlers, cigarettes, or open flames.

3. Pregnant and nursing mothers should only use Malathion after consulting their physician.

Are treatment failures common?

No, however reinfestation is common.

Is a second treatment needed?

Maybe. If crawling lice are still found, a second treatment may be given in 7–9 days. Other family members should be checked for signs of infestation.

Does Malathion kill head lice eggs?

Yes. Some medication remains on the hair for several days to kill any eggs that may hatch.

Chapter 38

Scabies (Itch Mite Infestation)

What is scabies?

Scabies is a skin infection.

What causes scabies?

A tiny insect called a mite causes scabies. Mites burrow under the skin to live and reproduce. The symptoms of scabies are caused by an allergic reaction to the mites.

Who can get scabies?

Anyone can get scabies. Being unclean or dirty does not cause infection. Children are more likely than adults to get scabies because they play close to one another. Pets can't get scabies or spread the infection.

What are the symptoms of scabies?

The most typical sign of scabies is an itchy rash or small, itchy blisters. Blisters may break when your child scratches them. Skin may become thick, scaly, and have scratch marks. Young children usually get the rash on their hands, feet, armpits, and sometimes their scalp and face. Older children usually get the rash on their wrists, elbows, armpits, breasts, groin, genitals, and between the fingers.

The mite's burrows look like short, dark, wavy lines on the skin. These are usually found between the fingers and around the wrists. Itching is worst at night or after a bath. Itching can make it hard to sleep. Scabies does not cause fever.

Is scabies contagious?

Yes. Scabies is contagious. Tell your child's school or daycare if your child has scabies. Other children should be checked and treated if needed. Scabies is spread through direct contact (skin to skin) with a person who has scabies. It can also be spread by sharing the same bed or through sexual contact. Scabies can live on items used by an infected person. Contact with these items can spread infection.

A person with scabies can spread the infection before his symptoms have started. After treatment, a person is still contagious for 2–4 hours.

How is scabies treated?

Everyone in your house should be treated for scabies at the same time whether they have symptoms or not. Scabies is treated with medicated cream prescribed by a doctor. It must be put on correctly to work. Rub the medicated cream over the entire body except the face and scalp. Rub the cream between fingers, toes, on the genitals, and under the fingernails. Wash the cream off with soap and water 8–12 hours after putting it on. The medicated cream could make the skin dry and cause itching. The day after treatment, you can use lotion (such as Lubriderm or Aveeno) for dry skin.

Oatmeal baths and mild soap (such as Dove) can also help ease itching. Anti-itch medications (such as Benadryl or Antarax) can help ease itching. These may help children sleep if given just before bedtime.

Keep your child's fingernails short to cut down on scratching. Put mittens or socks on your child's hands before he goes to bed, especially if he sucks his thumb.

How long does scabies last?

One treatment will usually cure the infection. Your child can go back to school or daycare the day after treatment. Itching may last for several weeks while the skin heals. Don't put medicated cream on again unless directed by the doctor. Scratch marks will usually go away one or two weeks after treatment. It may take up to 2 months.

Can I prevent scabies?

There are a number of things you can do to prevent the spread of scabies.

Personal and household items should be washed to keep scabies from spreading. Items should be washed in hot water, put in a hot dryer, or dry cleaned. Seal items that can't be washed in plastic bags for two weeks. Mites will usually die after 3 or 4 days off the skin. Vacuum furniture and carpeting. Do not spray the house with chemicals. Teach your child not to share personal items with an infected person.

If scabies is not treated it can lead to more infections.

When should I call the doctor?

- Call the doctor if your child has a skin itch.

- Call the doctor if you're worried about your child's infection.

- Call the doctor if skin looks infected or if the itchy rash has spread.

- Call the doctor if your child's symptoms have worsened or not improved after 2 weeks.

- Pregnant women and children under 2 years old may not be able to use medicated cream. Talk to the doctor about treatment.

References

The Children's Hospital, Boston, "Scabies," (Virtual Children's Hospital) 1993. URL: http://www.vh.org/Patients/IHB/Peds/Infectious/Scabies1.html

KidsHealth, "Scabies," 1995-2000. URL: http://www.kidshealth.org/PageManager.jsp?dn=KidsHealth&lic=1&ps=107&cat_id=&article_set=22947

Pediatric Infectious Diseases Journal, "Scabies (Itch Mite Infestation)," (Virtual Children's Hospital). URL: http://www.vh.org/Patients/IHB/Peds/Infectious/Scabies2.html

Chapter 39

Warts

What are warts?

Warts are non-cancerous skin growths caused by a viral infection in the top layer of the skin. Viruses that cause warts are called human papillomavirus (HPV). Warts are usually skin-colored and feel rough to the touch, but they can be dark, flat and smooth. The appearance of a wart depends on where it is growing.

How many kinds of warts are there?

There are several different kinds of warts including:

- common warts
- foot (plantar) warts
- flat warts

Common warts. Usually grow on the fingers, around the nails and on the backs of the hands. They are more common where skin has been broken, for example where fingernails are bitten or hangnails picked. These are often called seed warts because the blood vessels to the wart produce black dots that look like seeds.

Foot warts. Are usually on the soles (plantar area) of the feet and are called plantar warts. When plantar warts grow in clusters they are known as mosaic warts. Most plantar warts do not stick up above the surface like common warts because the pressure of walking flattens them and pushes them back into the skin. Like common warts, these warts may have black dots. Plantar warts have a bad reputation because they can be painful, feeling like a stone in the shoe.

Flat warts. Are smaller and smoother than other warts. They tend to grow in large numbers—20 to 100 at any one time. They can occur anywhere, but in children they are most common on the face. In adults they are often found in the beard area in men and on the legs in women. Irritation from shaving probably accounts for this.

How do you get warts?

Warts are passed from person to person, sometimes indirectly. The time from the first contact to the time the warts have grown large enough to be seen is often several months. The risk of catching hand, foot, or flat warts from another person is small.

Why do some people get warts and others don't?

Some people get warts depending on how often they are exposed to the virus. Wart viruses occur more easily if the skin has been damaged in some way, which explains the high frequency of warts in children who bite their nails or pick at hangnails. Some people are just more likely to catch the wart virus than are others, just as some people catch colds very easily. Patients with a weakened immune system also are more prone to a wart virus infection.

Do warts need to be treated?

In children, warts can disappear without treatment over a period of several months to years. However, warts that are bothersome, painful, or rapidly multiplying should be treated. Warts in adults often do not disappear as easily or as quickly as they do in children.

How do dermatologists treat warts?

Dermatologists are trained to use a variety of treatments, depending on the age of the patient and the type of wart.

Common warts. In young children, common warts can be treated at home by their parents on a daily basis by applying salicylic acid gel, solution or plaster. There is usually little discomfort but it can take many weeks of treatment to obtain favorable results. Treatment should be stopped at least temporarily if the wart becomes sore. Warts may also be treated by painting with cantharidin in the dermatologist's office. Cantharidin causes a blister to form under the wart. The dermatologist can then clip away the dead part of the wart in the blister roof in a week or so.

For adults and older children cryotherapy (freezing) is generally preferred. This treatment is not too painful and rarely results in scarring. However, repeat treatments at one to three week intervals are often necessary. Electrosurgery (burning) is another good alternative treatment. Laser treatment can also be used for resistant warts that have not responded to other therapies.

Foot warts. These are difficult to treat because the bulk of the wart lies below the skin surface. Treatments include the use of salicylic acid plasters, applying other chemicals to the wart, or one of the surgical treatments including laser surgery, electrosurgery, or cutting. The dermatologist may recommend a change in footwear to reduce pressure on the wart and ways to keep the foot dry since moisture tends to allow warts to spread.

Flat warts. These are often too numerous to treat with methods mentioned above. As a result, peeling methods using daily applications of salicylic acid, tretinoin, glycolic acid, or other surface peeling preparations are often recommended. For some adults, periodic office treatments for surgical treatments are sometimes necessary.

What are some of the other treatments for warts?

There are several different lasers used for the treatment of warts. Laser therapy is used to destroy some types of warts. Lasers are more expensive and require the injection of a local anesthesia to numb the area treated.

Another treatment is to inject each wart with an anti-cancer drug called bleomycin. The injections may be painful and can have other side effects.

Immunotherapy, which attempts to use the body's own rejection system is another method of treatment. Several methods of immunotherapy are being used. With one method the patient is made allergic to a certain chemical which is then painted on the wart. A mild allergic reaction occurs around the treated warts, and may result in the disappearance of the warts.

Warts may also be injected with interferon, a treatment to boost the immune reaction and cause rejection of the wart.

Can I treat my own warts without seeing a doctor?

There are some wart remedies available without a prescription. However, you might mistake another kind of skin growth for a wart, and end up treating something more serious as though it were a wart. If you have any questions about either the diagnosis or the best way to treat a wart, you should seek your dermatologist's advice.

What about the use of hypnosis or folk remedies?

Many people, patients and doctors alike, believe folk remedies and hypnosis are effective. Since warts, especially in children, may disappear without treatment, it's hard to know whether it was a folk remedy or just the passage of time that led to the cure. Since warts are generally harmless, there may be times when these treatments are appropriate. Medical treatments can always be used if necessary.

What about the problem of recurrent warts?

Sometimes it seems as if new warts appear as fast as old ones go away. This may happen because the old warts have shed virus into the surrounding skin before they were treated. In reality new baby warts are growing up around the original mother warts. The best way to limit this is to treat new warts as quickly as they develop so they have little time to shed virus into nearby skin. A check by your dermatologist can help assure the treated wart has resolved completely.

Is there any research going on about warts?

Research is moving along very rapidly. There is great interest in new treatments, as well as the development of a vaccine against warts. We hope there will be a solution to the annoying problem of warts in the not too distant future.

Chapter 40

Tinea Infections: Athlete's Foot, Jock Itch, and Ringworm

What is tinea?

Tinea is a fungus that can grow on your skin, hair, or nails. As it grows, it spreads out in a circle, leaving normal-looking skin in the middle. This makes it look like a ring. At the edge of the ring, the skin is lifted up by the irritation and looks red and scaly. To some people, the infection looks like a worm is under the skin. Because of the way it looks, tinea infection is often called ringworm. However, there really isn't a worm under the skin.

How did I get a fungal infection?

You can get a fungal infection by touching a person who has one. Some kinds of fungi live on damp surfaces, like the floors in public showers or locker rooms. You can easily pick up a fungus there. You can even catch a fungal infection from your pets. Dogs and cats, as well as farm animals, can be infected with a fungus. Often this infection looks like a patch of skin where fur is missing.

What areas of the body are affected by tinea infections?

Fungal infections are named for the part of the body they infect. Tinea corporis is a fungal infection of the skin on the body (corporis is the Latin word for body). If you have this infection, you may see small, red spots that grow into large rings almost anywhere on your arms, legs or chest.

Tinea pedis is usually called athlete's foot (pedis is the Latin word for foot). The moist skin between your toes is a perfect place for a fungus to grow. The skin may become itchy and red, with a white, wet surface. The infection may spread to the toenails (this is called tinea unguium—unguium comes from the Latin word for nail). Here it causes the toenails to become thick and crumbly. It can also spread to your hands and fingernails.

When a fungus grows in the moist, warm area of the groin, the rash is called tinea cruris (cruris comes from the Latin for leg). The common name for this infection is jock itch. Tinea cruris generally occurs in men, especially if they often wear athletic equipment.

Tinea capitis, which is called ringworm, causes itchy, red areas, usually on the head (capitis comes from the Latin for head). The hair is destroyed, leaving bald patches. This tinea infection is most common in children.

How do I know if I have a fungal infection?

The best way to know for sure is to ask your doctor. Other skin problems can look just like a fungal infection but have very different treatments. To find out what is causing your rash, your doctor may scrape a small amount of the irritated skin onto a glass slide (or clip off a piece of nail or hair). Then he or she will look at the skin, nail, or hair under a microscope. After doing this, your doctor will usually be able to tell if your skin problem is caused by a fungus.

Sometimes a piece of your skin, hair, or nail will be sent to a lab to grow the fungus in a test tube. This is another way the lab can tell if your skin problem is caused by a fungus. They can also find out the exact type of fungus. This process takes a while because a fungus grows slowly.

How do I get rid of a tinea infection?

Once your doctor decides that you have a tinea infection, medicine can be used to get rid of it. You may only need to put a special cream on the rash for a few weeks. This is especially true for jock itch.

It can be harder to get rid of fungal infections on other parts of the body. Sometimes you have to take medicine by mouth. This medicine usually has to be taken for a long time, maybe even for months.

Irritated skin takes time to heal. New hair or nails will have to grow back.

Some medicines can have unpleasant effects on the rest of your body, especially if you're also taking other medicines. There are some newer medicines that seem to work better with fewer side effects. You may need to have blood tests to make sure that your body is not having a bad reaction to the medicine.

What can I do to prevent tinea infections?

Skin that is kept clean and dry is your best defense. However, you're also less likely to get a tinea infection if you do the following things:

- When you're at home, take your shoes off and expose your feet to the air.

- Change your socks and underwear every day, especially in warm weather.

- Dry your feet carefully (especially between the toes) after using a locker room or public shower.

- Avoid walking barefoot in public areas. Instead, wear flip-flops, sandals, or water shoes.

- Don't wear thick clothing for long periods of time in warm weather. It will make you sweat more.

- Throw away worn-out exercise shoes. Never borrow other people's shoes.

- Check your pets for areas of hair loss. Ask your veterinarian to check them too. It's important to check pets carefully, because if you don't find out whether they're causing your fungal infection, you may get it again from them, even after treatment.

Can tinea cause serious illness?

A fungus rarely spreads below the surface of the body to cause serious illness. Your body usually prevents this. However, people with weak immune systems, such as people with AIDS (acquired immunodeficiency syndrome) may have a hard time getting well from a fungal infection.

Tinea infections usually don't leave scars after the fungus is gone. Sometimes, people don't even know they have a fungal infection and get better without any treatment.

271

Chapter 41

Impetigo

What is impetigo?

Impetigo is a skin infection caused by *Streptococcus* (strep) and *Staphylococcus* (staph) bacteria. The infection is common in children and occurs when the bacteria gets into scrapes and insect bites. Impetigo often occurs in the summer. Some people think that children get impetigo because they have not been washed properly. However, impetigo does not result from a lack of cleanliness.

Impetigo is a skin rash that is characterized by a cluster of blisters or red bumps. The blisters may ooze or be covered with a honey-colored crust. The rash usually appears around the nose, mouth, and parts of the skin not covered by clothes.

How is impetigo transmitted?

The infection is spread when someone touches an impetigo rash and then touches another person. The spread can be prevented by washing hands after touching infected skin. Treatment of impetigo with antibiotics can also prevent the spread of infection.

How is it diagnosed?

A physician diagnoses impetigo by examining the child and taking a culture for infection (or swab). The infection is treated with antibiotics, which may be given by mouth or applied on the skin in the form of an ointment.

What can parents do?

- Watch your child for signs of impetigo if another child has it.

- If you think your child has impetigo, contact your physician for diagnosis and treatment.

- Make sure that all household members wash their hands thoroughly with soap and running water after touching infected skin. Family members should not share face cloths or hand and bath towels.

- If your child has impetigo, he or she should not return to the child care facility or school until the antibiotic prescribed by your physician has been taken for at least one full day. It is important for the child to take all the medication prescribed by the physician, even after the signs of infection have gone away.

Chapter 42

Cellulitis

What is cellulitis?

Cellulitis is a spreading infection of the skin that usually begins as a small area of tenderness, swelling, and redness on the skin. As this red area begins to spread, the person may develop a fever, sometimes with chills and sweats, and swollen lymph nodes (swollen glands) near the area of infected skin.

Unlike impetigo, which is a very superficial skin infection, cellulitis refers to an infection involving the skin's deeper layers; the dermis and subcutaneous tissue. The main bacteria involved in cellulitis is *Staphylococcus* (staph), the same bacteria that causes many cases of impetigo. Occasionally, other bacteria may cause cellulitis as well.

Where does cellulitis occur?

Some cases of cellulitis appear on areas of trauma, where the skin has broken open, such as the skin near ulcers or surgical wounds. Many times, however, cellulitis occurs where there has been no break in the skin at all. In such cases, it is anyone's guess where the bacteria came from. Patients who have diabetes or impairment of the immune system (for example, from HIV [human immunodeficiency virus] or AIDS [acquired immunodeficiency syndrome] or from drugs that depress the immune system) are particularly prone to developing cellulitis.

Excerpted from "Cellulitis," reviewed April 2002, © 2002 MedicineNet, Inc. (http://www.medicinenet.com); reprinted with permission.

What does cellulitis look like?

The signs of cellulitis are those of any inflammation; redness, warmth, swelling, and pain. Any skin wound or ulcer that exhibits these signs may be developing cellulitis.

Other forms of noninfected inflammation may mimic cellulitis. People with poor leg circulation, for instance, often develop scaly redness on the shins and ankles; this is called stasis dermatitis and is often mistaken for the bacterial infection of cellulitis.

What causes cellulitis?

Staph (*Staphylococcus aureus*) is the most common bacteria that causes cellulitis.

Strep (Group A *Streptococcus*) is next most common bacteria that causes cellulitis. A form of rather superficial cellulitis caused by strep is called erysipelas; it is characterized by spreading hot, bright red circumscribed area on the skin with a sharp raised border. The so-called flesh-eating bacteria are, in fact, also a strain of strep which can in severe cases destroy tissue almost as fast as surgeons can cut it out.

Cellulitis can be caused by many other types of bacteria. In children under six, *H. flu* (*Haemophilus influenzae*) bacteria can cause cellulitis, especially on the face, arms, and upper torso. Cellulitis from a dog or cat bite or scratch may be caused by the *Pasteurella multocida* bacteria, which has a very short incubation period of only four to 24 hours. Cellulitis after an injury from a saltwater fish or shellfish (like a fish bite, a puncture from a fish spine, or a crab pinch) can be due to the *Erysipelothrix rhusiopathiae* bacteria. These same bacteria can also cause cellulitis after a skin injury on the farm, especially if it happened while working with pigs or poultry.

Is cellulitis contagious?

Cellulitis is not contagious because it is an infection of the skin's deeper layers, the dermis and subcutaneous tissue, and the skin's top layer (the epidermis) provides a cover over the infection. In this regard, cellulitis is different from impetigo in which there is a very superficial skin infection that can be contagious.

How is cellulitis treated?

First, it is crucial for the doctor to distinguish whether or not the inflammation is due to an infection. The history and physical exam can provide clues in this regard, as can sometimes the white blood cell count. A culture for bacteria may also be of value.

When it is difficult or impossible to distinguish whether or not the inflammation is due to an infection, doctors sometimes treat with antibiotics just to be sure. If the condition does not respond, it may need to be addressed by different methods dealing with types of inflammation that are not infected. For example, if the inflammation is thought to be due to an autoimmune disorder, treatment may be with a corticosteroid.

Antibiotics such as derivatives of penicillin or other types of antibiotics that are effective against the staph germ are used to treat cellulitis. If other bacteria, as determined by culture tests, turn out to be the cause, or if patients are allergic to penicillin, other appropriate antibiotics can be substituted.

Chapter 43

Fifth Disease

What is fifth disease?

Fifth disease is a viral infection caused by human Parvovirus B19. In most instances, fifth disease is a relatively mild, self-limited rash illness of childhood; recent studies indicate, however, that infection with Parvovirus B19 in rare instances can lead to serious complications.

Who gets fifth disease?

Anyone can become infected with the virus which causes fifth disease, but the disease is most often recognized in elementary school-aged children. Occurrence of B19 infection is worldwide and can occur throughout the year in all age groups as either sporadic cases or as clusters of cases of fifth disease.

What are the symptoms of fifth disease and when do they appear?

Four to fourteen days after exposure to the virus, an individual may experience low grade fever and tiredness. This is often followed by a distinctive facial rash often referred to as slapped cheeks. The facial

"Fifth Disease," *MCW HealthLink*, May 2000, available at http://health link.mcw.edu/article/954994100.html. © 2000 Medical College of Wisconsin. Reprinted with permission of the Medical College of Wisconsin/MCW HealthLink, http://healthlink.mcw.edu.

rash may then progress to a lace-like rash on the trunk, legs, and arms; this rash tends to fade and reappear with changes in temperature, sunlight, and emotional stress.

Approximately 20 percent of infected children and adults do not have any symptoms. Some adults do not develop rash but may complain of painful and swollen joints.

How is fifth disease spread?

The virus is spread by exposure to airborne droplets from the nose and throat of infected individuals. Approximately 50 percent of susceptible (have not been previously infected) household contacts of a case of fifth disease will become infected. In school outbreaks of fifth disease, about 30 percent of susceptible staff and as many as 60 percent of susceptible children will become infected with the virus.

When and for how long is a person able to spread fifth disease?

Persons with fifth disease appear to be contagious during the week before the appearance of their rash. By the time their rash is evident, the individual is probably beyond the contagious period.

How is fifth disease diagnosed?

In most cases, fifth disease is diagnosed based on the appearance of the characteristic rash. In addition, a specific blood test (which is not widely available) can confirm the diagnosis; this blood test is available through your local public health agency for those individuals who are at risk of serious consequences (severe anemia or miscarriage) if infected with B19 virus.

Does past infection with the virus make a person immune?

It is thought that persons who have previously been infected acquire long-term or lifelong immunity. Studies have shown that approximately 50 percent of adults are immune to Parvovirus B19 and therefore are not susceptible.

What are the complications associated with fifth disease?

While most individuals infected with Parvovirus B19 virus will experience a mild, self-limited infection, newly emerging information suggests that some individuals may be at increased risk if they become infected with this virus. While most women infected during pregnancy will not be affected, limited studies have shown that Parvovirus B19 may infect the fetus and increase the risk of miscarriage within the first 20 weeks of pregnancy. In individuals with impaired immune function (e.g. leukemia or cancer) or with chronic red blood cell disorders, such as sickle-cell disease, infection may result in severe anemia.

Persons who are exposed to Parvovirus B19 and are either pregnant or have an impaired immune function or a chronic red blood cell disorder should consult with their physician.

Where can I call for additional information regarding fifth disease during pregnancy? How can I arrange to have a blood test done if I am pregnant and have been exposed to a case of fifth disease?

In addition to your physician, further information about fifth disease and arrangements for blood testing can be obtained from your local public health department.

What is the treatment for fifth disease?

At this time there is no specific treatment beyond the supportive blood transfusions which are sometimes necessary for those with impaired immune function or chronic red blood cell disorders.

Is there a vaccine against the virus which causes fifth disease?

There is currently no vaccine to prevent infection with this virus.

What can be done to prevent the spread of fifth disease?

Measures to effectively control fifth disease have not been developed yet. When outbreaks of fifth disease occur in a school or community, options for preventing transmission are limited. Because the risk of transmitting B19 virus to others is greatest before signs and symptoms develop, transmission cannot be prevented by identifying and excluding symptomatic individuals. Individuals with fifth disease should not be excluded from schools or daycare centers; when their fever subsides and they feel well, they can return to school. Good hand washing may be a practical and effective method to reduce spread of virus in schools or daycare centers where there are known cases.

Should pregnant women and employees or children who have chronic hemolytic anemias or immunodeficiency be excluded from settings where there are known cases of fifth disease?

Routine exclusion is not recommended for the following reasons: 1) many women of childbearing age are immune and 90 percent of maternal infections do not result in adverse fetal outcome; 2) outbreaks of fifth disease often persist for many months in a community and thus there are many settings besides schools or daycare centers where an individual may be exposed to the virus; 3) Parvovirus B19 infection can occur in the absence of apparent outbreaks from exposure to sporadic cases; 4) risk to individuals with impaired immune function or red blood cell metabolism defect is minimal if the individual is managed appropriately by a physician.

Part Six

Other Infectious Diseases

Chapter 44

Chickenpox

Chickenpox is a very common and highly contagious disease. Although the symptoms can be annoying and uncomfortable and limit normal activities, the disease is usually mild and rarely serious. In otherwise healthy children, chickenpox lasts two weeks or less and does not cause complications. In adults, newborn babies, and children with weakened immune systems, however, it can be a serious, long-lasting disease.

Chickenpox is caused by a type of herpes virus called varicella-zoster virus (VZV). After the initial chickenpox infection, VZV hides in nerve cells and is sometimes reactivated later in life. This reactivated, often very painful, disease is called herpes zoster or shingles. Researchers are trying to learn what causes the virus to become active again after being dormant for many years.

Chickenpox epidemics can occur anytime of the year, but are most common in late winter and early spring. Doctors estimate that each year 3.5 to 4 million people, mostly children, get chickenpox. Ninety percent of cases are in people under 15 years of age. The U.S. Centers for Disease Control and Prevention (CDC) reports that there are approximately 100 deaths and 9,300 hospitalizations due to the complications of chickenpox each year. A vaccine to prevent chickenpox became available in 1995. The numbers of cases should decline as more people get immunized with this vaccine.

Excerpted from "Chickenpox," National Institute of Allergy and Infectious Diseases (NIAID), National Institutes of Health (NIH), January 1998.

Symptoms and Diagnosis

The most common signs and symptoms of chickenpox include a rash, fever, tiredness, and loss of appetite. The fever begins a day or two before the rash in about half of patients and is usually less than 101.5° Fahrenheit (F), but may be as high as 106° F. The rash consists of many (usually less than 300) fluid-filled vesicles surrounded by red sores. Although the rash can involve the entire body, it typically is found on the back, chest, face, and abdomen. The effects of the rash may be mild and barely noticeable or severe and accompanied by intense itching. As the disease spreads from child to child within a family, the intensity and extent of the rash may increase.

A doctor can easily diagnose chickenpox by examining the characteristic rash, with healed and unhealed sores on the body, and by noting the presence of other symptoms mentioned above.

Transmission

It is virtually impossible for a susceptible person to avoid getting chickenpox. It is highly contagious and spreads quickly in settings like day-care facilities and schools and within families. The virus is transmitted by direct contact with the rash on an infected person or by droplets dispersed into the air by coughing or sneezing.

The time between exposure to the virus and the development of symptoms is usually about two weeks, but can range from 10 to 21 days. A person can transmit the disease for up to 48 hours before the telltale rash of chickenpox appears. The period of transmission lasts for four to five days after the rash begins until the sores have crusted over. Therefore, staying away from someone only after they have visible signs of chickenpox is probably too late to prevent transmission.

Rarely, a susceptible person can get chickenpox from someone who has a reactivated VZV infection (shingles).

Treatment

Unless the infection is severe, children with chickenpox usually are not treated.

Scratching can make the lesions harder to heal, cause scarring and increase the risk of bacterial skin infections. The doctor may recommend anti-itch drugs, such as over-the-counter antihistamines, to control this troublesome symptom. Warm baths with uncooked oatmeal or cornstarch added also can help relieve the itching. Fingernails should be kept clean and cut short.

Fever can be reduced with acetaminophen. Aspirin should not be taken by anyone with chickenpox because it can lead to a serious disease called Reye syndrome. Cool baths also can help bring down a fever.

Acyclovir (Zovirax) is an antiviral drug that attacks the virus. When treatment is started very soon after the first sores appear, it shortens the duration of rash formation by about one day and reduces the number of new sores. The American Academy of Pediatrics recommends it for use in premature babies, adolescents, adults, and other high-risk populations.

Complications

Because chickenpox most often is an uncomplicated infection, it ordinarily does not require a visit to the doctor.

It is wise, however, to visit a doctor if symptoms other than the rash, low fever, and fatigue are present. Symptoms that require immediate medical attention are fever of more than 103° F, dizziness, rapid heartbeat, shortness of breath, tremors, loss of muscle coordination, vomiting, and/or stiff neck.

If the lesions become infected with bacteria such as *Staphylococcus* or *Streptococcus*, a doctor can prescribe an appropriate antibiotic.

In children and adults whose immune systems are impaired by disease or suppressed by drugs (including steroids), chickenpox can affect internal organs. Also, people with impaired immune systems are more likely to develop bacterial skin infections, and their sores take longer to heal. In children with leukemia, chickenpox can be life-threatening.

Infrequently, chickenpox can cause central nervous system complications of which the most serious is encephalitis (inflammation of the brain). Encephalitis can be life-threatening in adults and usually lasts for a minimum of two weeks. Of those patients who survive, 15 percent continue to have neurologic symptoms after the initial infection has cleared. Other nervous system complications include meningitis and Reye syndrome.

Another serious complication, which occurs mainly in adults, is varicella pneumonitis (inflammation of the lungs). This complication can be life-threatening to women during the second or third trimester of pregnancy.

If a pregnant woman develops chickenpox five days before or up to 48 hours after delivery, the baby can be born with complications from the infection. Serious disease in the newborn, however, is uncommon.

A pregnant woman who is not immune to chickenpox and has a prolonged exposure to a person with the disease should consult with her physician about the risk to herself and her unborn child.

Prevention

The use of varicella vaccine (Varivax) is the best way to prevent chickenpox. According to CDC, the vaccine protects about 70 to 90 percent of people who receive it. CDC's Advisory Committee on Immunization Practices recommends that a single dose of the vaccine be given routinely to children ages 12 months to 12 years old who have not had chickenpox and who have not been vaccinated. It also recommends that persons older than 13 years of age who have not had chickenpox receive two injections of the vaccine, especially those in high-risk groups such as:

- Teachers of young children, day care employees, and residents and staff in institutional settings.

- College students and military personnel.

- Nonpregnant women of childbearing age.

- Family and health care workers who have not had chickenpox and who are in close contact with persons who may suffer serious complications if infected with chickenpox.

- International travelers, especially if they expect to have close contact with local populations.

A question remains about how long the vaccine's protection will last. Recent studies show that protection should last at least ten years, but it is still not known if a booster will be needed later in life.

Chapter 45

Cytomegalovirus (CMV)

General Information

Cytomegalovirus, or CMV, is found universally throughout all geographic locations and socioeconomic groups, and infects between 50% and 85% of adults in the United States by 40 years of age. CMV is also the virus most frequently transmitted to a developing child before birth. CMV infection is more widespread in developing countries and in areas of lower socioeconomic conditions. For most healthy persons who acquire CMV after birth there are few symptoms and no long-term health consequences. Some persons with symptoms experience a mononucleosis-like syndrome with prolonged fever, and a mild hepatitis. Once a person becomes infected, the virus remains alive, but usually dormant within that person's body for life. Recurrent disease rarely occurs unless the person's immune system is suppressed due to therapeutic drugs or disease. Therefore, for the vast majority of people, CMV infection is not a serious problem.

However, CMV infection is important to certain high-risk groups. Major areas of concern are (1) the risk of infection to the unborn baby during pregnancy, (2) the risk of infection to people who work with children, and (3) the risk of infection to the immunocompromised person, such as organ transplant recipients and persons infected with human immunodeficiency virus (HIV).

"Cytomegalovirus (CMV) Infection," National Center for Infectious Diseases, Centers for Disease Control and Prevention (CDC), http://www.cdc.gov/ncidod/diseases/cmv.htm, October 2002.

Transmission and Prevention

Transmission of CMV occurs from person to person. Infection requires close, intimate contact with a person excreting the virus in their saliva, urine, or other bodily fluids. CMV can be sexually transmitted and can also be transmitted via breast milk, transplanted organs, and rarely from blood transfusions.

Although the virus is not highly contagious, it has been shown to spread in households and among young children in day care centers. Transmission of the virus is often preventable because it is most often transmitted through infected bodily fluids that come in contact with hands and then are absorbed through the nose or mouth of a susceptible person. Therefore, care should be taken when handling children and items like diapers. Simple hand washing with soap and water is effective in removing the virus from the hands.

CMV infection without symptoms is common in infants and young children; therefore, it is unjustified and unnecessary to exclude from school or an institution a child known to be infected. Similarly, hospitalized patients do not need separate or elaborate isolation precautions.

Screening children and patients for CMV is of questionable value. The cost and management of such procedures are impractical. Children known to have CMV infection should not be singled out for exclusion, isolation, or special handling. Instead, staff education and effective hygiene practices are advised in caring for all children.

People Who Work with Infants and Children

Most healthy people working with infants and children face no special risk from CMV infection. However, for women of child-bearing age who previously have not been infected with CMV, there is a potential risk to the developing unborn child. Contact with children who are in day care, where CMV infection is commonly transmitted among young children (particularly toddlers), may be a source of exposure to CMV. Since CMV is transmitted through contact with infected body fluids, including urine and saliva, child care providers (meaning day care workers, special education teachers, therapists, as well as mothers) should be educated about the risks of CMV infection and the precautions they can take. Day care workers appear to be at a greater risk than hospital and other health care providers, and this may be due in part to the increased emphasis on personal hygiene in the health care setting.

Recommendations for individuals providing care for infants and children:

1. Female employees should be educated concerning CMV, its transmission, and hygienic practices, such as hand washing, which minimize the risk of infection.

2. Susceptible nonpregnant women working with infants and children should not routinely be transferred to other work situations.

3. Pregnant women working with infants and children should be informed of the risk of acquiring CMV infection and the possible effects on the unborn child.

4. Routine laboratory testing for CMV antibody in female workers is not recommended, but can be performed to determine their immune status.

Diagnosis of CMV Infection

Most infections with CMV are not diagnosed because the virus usually produces few, if any, symptoms and tends to reactivate intermittently without symptoms. However, persons who have been infected with CMV develop antibodies to the virus, and these antibodies persist in the body for the lifetime of that individual. A number of laboratory tests that detect these antibodies to CMV have been developed to determine if infection has occurred and are widely available from commercial laboratories. In addition, the virus can be cultured from specimens obtained from urine, throat swabs, and tissue samples to detect active infection.

CMV should be suspected if a patient:

*   has symptoms of infectious mononucleosis but has negative test results for mononucleosis and Epstein Barr virus, or,

*   shows signs of hepatitis, but has negative test results for hepatitis A, B, and C.

For best diagnostic results, laboratory tests for CMV antibody should be performed by using paired serum samples. One blood sample should be taken upon suspicion of CMV, and another one taken within 2 weeks. A virus culture can be performed at any time the patient is symptomatic.

Laboratory testing for antibody to CMV can be performed to determine if a woman has already had CMV infection. However, routine laboratory testing of all pregnant women is costly and the need for testing should therefore be evaluated on a case-by-case basis.

Serologic Testing

The enzyme-linked immunosorbent assay (or ELISA) is the most commonly available serologic test for measuring antibody to CMV. The result can be used to determine if acute infection, prior infection, or passively acquired maternal antibody in an infant is present. Other tests include various fluorescence assays, indirect hemagglutination, and latex agglutination.

An ELISA technique for CMV-specific IgM (immunoglobulin M) is available, but may give false-positive results unless steps are taken to remove rheumatoid factor or most of the IgG (immunoglobulin G) antibody before the serum sample is tested. Because CMV-specific IgM may be produced in low levels in reactivated CMV infection, its presence is not always indicative of primary infection. Only virus recovered from a target organ, such as the lung, provides unequivocal evidence that the current illness is caused by acquired CMV infection. If serologic tests detect a positive or high titer of IgG, this result should not automatically be interpreted to mean that active CMV infection is present. However, if antibody tests of paired serum samples show a fourfold rise in IgG antibody and a significant level of IgM antibody, meaning equal to at least 30% of the IgG value, or virus is cultured from a urine or throat specimen, the findings indicate that an active CMV infection is present.

Treatment

Currently, no treatment exists for CMV infection in the healthy individual. Antiviral drug therapy is now being evaluated in infants. Ganciclovir treatment is used for patients with depressed immunity who have either sight-related or life-threatening illnesses. Vaccines are still in the research and development stage.

Chapter 46

Encephalitis and Meningitis

Questions and Answers about Encephalitis

What is encephalitis?

Encephalitis is an inflammation of the brain. There are many types of encephalitis, most of which are caused by viral infection. Symptoms include sudden fever, headache, vomiting, photophobia (abnormal visual sensitivity to light), stiff neck and back, confusion, drowsiness, clumsiness, unsteady gait, and irritability. Symptoms that require emergency treatment include loss of consciousness, poor responsiveness, seizures, muscle weakness, sudden severe dementia, memory loss, withdrawal from social interaction, and impaired judgment. Anyone experiencing symptoms of encephalitis should see a doctor immediately.

Is there any treatment?

Antiviral medications may be prescribed for herpes encephalitis or other severe viral infections. Antibiotics may be prescribed for bacterial infections. Anticonvulsants are used to prevent or treat seizures. Corticosteroids are used to reduce brain swelling and inflammation. Sedatives may be needed for irritability or restlessness. Over-the-counter medications may be used for fever and headache. Individuals

This chapter contains text from "Encephalitis and Meningitis," National Institute of Neurological Disorders and Stroke (NINDS), reviewed April 2001, and "Meningococcal Disease," Centers for Disease Control and Prevention (CDC), reviewed October 2002.

with bacterial meningitis are usually hospitalized and treated with antibiotics. Antiviral drugs may also be prescribed.

What is the prognosis?

The prognosis for encephalitis varies. Some cases are mild, short and relatively benign, and patients have full recovery. Other cases are severe, and permanent impairment or death is possible. The acute phase of encephalitis may last for 1 to 2 weeks, with gradual or sudden resolution of fever and neurological symptoms. Neurological symptoms may require many months before full recovery. With early diagnosis and prompt treatment, most patients recover from meningitis. However, in some cases, the disease progresses so rapidly that death occurs during the first 48 hours, despite early treatment.

Questions and Answers about Meningitis

What is meningitis?

Meningitis is an infection of the membranes (called meninges) that surround the brain and spinal cord. Symptoms, which may appear suddenly, often include high fever, severe and persistent headache, stiff neck, nausea, and vomiting. Changes in behavior such as confusion, sleepiness, and difficulty waking up are extremely important symptoms and may require emergency treatment. In infants symptoms of meningitis may include irritability or tiredness, poor feeding, and fever. Some types of meningitis can be deadly if not treated promptly. Anyone experiencing symptoms of meningitis should see a doctor immediately.

What causes meningitis?

Meningitis may be caused by many different viruses and bacteria. Knowing whether meningitis is caused by a virus or bacterium is important because the severity of illness and the treatment differ. Viral meningitis is generally less severe and resolves without specific treatment, while bacterial meningitis can be quite severe and may result in brain damage, hearing loss, or learning disability. For bacterial meningitis, it is also important to know which type of bacteria is causing the meningitis because antibiotics can prevent some types from spreading and infecting other people. Before the 1990s, *Haemophilus influenzae* type b (Hib) was the leading cause of bacterial meningitis, but new vaccines being given to all children as part of their routine immunizations have reduced the occurrence of invasive disease due to *H. influenzae*. Today, *Streptococcus pneumoniae* and *Neisseria meningitidis* are the leading causes of bacterial meningitis.

What are the signs and symptoms of meningitis?

High fever, headache, and stiff neck are common symptoms of meningitis in anyone over the age of 2 years. These symptoms can develop over several hours, or they may take 1 to 2 days. Other symptoms may include nausea, vomiting, discomfort looking into bright lights, confusion, and sleepiness. In newborns and small infants, the classic symptoms of fever, headache, and neck stiffness may be absent or difficult to detect, and the infant may only appear slow or inactive, or be irritable, have vomiting, or be feeding poorly. As the disease progresses, patients of any age may have seizures.

How is meningitis diagnosed?

Early diagnosis and treatment are very important. If symptoms occur, the patient should see a doctor immediately. The diagnosis is usually made by growing bacteria from a sample of spinal fluid. The spinal fluid is obtained by performing a spinal tap, in which a needle is inserted into an area in the lower back where fluid in the spinal canal is readily accessible. Identification of the type of bacteria responsible is important for selection of correct antibiotics.

Can meningitis be treated?

Bacterial meningitis can be treated with a number of effective antibiotics. It is important, however, that treatment be started early in the course of the disease. Appropriate antibiotic treatment of most common types of bacterial meningitis should reduce the risk of dying from meningitis to below 15%, although the risk is higher among the elderly.

Is meningitis contagious?

Yes, some forms are bacterial meningitis are contagious. The bacteria are spread through the exchange of respiratory and throat secretions (i.e., coughing, kissing). Fortunately, none of the bacteria that cause meningitis are as contagious as things like the common cold or the flu, and they are not spread by casual contact or by simply breathing the air where a person with meningitis has been.

However, sometimes the bacteria that cause meningitis have spread to other people who have had close or prolonged contact with a patient with meningitis caused by *Neisseria meningitidis* (also called meningococcal meningitis) or Hib. People in the same household or day-care center, or anyone with direct contact with a patient's oral secretions (such as a boyfriend or girlfriend) would be considered at increased risk of acquiring the infection. People who qualify as close contacts of a person with meningitis caused by *N. meningitidis* should receive antibiotics to prevent them from getting the disease. Antibiotics for contacts of a person with Hib meningitis disease are no longer recommended if all contacts 4 years of age or younger are fully vaccinated against Hib disease (see below).

Are there vaccines against meningitis?

Yes, there are vaccines against Hib and against some strains of *N. meningitidis* and many types of *Streptococcus pneumoniae*. The vaccines against Hib are very safe and highly effective.

There is also a vaccine that protects against four strains of *N. meningitidis*, but it is not routinely used in the United States and is not effective in children under 18 months of age. The vaccine against *N. meningitidis* is sometimes used to control outbreaks of some types of meningococcal meningitis in the United States. Meningitis cases should be reported to state or local health departments to assure follow-up of close contacts and recognize outbreaks. Although large epidemics of meningococcal meningitis do not occur in the United States, some countries experience large, periodic epidemics. Overseas travelers should check to see if meningococcal vaccine is recommended for their destination. Travelers should receive the vaccine at least 1 week before departure, if possible. Information on areas for which meningococcal vaccine is recommended can be obtained by calling the Centers for Disease Control and Prevention (CDC) at (404)-332-4565.

A vaccine to prevent meningitis due to *S. pneumoniae* (also called pneumococcal meningitis) can also prevent other forms of infection due to *S. pneumoniae*. The pneumococcal vaccine is not effective in children under 2 years of age but is recommended for all persons over 65 years of age and younger persons with certain chronic medical problems.

The Advisory Committee on Immunization Practices (ACIP) has modified its guidelines for use of the polysaccharide meningococcal vaccine to prevent bacterial meningitis, particularly for college freshmen who live in dormitories, a group found to be at a modestly increased risk of meningococcal disease relative to other persons their age. See http://www.cdc.gov/mmwr/preview/mmwrhtml/rr4907a2.htm for more information.

Chapter 47

Hand, Foot, and Mouth Disease (HFMD)

What is hand, foot, and mouth disease?

Hand, foot, and mouth disease (HFMD) is a common illness of infants and children. It is characterized by fever, sores in the mouth, and a rash with blisters. HFMD begins with a mild fever, poor appetite, malaise (feeling sick), and frequently a sore throat. One or 2 days after the fever begins, sores develop in the mouth. They begin as small red spots that blister and then often become ulcers. They are usually located on the tongue, gums, and inside of the cheeks. The skin rash develops over 1 to 2 days with flat or raised red spots, some with blisters. The rash does not itch, and it is usually located on the palms of the hands and soles of the feet. It may also appear on the buttocks. A person with HFMD may have only the rash or the mouth ulcers.

Is HFMD the same as foot-and-mouth disease?

No. HFMD is a different disease than foot-and-mouth disease of cattle, sheep, and swine. Although the names are similar, the two diseases are not related at all and are caused by different viruses.

What causes HFMD?

Several different viruses cause HFMD. The most common cause is coxsackievirus A16; sometimes, enterovirus 71 (EV71) or other strains

"Hand, Foot, and Mouth Disease," Respiratory and Enteric Viruses Branch, National Center for Infectious Diseases, Centers for Disease Control and Prevention (CDC), reviewed August 2001.

of enteroviruses cause HFMD. The enterovirus group includes polio-viruses, coxsackieviruses, and echoviruses.

Is HFMD serious?

Usually not. HFMD caused by coxsackievirus A16 infection is a mild disease and nearly all patients recover without medical treatment in 7 to 10 days. There are no common complications. Rarely, this illness may be associated with aseptic or viral meningitis, in which the person has fever, headache, stiff neck, or back pain, and may need to be hospitalized for a few days. Another cause of HFMD, EV71 may also cause viral meningitis and, rarely, more serious diseases, such as encephalitis, or a poliomyelitis-like paralysis. EV71 encephalitis may be fatal. Cases of fatal encephalitis occurred during outbreaks of HFMD in Malaysia in 1997 and in Taiwan, 1998.

Is it contagious?

Yes, HFMD is moderately contagious. Infection is spread from person to person by direct contact with nose and throat discharges or the stool of infected persons. A person is most contagious during the first week of the illness. HFMD is not transmitted to or from pets or other animals.

How soon will someone become ill after getting infected?

The usual period from infection to onset of symptoms is 3 to 7 days. Fever is often the first symptom of HFMD.

Who is at risk for HFMD?

HFMD occurs mainly in children under 10 years old, but adults may also be at risk. Everyone is susceptible to infection. Infection results in immunity to the specific virus, but a second episode may occur following infection with a different member of the enterovirus group.

When and where does HFMD occur?

Individual cases and outbreaks of HFMD occur worldwide, more frequently in summer and early autumn. In the recent past, major outbreaks of HFMD attributable to enterovirus 71 have been reported in some South East Asian countries (Malaysia in 1997, Taiwan in 1998).

How is HFMD diagnosed?

HFMD is one of many infections that result in mouth sores. Another common cause is oral herpesvirus infection, which produces an inflammation of the mouth and gums (sometimes called stomatitis). Usually, the physician can distinguish between HFMD and other causes of mouth sores based on the age of the patient, the pattern of symptoms reported by the patient or parent, and the appearance of the rash and sores on examination. A throat swab or stool specimen may be sent to a laboratory to determine which enterovirus caused the illness. Since the testing often takes 2 to 4 weeks to obtain a final answer, the physician usually does not order these tests.

How is HFMD treated? Can it be prevented?

No specific treatment is available for this or other enterovirus infections. Symptomatic treatment is given to provide relief from fever, aches, or pain from the mouth ulcers. Preventive measures include frequent hand washing, especially after diaper changes; disinfection of contaminated surfaces by household cleaners (such as diluted bleach solution made by mixing 1 capful of household bleach containing chlorine with 1 gallon water), and washing soiled articles of clothing. Children are often excluded from child care programs, schools, or other group settings during the first few days of the illness. These measures may reduce the spread of infection, but they will not completely interrupt it.

Chapter 48

Hepatitis in Children

Questions and Answers about Hepatitis

What is hepatitis A?

Hepatitis A is a liver disease caused by the hepatitis A virus (HAV). Hepatitis A can affect anyone. In the United States, hepatitis A can occur in situations ranging from isolated cases of disease to widespread epidemics.

What are the signs and symptoms of hepatitis A?

Persons with hepatitis A virus infection may not have any signs or symptoms of the disease. Older persons are more likely to have symptoms than children. If symptoms are present, they usually occur abruptly and may include fever, tiredness, loss of appetite, nausea, abdominal discomfort, dark urine, and jaundice (yellowing of the skin and eyes). Symptoms usually last less than 2 months; a few persons are ill for as long as 6 months. The average incubation period for hepatitis A is 28 days (range: 15–50 days).

This chapter contains "Questions and Answers about Hepatitis," excerpted and adapted from the Centers for Disease Control and Prevention (CDC)'s Hepatitis Home Page at www.cdc.gov/ncidod/diseases/hepatitis/index.htm, cited February 2003, and text from "Hepatitis A in the Child Care Setting," and "Hepatitis B in the Child Care Setting," 1997. These two documents were updated in June 2002 by Dr. David A. Cooke, MD, Diplomate, American Board of Internal Medicine.

How is hepatitis A virus transmitted?

Hepatitis A virus is spread from person to person by putting something in the mouth that has been contaminated with the stool of a person with hepatitis A. This type of transmission is called "fecal-oral." For this reason, the virus is more easily spread in areas where there are poor sanitary conditions or where good personal hygiene is not observed.

Most infections result from contact with a household member or sex partner who has hepatitis A. Casual contact, as in the usual office, factory, or school setting, does not spread the virus.

Does CDC recommend that children be vaccinated against hepatitis A?

Hepatitis A vaccine has been licensed in the United States for use in persons 2 years of age and older. The vaccine is recommended (before exposure to hepatitis A virus) for persons who are more likely to get hepatitis A virus infection or are more likely to get seriously ill if they do get hepatitis A. Because of the limited experience with hepatitis A vaccination among children under 2 years of age, the vaccine is not currently licensed for this age-group in the United States.

Children living in states, counties, and communities that have consistently increased rates of hepatitis A and periodic outbreaks should be routinely vaccinated beginning at 2 years of age. High rates of hepatitis A can be found in these populations, both in urban and rural settings. In addition, to effectively prevent epidemics of hepatitis A, vaccination of previously unvaccinated older children is recommended within 5 years of initiation of routine childhood vaccination programs. Although rates differ among areas, available data indicate that a reasonable cutoff age in many areas is 10-15 years of age because older persons have often already had hepatitis A. Vaccination of children before they enter school should receive highest priority, followed by vaccination of older children who have not been vaccinated.

Hepatitis A vaccine is generally not recommended for children solely because of day care center attendance. The frequency of outbreaks of hepatitis A is not high enough in this setting to warrant routine hepatitis A vaccination. In some communities, however, day care centers play a role in sustaining community-wide outbreaks. In this situation, consideration should be given to adding hepatitis A vaccine to the prevention plan for children and staff in the involved center(s).

What is hepatitis B?

Hepatitis B is a serious disease caused by a virus that attacks the liver. The virus, which is called hepatitis B virus (HBV), can cause life-long infection, cirrhosis (scarring) of the liver, liver cancer, liver failure, and death. People of all ages get hepatitis B and about 5,000 die per year of sickness caused by HBV.

How do you get hepatitis B?

You get hepatitis B by direct contact with the blood or body fluids of an infected person; for example, you can become infected by having sex or sharing needles with an infected person. A baby can get hepatitis B from an infected mother during childbirth. Hepatitis B is not spread through food or water or by casual contact.

How can you prevent hepatitis B?

One out of 20 people in the United States will get infected with HBV some time during their lives. The CDC recommends that all babies be vaccinated against hepatitis at birth. CDC also recommends vaccinations for all children between the ages of 0-18 years of age who have not been vaccinated. Others who should be vaccinated include persons of any age whose behavior puts them at high risk for HBV infection and persons whose jobs expose them to human blood.

What is hepatitis C?

Hepatitis C is a liver disease caused by the Hepatitis C virus (HCV), which is found in the blood of persons who have the disease. HCV is spread primarily by direct contact with human blood. For example, you may have gotten infected with HCV if:

- you ever injected street drugs, as the needles and/or other drug "works" used to prepare or inject the drug(s) may have had someone else's blood that contained HCV on them.

- you received blood, blood products, or solid organs from a donor whose blood contained HCV.

- you were ever on long-term kidney dialysis as you may have unknowingly shared supplies/equipment that had someone else's blood on them.

- you were ever a healthcare worker and had frequent contact with blood on the job, especially accidental needlesticks.

- your mother had hepatitis C at the time she gave birth to you. During the birth her blood may have gotten into your body.

- you ever had sex with a person infected with HCV.

- you lived with someone who was infected with HCV and shared items such as razors or toothbrushes that might have had his/ her blood on them.

HCV is not spread by sneezing, hugging, coughing, food or water, sharing eating utensils or drinking glasses, or casual contact. Persons should not be excluded from work, school, play, child-care or other settings on the basis of their HCV infection status.

What is hepatitis D?

Hepatitis D is a defective virus that needs the hepatitis B virus to exist. Hepatitis D virus (HDV) is found in the blood of persons infected with the virus.

What is hepatitis E?

Hepatitis E is a virus (HEV) transmitted in much the same way as hepatitis A virus. Hepatitis E, however, does not often occur in the United States.

Hepatitis A in the Child Care Setting

Outbreaks of hepatitis A among children attending child care centers and persons employed at these centers have been recognized since the 1970s. Because infection among children is usually mild or asymptomatic and people are infectious before they develop symptoms, outbreaks are often only recognized when adult contacts (usually parents) become ill. Poor hygienic practices among staff who change diapers and also prepare food contribute to the spread of hepatitis A. Children in diapers are likely to spread the diseases because of contact with contaminated feces. Outbreaks rarely occur in child care settings serving only toilet-trained children.

A vaccine is available to prevent hepatitis A, and is licensed for children over 2 years of age. Although the vaccine is extremely safe, current guidelines do not recommend it for all children at this point. Experts are focusing on vaccinating the children who are at the highest risk of catching hepatitis A disease. These include children who live in certain states and counties where the disease is very common, as well as children who live on Indian Reservations. Your child's pediatrician will know whether you live in a high-risk area; you can also get this information by calling your local health department. Children with certain conditions such as HIV infection or liver disease are also strongly recommended to get the vaccine. It may be considered for other children, such as those who attend day care, but it is not considered mandatory. There are very few children for whom hepatitis A vaccination would not be safe, so any parent who wishes to have their child vaccinated may request it.

Although hepatitis A outbreaks sometimes occur in child care settings, they do not happen often enough to require child care providers or children attending child care to be routinely vaccinated against hepatitis A. Some medical authorities feel that vaccinating these populations may be wise, however. When outbreaks occur in child care settings, gamma globulin may be administered to children, providers, and families of child care attendees to limit transmission of hepatitis A.

If a child or adult is diagnosed with hepatitis A:

- Exclude the child or adult from the child care setting until 1 week after onset of symptoms.

- Immediately notify your local health department and request advice.

- Gamma globulin, if administered within the first 2 weeks after exposure, can prevent the infection from spreading to other children and families.

- Use good handwashing and hygiene practices.

Hepatitis B in the Child Care Setting

The hepatitis B virus (HBV) is completely different from hepatitis A. Only about 10 percent of children who become infected with HBV show any symptoms. When children do have symptoms, they may be similar to those for hepatitis A: fatigue, loss of appetite, jaundice, dark urine, light stools, nausea, vomiting, and abdominal pain. However, hepatitis B is a much more serious infection. After infection with HBV, chronic infection develops in 70% to 90% of infants, 15% to 25% of 1- to 4-year-old children, and 5% to 10% of older children and adults. Premature death from cirrhosis or liver cancer occurs in 15% to 25% of persons with chronic infection. Persons who develop chronic HBV infection may remain infectious for the rest of their lives.

HBV infection is most commonly spread by:

- infected mothers to newborn infants through blood exposure at birth

- sharing contaminated needles during intravenous drug abuse

- sexual intercourse

- exposure of cuts or mucous membranes to contaminated blood

- infected blood or body fluids which come in contact with non-intact skin of an uninfected person, such as by biting, if the skin is broken. However, this is rare.

Hepatitis B is vaccine-preventable, and efforts are underway to try to eliminate it in the United States by vaccinating all children against the disease. All infants should be vaccinated with three doses of hepatitis B vaccine during the first 18 months of life. Children who receive certain forms of combination vaccines containing the hepatitis B vaccine may need four doses. A child not previously vaccinated should receive three doses of vaccine by the age of 11 or 12 years. Child care providers should discuss with their doctor whether it is appropriate for them to receive hepatitis B vaccine.

To reduce the spread of hepatitis B:

- Ensure that all immunizations for children are up-to-date.

- Make sure that all children and adults use good handwashing practices.

- Do not allow children to share toothbrushes.

- Clean up blood spills immediately.

- Wear gloves when cleaning up blood spills unless the spill is so small it can be contained in the cloth or towel being used to clean it up.

- Wear gloves when changing a diaper soiled with bloody stools.

- Disinfect any surfaces on which blood has been spilled, using freshly prepared bleach solution.

- If a child care provider has open sores, cuts, or other abrasions on the hands, the provider should wear gloves when changing diapers or cleaning up blood spills.

- Observe children for aggressive behavior, such as biting.

• A child who is a chronic HBV carrier should be evaluated by a team that includes the child's parents or guardians, the child's physician, public health personnel, the proposed child care provider, and others to determine the most appropriate child care setting. This evaluation should consider the behavior, neurologic development, and physical condition of the child and the expected type of interaction with others in the child care setting. In each case, risks and benefits to both the infected child and to others in the child care setting should be weighed.

Chapter 49

Kawasaki Disease

Toddlers with fevers? Only about as common as sand on the beach. But for toddlers with Kawasaki syndrome, fever is just one of the early signs of a very serious illness.

Kawasaki disease, or Kawasaki syndrome, is an infectious inflammatory disease that affects mainly infants and young children. At first, the symptoms—fever, rash, watery eyes, swollen lymph nodes—look like those seen with many of the bugs kids pick up all the time.

But this is no simple bug. It affects many systems in youngsters' bodies, but damage to the heart and surrounding tissue is of the greatest concern. Left untreated, Kawasaki syndrome can damage the coronary arteries that feed the heart, possibly causing a massive heart attack.

Although there have been rare reports of Kawasaki syndrome in adults, the disease primarily affects children under 5 years old, with most cases affecting 1- to 2-year-olds. The disease affects boys about 50 percent more often than girls, and seems to affect children of Asian descent at a much higher rate than children of African or European descent. "The typical patient would be a 2-year-old boy with high fever," says Stanford Shulman, MD, Chief of Infectious Diseases at Children's Memorial Hospital in Chicago.

The disease was first described by Tomisaku Kawasaki, MD, a Tokyo pediatrician, in 1967, but wasn't reported in English literature

"New Treatment Lessens Threat of Kawasaki Syndrome," by Amy Roffmann, *FDA Consumer*, November 1992, updated in May 2001 by Dr. David A. Cooke, MD, Diplomate, American Board of Internal Medicine.

until 1974. Fever develops within the first few days of onset of the disease. Many Kawasaki patients experience abrupt spikes in temperature—several spikes a day for five or more days—as the disease begins. Left untreated, the spiking can continue for as long as four weeks.

A measles-like rash usually accompanies the fever, and lymph nodes in the neck swell. Conjunctivitis, characterized by red eyes and swollen eyelids, may also develop in the first few days. The lips, tongue, and throat may become red and swollen. One of the most distinguishing symptoms of Kawasaki disease is the redness and swelling of palms and soles within a few days of onset. After a couple of weeks, the skin of the hands and feet begins to peel. Less obviously, but more seriously, the child may develop heart damage. Intense inflammation in the blood vessels leads to aneurysms, which are bulging weak spots in arteries. This often occurs during the time that the child appears to be recovering from the disease.

A Mysterious Disorder

The cause of Kawasaki disease is unknown. There is persistent debate about whether it is infectious, or has some other cause. No responsible organism has ever been identified, and it does not appear to be contagious. However, outbreaks tend to occur in certain geographic regions. The disease is most common in Asia, particularly in Japan and Korea. There have been three epidemics of the disease in Japan: in 1979, 1982 and 1986. In the United States, the incidence in children of Japanese or Korean background is four times greater than in children of European background. This link puzzles researchers. The disease is more prevalent even in Asian children with little or no exposure to the foods or customs of Asian culture.

In Hawaii, the disease is far more common among Japanese-American children. While Japanese-Americans compose one-third of Hawaii's population, Japanese-American children account for 85 to 90 percent of the cases of Kawasaki syndrome in that state. Most of these children are third- or fourth-generation Americans with little or no Japanese cultural influence in their daily lives. These statistics appear to indicate a genetic factor that researchers are not yet able to explain.

Inexplicably, a possible connection has been made by some studies between children contracting Kawasaki syndrome and recently cleaned carpets. Researchers at Cornell University Medical Center were the first to find the apparent association in a survey of the families of

Kawasaki patients and a separate control group. Researchers asked questions about other family members with the disease, the type of foods the patient had been eating, and whether or not the child was breast-fed. The only factor that clearly differed between the two groups is that children with Kawasaki disease were more likely to have been exposed to carpets and rugs that had been shampooed, beaten, or vigorously cleaned within a month of the onset of illness. Most cases of Kawasaki syndrome occur between December and May, prompting some experts to recommend that families with infants and toddlers not clean carpets during winter and early spring.

Since the Cornell study, 13 additional studies have tested the connection. "Four studies have found an association between exposure to shampooed carpets and development of Kawasaki," says Shulman. "Nine of the studies failed to find an association." Shulman explains that while the association is generally unproved, it may be valid in certain geographic locations. To be on the safe side, he recommends keeping children away from just-shampooed carpets for 24 to 48 hours.

Diagnosis Critical

Early and accurate diagnosis is critical to successful treatment, as the disease can start to damage the heart after just one week of illness. But diagnosis is difficult. One problem is that the symptoms don't always appear together. Some patients experience all of the symptoms, and some have only a few. Infants are less likely than toddlers to have all symptoms. Fever and swollen glands are a source of concern for any parent, but "cardiac involvement is the only long-term issue in Kawasaki disease," says Shulman, "It's the only thing of real importance."

The acute phase of Kawasaki syndrome is followed by a convalescent stage, which can be misleading. Often patients' families see improvement, even without treatment. Fever is reduced—sometimes temperature even returns to normal—skin redness subsides, and skin begins to peel. "The worrisome thing [during this stage]," says Shulman, "is that in those children who are destined to develop heart involvement, this is the period of time it begins to show up."

According to a study by the Division of Pediatric Cardiology of Columbia University's College of Physicians and Surgeons, 25 percent of Kawasaki patients show some signs of heart inflammation—such as fast or irregular heartbeat—during this stage. Heart inflammation is a warning sign indicating the possibility of damage to the cardiovascular system.

Kawasaki disease appears to trigger an inappropriate immune response. Children with the disease produce an unusually large number of immune cells. The immune cells go haywire and begin to attack artery walls. Once the artery wall is damaged, it becomes a dam where platelets can form a blood clot. This clot, combined with the damage to the artery wall, further enlarges the artery, causing an aneurysm. Once this happens, blood flow is severely restricted, and a heart attack is possible. Aneurysms can also burst, with catastrophic results. According to surveys in Japanese epidemics, 1 in 250 children with the disease died from it, and 15 to 20 percent developed heart aneurysms.

Ultrasound of the heart, known as echocardiography, is used in children diagnosed with Kawasaki disease. It can accurately determine whether aneurysms have formed, and it can be used to follow the course of the disease.

"The peak size of an aneurysm is typically reached three to four weeks after the onset of fever," says Jane Newburger, MD, a pediatric cardiologist with Children's Hospital in Boston. This makes it important to monitor Kawasaki patients carefully. Once an aneurysm has formed, there is no guarantee that the damage can be reversed. However, treatment is aimed at preventing the formation of aneurysms.

Aspirin and IVIG (Intravenous Immune Globulin)

Early diagnosis and treatment helps minimize the danger from Kawasaki syndrome. Although the cause is unknown, it can be treated effectively, says Mary Glode, MD, an infectious disease specialist with the Department of Pediatrics of the University of Colorado in Denver.

Researchers have found that a combination of aspirin and intravenous immune globulin (often abbreviated IVIG) is highly effective in preventing long-term coronary artery problems from Kawasaki syndrome. Comparative studies of IVIG and aspirin found a reduction in risk of coronary artery aneurysms from 20% to 3–4% when the combination is used.

How IVIG helps is unclear. IVIG is a product made by purifying the naturally occurring antibodies in human blood plasma. Several pharmaceutical companies produce IVIG, but only one product, produced by Oesterreichisches Institut fuer Haemoderizate (OIH), a pharmaceutical company based in Austria, has been approved by the Food and Drug Administration (FDA) for use in treatment of Kawasaki disease.

According to John Finlayson, Ph.D., a protein specialist with FDA, "We don't really understand why immune globulin works, but the major benefit is in minimizing coronary aneurysms."

The immune globulin is given intravenously in either a single large dose of 2 grams per kilogram of body weight over 12 hours, or four smaller daily doses of 400 milligrams per kilogram (1 kilogram is about 2.2 pounds).

Besides minimizing the potential for cardiac damage, this treatment seems to turn off the disease. If treatment starts within 24 hours of the onset of the disease, the child is usually feeling much better by the next day.

According to Newburger, aspirin provides both an anti-inflammatory and anti-platelet effect. The anti-inflammatory effect keeps the arteries from swelling, and the anti-platelet effect prevents clots from forming in arteries.

Aspirin is given is fairly high daily doses—from 30 to 180 milligrams per kilogram (for example, 405 to 2,430 milligrams per day for a 30-pound child) of the patient's body weight—for the first two weeks of the disease. (For comparison, one regular aspirin is 325 milligrams.) The dose is then lowered to 3 to 5 milligrams per kilogram for an additional six to eight weeks.

Patients who have some heart damage may be given low doses of aspirin for several months; those with more severe damage, for years.

Aspirin use in the treatment regimen for children is somewhat controversial. The association between aspirin and Reye syndrome in children with flu and chickenpox has made parents and doctors wary of using aspirin to treat children with any acute illness. However, no association has been reported between Reye syndrome and the use of aspirin in children with Kawasaki syndrome. Therefore, the benefits of its use in this instance, under a doctor's direction, outweigh its risks. Children who need to continue low doses of aspirin for long periods after the acute stage of the disease are monitored closely for signs of chickenpox or flu, and the aspirin can be stopped for a few days if a child develops symptoms of these illnesses.

Long-Term Outlook

According to Newburger, a Kawasaki patient's long-term outlook depends on how much damage is done to the heart. Patients who receive treatment early will likely suffer no damage to the arteries. More than half the children who do develop aneurysms recover within a year.

Patients who don't fare as well are those who don't receive treatment and develop extremely large aneurysms. "The most [severely affected] patients—those with aneurysms of at least 8 millimeters—those patients will probably not return to normal," says Newburger. Because the disease was so recently identified, doctors don't yet know if there are any long-term effects that aren't apparent when the acute phase of the disease ends.

While most childhood fevers, sniffles, and watery eyes are no reason for alarm, parents should be aware that accompanied by other symptoms, the illness may require immediate medical attention. Recognized and treated early, Kawasaki syndrome can be stopped before it becomes a life-threatening problem.

Chapter 50

Lyme Disease

Introduction

Lyme disease is an infection caused by the corkscrew-shaped bacteria *Borrelia burgdorferi* that are transmitted by the bite of deer ticks (*Ixodes scapularis*) and western black-legged ticks (*Ixodes pacificus*). The deer tick, which normally feeds on the white-footed mouse, the white-tailed deer, other mammals, and birds, is responsible for transmitting Lyme disease bacteria to humans in the northeastern and north-central United States. On the Pacific Coast, the bacteria are transmitted to humans by the western black-legged tick.

Natural History

Ixodes ticks are much smaller than common dog and cattle ticks. In their larval and nymphal stages, they are no bigger than a pinhead. Adult ticks are slightly larger. Ticks feed on blood by inserting their mouth parts (not their whole bodies) into the skin of a host animal. They are slow feeders: a complete blood meal can take several days. As they feed, their bodies slowly enlarge.

This chapter contains text from "Lyme Disease: Introduction," Division of Vector-Borne Infectious Diseases, Centers for Disease Control and Prevention (CDC) reviewed September 2001: "Lyme Disease: Questions and Answers," CDC, reviewed September 2001; and "Lyme Disease: Prevention and Control," CDC, September 2002. More information about Lyme disease is available on the CDC website at http://www.cdc.gov.

Risk

The number of annually reported cases of Lyme disease in the United States has increased about 25-fold since national surveillance began in 1982, and a mean of approximately 12,500 cases annually were reported by states to the Centers for Disease Control and Prevention (CDC) from 1993–1997. In the United States, the disease is mostly localized to states in the northeastern, mid-Atlantic, and upper north-central regions, and to several counties in northwestern California.

Most *B. burgdorferi* infections are thought to result from peri-residential exposure to infected ticks during property maintenance, recreation, and leisure activities. Thus, individuals who live or work in residential areas surrounded by woods or overgrown brush infested by vector ticks are at risk of getting Lyme disease. In addition, persons who participate in recreational activities away from home such as hiking, camping, fishing and hunting in tick habitat, and persons who engage in outdoor occupations, such as landscaping, brush clearing, forestry, and wildlife and parks management in endemic areas may also be at risk of getting Lyme disease.

Questions and Answers

How is Lyme disease transmitted?

Lyme disease is transmitted by ticks (deer ticks and western black-legged ticks) that become infected with bacteria that cause Lyme disease. Immature ticks become infected by feeding on small rodents, such as the white-footed mouse, and other mammals that are infected with the bacterium *Borrelia burgdorferi*. In later stages, these ticks then transmit the Lyme disease bacterium to humans and other mammals during the feeding process. Lyme disease bacteria are maintained in the blood systems of small rodents.

Lyme disease bacteria are NOT transmitted from person-to-person. For example, you cannot get infected from touching or kissing a person who has Lyme disease, or from a health care worker who has treated someone with the disease.

Lyme disease is the leading cause of vector-borne infectious illness in the U.S. with about 15,000 cases reported annually, though the disease is greatly underreported. Based on reported cases, during the past ten years 90% of cases of Lyme disease occurred in ten states: New York, Connecticut, Pennsylvania, New Jersey, Wisconsin, Rhode Island, Maryland, Massachusetts, Minnesota, and Delaware.

What are the signs and symptoms of Lyme disease?

Within days to weeks following a tick bite (usually 7 to 14 days), 80% of patients will have a red, slowly expanding "bull's-eye" rash (called erythema migrans), accompanied by general tiredness, fever, headache, stiff neck, muscle aches, and joint pain. If untreated, weeks to months later some patients may develop arthritis, including intermittent episodes of swelling and pain in the large joints; neurologic abnormalities, such as aseptic meningitis, facial palsy, motor and sensory nerve inflammation (radiculoneuritis) and inflammation of the brain (encephalitis); and, rarely, cardiac problems, such as atrioventricular block, acute inflammation of the tissues surrounding the heart (myopericarditis) or enlarged heart (cardiomegaly). Some patients exhibit later manifestations without having had early signs of disease. Lyme disease is rarely, if ever, fatal.

Can a person be reinfected with Lyme disease?

Yes. Having had Lyme disease doesn't protect against reinfection. Some persons have had Lyme disease more than once after re-exposure to infective tick bites. This stresses the need for continued tick bite prevention activities such as wearing appropriate clothing when in tick-infested areas, daily tick checks, and quick removal of attached ticks.

How is Lyme disease treated?

According to treatment experts, antibiotic treatment for 3–4 weeks with doxycycline or amoxicillin is generally effective in early disease. Cefuroxime axetil or erythromycin can be used for persons allergic to penicillin or who cannot take tetracyclines. Later disease, particularly with objective neurologic manifestations, may require treatment with intravenous ceftriaxone or penicillin for 4 weeks or more, depending on disease severity. In later disease, treatment failures may occur and retreatment may be necessary.

Should children be vaccinated against Lyme disease?

It is not recommended for children aged less than 15 years and pregnant women to receive the Lyme disease vaccine.

Lyme Disease: Prevention and Control

Avoid Tick Habitats

Whenever possible, avoid entering areas that are likely to be infested with ticks, particularly in spring and summer when nymphal ticks feed. Ticks favor a moist, shaded environment, especially areas with leaf litter and low-lying vegetation in wooded, brushy, or overgrown grassy habitat.

Use Personal Protection Measures

If you are going to be in areas that are tick infested, wear light-colored clothing so that ticks can be spotted more easily and removed before becoming attached. Wearing long-sleeved shirts and tucking pants into socks or boot tops may help keep ticks from reaching your skin. Ticks are usually located close to the ground, so wearing high rubber boots may provide additional protection.

The risk of tick attachment can also be reduced by applying insect repellents containing DEET to clothes and exposed skin, and applying permethrin (which kills ticks on contact) to clothes. DEET can be used safely on children and adults but should be applied according to Environmental Protection Agency (EPA) guidelines to reduce the possibility of toxicity.

Perform a Tick Check and Remove Attached Ticks

The transmission of *B. burgdorferi* (the bacteria that causes Lyme disease) from an infected tick is unlikely to occur before 36 hours of tick attachment. For this reason, daily checks for ticks and promptly removing any attached tick that you find will help prevent infection. Embedded ticks should be removed using fine-tipped tweezers. DO NOT use petroleum jelly, a hot match, nail polish, or other products. Grasp the tick firmly and as closely to the skin as possible. With a steady motion, pull the tick's body away from the skin. The tick's mouthparts may remain in the skin, but do not be alarmed. The bacteria that cause Lyme disease are contained in the tick's midgut or salivary glands. Cleanse the area with an antiseptic.

Taking Preventive Antibiotics after a Tick Bite

The relative cost-effectiveness of postexposure treatment of tick bites to avoid Lyme disease in endemic areas (areas where the disease is known to occur regularly) is dependent on the probability of *B. burgdorferi* infection after a tick bite. In most circumstances, treating persons who only have a tick bite is not recommended. Individuals who are bitten by a deer tick should remove the tick promptly, and may wish to consult with their health care provider. Persons should promptly seek medical attention if they develop any signs and symptoms of early Lyme disease, ehrlichiosis, or babesiosis.

Chapter 51

Measles

Measles is a respiratory disease caused by a virus. The virus normally grows in the cells that line the back of the throat and in the cells that line the lungs. The symptoms of measles include a rash, high fever, cough, runny nose, and red, watery eyes (which last about a week). These symptoms begin to appear about 10 to 12 days after exposure to the virus. The infected person first experiences a fever lasting about 2 to 4 days that can peak as high as 103° F to 105° F. This is followed by the onset of cough, runny nose, and/or conjunctivitis (pink eye). The rash usually appears about 14 days after exposure and lasts 5 to 6 days. It begins at the hairline, then involves the face and upper neck. Over the next 3 days, the rash gradually proceeds downward and outward, reaching the hands and feet.

Measles may cause complications, including diarrhea, ear infections, pneumonia, encephalitis, seizures, and death. Measles causes ear infections in nearly one out of every 10 children who get it. As many as one out of 20 children with measles gets pneumonia, and about one child in every 1,000 who get measles will develop encephalitis. (This is an inflammation of the brain that can lead to convulsions, and can leave your child deaf or mentally retarded.) For every

This chapter includes excerpts from "Measles: What You Need to Know," National Immunization Program (NIP), Centers for Disease control and Prevention (CDC), February 2001; "FAQs (frequently asked questions) about Measles," NIP, CDC, February 2001; "Recommendations for Prevention," NIP, CDC, February 2001; "MMR Vaccine and Autism," NIP, CDC, May 2002; and "Measles Vaccine and Inflammatory Bowel Disease," NIP, CDC, May 2002.

1,000 children who get measles, one or two will die from it. Measles can also make a pregnant woman have a miscarriage, give birth prematurely, or have a low-birth-weight baby.

Measles is spread by coughing and sneezing. The disease is highly contagious, and can be transmitted from 4 days prior to the onset of the rash to 4 days after the onset. If one person has it, 90% of their susceptible close contacts will also become infected with the measles virus.

Measles can be prevented by a vaccine. The MMR vaccine is a live, attenuated (weakened), combination vaccine that protects against the measles, mumps, and rubella viruses. It was first licensed in the combined form in 1971 and contains the safest and most effective forms of each vaccine. It is made by taking the measles virus from the throat of an infected person and adapting it to grow in chick embryo cells in a laboratory. As the virus becomes better able to grow in the chick embryo cells, it becomes less able to grow in a child's skin or lungs. When this vaccine virus is given to a child it replicates only a little before it is eliminated from the body. This replication causes the body to develop an immunity that, in 95% of children, lasts for a lifetime. A second dose of the vaccine is recommended to protect those 5% who did not develop immunity in the first dose and to give "booster" effect to those who did develop an immune response.

Questions and Answers about Measles

How does someone catch measles?

Measles is highly contagious. Infected people are usually contagious from about 4 days before their rash starts to 4 days afterwards. The measles virus resides in the mucus in the nose and throat of infected people. When they sneeze or cough, droplets spray into the air and the droplets remain active and contagious on infected surfaces for up to two hours.

Why is vaccination necessary?

Before the measles vaccine became available, there were approximately 450,000 measles cases and an average of 450 measles-associated deaths were reported each year. Widespread use of measles vaccine has led to a greater than 99% reduction in measles cases in the U.S. compared with the pre-vaccine era. However, measles is common in other countries where it spreads rapidly and can be easily brought into the U.S. If vaccinations were stopped, measles would return to pre-vaccine levels in the U.S. and hundreds of people would die from measles-related illnesses.

In developing countries, where malnutrition and vitamin A deficiency are prevalent, measles has been known to kill as many as one out of four people. It is the leading cause of blindness among African children. Measles kills almost one million children in the world each year.

If measles is rare in the United States, why is vaccination still recommended?

It is true that vaccination has enabled us to reduce measles and most other vaccine-preventable diseases to very low levels in the United States. However, measles is still very common—even epidemic—in other parts of the world. Visitors to our country and U.S. travelers returning from other countries can unknowingly bring this disease into the United States, and if we were not protected by vaccinations, it would quickly spread causing an epidemics here. The disease is very contagious.

We should be vaccinated protect ourselves and our children. Even if we think our chances of getting measles is small, the disease still exists and can still infect anyone who is not protected.

What kind of vaccine is given to prevent measles and when is it given?

The MMR vaccine prevents measles and two other viral diseases—mumps and rubella. These three vaccines are safe given together. MMR is a attenuated (weakened) live virus vaccine. This means that after injection, the viruses grows, and causes a harmless infection in the vaccinated person with very few, if any symptoms. The person's immune system fights the infection caused by these weakened viruses and immunity develops which lasts throughout that person's life. More than 95% of the people who receive a single dose of MMR will develop immunity to all three viruses. A second gives immunity to almost all of those who did not respond to the first dose.

Most infants born in the United States will receive passive protection against measles, mumps, and rubella in the form of antibodies from their mothers. These antibodies can destroy the vaccine virus if they are present when the vaccine is administered and cause it to be ineffective. By 12 months of age, almost all infants have lost this passive protection. For this reason, the first dose is usually given after the first birthday.

The second dose of MMR can be given anytime, as long as the child is at least 12 months old and it has been at least a month since the first dose. However, the second dose is usually administered before the child begins kindergarten or first grade (4–5 years of age) or before entry to middle school (11–12 years of age). The age at which the second dose is required is generally mandated by state school entry requirements.

Recommendations for Measles Prevention

Children

The MMR vaccine is the safest protection you can give your child against measles. Children should be given the first dose of MMR vaccine soon after the first birthday (12 to 15 months of age). The second dose is recommended before the start of the kindergarten.

Teens

Students entering middle school, high school, or college should have their vaccination records reviewed to make sure they have received both doses of the MMR vaccine.

Outbreaks continue to occur in high schools (one or two per year) and on college campuses (less than 1 per year). These educational institutions are potential high-risk areas for measles transmission because of large concentrations of susceptible people. That is why the Centers for Disease Control and Prevention (CDC) recommends that all states require proof of either two doses of the measles vaccine or evidence of past measles infection at the time of college or other post–high school entry.

Note: Pregnant women should not receive the MMR vaccine. Also, pregnancy should be avoided one month following the receipt of the measles vaccine and three months following the MMR vaccine.

Questions about Adverse Effects of the MMR Vaccine

What is the most common reaction following MMR vaccine?

Most people have no reaction. However, 5 percent to 10 percent of the people receiving the MMR vaccine experience a low grade fever and a mild rash.

Can the MMR vaccine cause autism?

Because signs of autism may appear at around the same time children receive the MMR vaccine, some parents may worry that the vaccine causes autism. Carefully performed scientific studies have found no relationship between MMR vaccine and autism, and the CDC continues to recommend two doses of MMR vaccine for all children.

In 1998, a study of autistic children raised the question of a connection between MMR vaccine and autism. The 1998 study has a number of limitations. For example, the study was very small, involving only 12 children. This is too few cases to make any generalizations about the causes of autism. In addition, the researchers suggested that MMR vaccination caused bowel problems in the children, which then led to autism. However, in some of the children studied, symptoms of autism appeared before symptoms of bowel disease. Other larger studies have found no relationship between MMR vaccine and autism.

Groups of experts, including the American Academy of Pediatrics, agree that MMR vaccine is not responsible for recent increases in the number of children with autism.

Can the MMR vaccine cause inflammatory bowel disease (IBD)?

Scientific studies have found no relationship between measles vaccine and inflammatory bowel disease. The CDC recommends two doses of MMR vaccine for all children.

Inflammatory bowel disease, or IBD, refers to diseases (including ulcerative colitis and Crohn's disease) that inflame the intestines and cause symptoms such as bloody diarrhea, pain, and weight loss. The cause of IBD is not known.

Studies conducted since 1998 by one group of researchers suggest that MMR vaccine may cause IBD. However, other scientists have concerns about the way these studies were done. For example, in one study researchers found parts of measles virus in the intestines of children with IBD. However, they did not compare the virus found in the children with the virus used in the MMR vaccine, nor did they provide information to indicate whether or not the children had ever received the MMR vaccine or had ever gotten measles disease.

Other scientists have done studies that provide strong scientific evidence that there is no association between measles vaccine and IBD. For instance, the CDC compared the vaccination histories of patients with IBD to those without IBD. The scientists found that vaccination with MMR does not increase the likelihood that a person will develop IBD.

Chapter 52

Mumps

Before vaccines, mumps was a common childhood disease. The most obvious sign of mumps is swelling of the cheeks and jaw, which is caused by inflammation in the salivary glands. Children with mumps usually also get a fever and headache. Generally, mumps is a mild disease, but it does have its serious side:

- About one child in every ten who get mumps also gets meningitis (an inflammation of the covering of the brain and spinal cord).

- Occasionally mumps also causes encephalitis, which is inflammation of the brain itself. Usually the child recovers without permanent damage.

- About one out of every four teenage or adult men who gets mumps develops a painful swelling of the testicles.

- Mumps can, rarely, cause deafness (about 1 in 20,000 cases) or death (about 1 in 10,000 cases).

Children get mumps through contact with others who are already infected with the mumps virus. The virus is spread through the air by coughing, sneezing, or simply talking.

This chapter contains excerpts from "Parents Guide to Childhood Immunization," National Immunization Program, Centers for Disease Control and Prevention, 2001; and *Epidemiology and Prevention of Vaccine-Preventable Diseases, 7th Edition*, Centers for Disease Control and Prevention, April 2002.

Children start to show signs of mumps 2 to 3 weeks after they are exposed. They are contagious from about 12 to 24 days after exposure.

The Mumps Virus

Mumps virus is a paramyxovirus in the same group as parainfluenza and Newcastle disease virus. It is acquired by respiratory droplets and it grows in the nasopharynx and regional lymph nodes. Inflammation in infected tissues leads to the characteristic symptoms.

The incubation period of mumps is 14–18 days (range, 14-25 days). Early symptoms are nonspecific, and include myalgia, anorexia, malaise, headache, and low-grade fever. Parotitis (inflammation of the salivary glands) is the most common manifestation, and occurs in 30%–40% of infected persons. Parotitis may be unilateral (on one side) or bilateral (on both sides) and any combination of single or multiple salivary glands may be affected. Parotitis tends to occur within the first two days and may first be noted as earache and jaw tenderness. Symptoms tend to decrease after one week and have usually resolved after 10 days.

Up to 20% of mumps infections produce no symptoms. An additional 40%–50% may have only nonspecific or primarily respiratory symptoms.

Complications of Mumps

Central nervous system (CNS) involvement in the form of aseptic meningitis is common, occurring without outward symptoms (inflammatory cells in cerebrospinal fluid) in 50%–60% of patients. Symptomatic meningitis (headache, stiff neck) occurs in up to 15% of patients. Adults are at higher risk for this complication than children, and boys are more commonly affected than girls (3:1 ratio). Encephalitis is rare (less than 2 per 100,000). In the pre-vaccine era, mumps virus was one of the most common causes of aseptic meningitis.

Orchitis (testicular inflammation) is the most common complication in postpubertal males. It occurs in up to 50% of postpubertal males, usually after parotitis, but may precede it, begin simultaneously, or occur alone. It is bilateral in up to 30% of affected males. There is usually abrupt onset of testicular swelling, tenderness, nausea, vomiting, and fever. Pain and swelling may subside in one week, but tenderness may last for weeks. Approximately 50% of patients with orchitis have some degree of testicular atrophy, but sterility is rare.

Oophoritis (ovarian inflammation) occurs in 5% of postpubertal females. It may mimic appendicitis. There is no relationship to impaired fertility.

Pancreatitis is infrequent, but occasionally occurs without parotitis; the hyperglycemia is transient and is reversible. While some single instances of diabetes mellitus have been reported, a causal relationship has yet to be conclusively demonstrated.

Deafness caused by mumps was a leading cause of acquired sensorineural deafness in childhood in the pre-vaccine era. The estimated incidence is approximately 1 per 20,000 reported cases of mumps. Hearing loss is unilateral in approximately 80% of cases and may be associated with vestibular reactions. Onset is usually sudden and results in permanent hearing impairment.

Electrocardiogram (EKG) changes compatible with inflammation of the muscles that make up the walls of the heart (a condition called myocarditis) are seen in 3%–15% of patients with mumps, but symptomatic involvement is rare. Complete recovery is the rule, but deaths have been reported.

Other less common complications of mumps include arthralgia, arthritis, and nephritis. An average of one death from mumps per year was reported in 1980–1999.

Mumps Immunization

The mumps vaccine we use today was licensed in 1967, and is a live, attenuated (weakened) vaccine. The number of reported cases has dropped from over 150,000 in 1968 to only 666 in 1998.

Mumps vaccine is usually given together with measles and rubella vaccines in a shot called MMR (measles, mumps, rubella).

MMR Vaccine

Most children get measles, mumps and rubella vaccines all together in one shot called MMR. All three of these vaccines work very well, and will protect most children for the rest of their lives.

Children should get two doses of MMR vaccine. The first is given between 12 and 15 months of age. The second may be given at any time, as long as it is at least 28 days after the first. It is usually given at 4–6 years of age, before the child enters kindergarten or first grade.

Measles, mumps, and rubella vaccines can be given separately, too. But this is not usually done because it means giving a child three shots instead of one. Sometimes—usually during a measles outbreak—children might be given measles or MMR vaccine before their first birthday. This is for short-term protection only. These children should still be given two doses of MMR vaccine at the usual ages.

Side Effects from Immunization

Very few children suffer any ill effects from mumps vaccine. Occasionally a child will get a mild fever one or two weeks after vaccination, or swollen glands in the cheeks or under the jaw. More serious reactions are extremely rare.

Febrile seizures (seizures caused by a fever) have occasionally been reported among children who have gotten MMR vaccine. These usually happen 1 or 2 weeks after the shot and are caused by the fever that can accompany vaccination rather than the vaccine itself. Children recover from febrile seizures quickly, and they do not cause permanent harm.

There have been reports of children getting encephalitis (inflammation of the brain) after an MMR shot. This happens so rarely—less than once in a million shots—that experts are not sure whether the MMR vaccine causes this problem or whether it simply happens by chance.

MMR, like any vaccine or medicine, could trigger a severe allergic reaction in a child who was allergic to one of the vaccine's components. But severe allergic reactions to childhood vaccines are very rare (estimated at around one per million doses), and no child is ever known to have died from an allergic reaction to a vaccine.

Precautions

There are several reasons a doctor might want to delay giving a child an MMR vaccination or not give it at all:

- A child who is known to have a severe allergy to gelatin or the antibiotic neomycin should not get MMR.

- A child who has had a severe (life-threatening) allergic reaction after a dose of MMR should not get another dose.

- A child whose immune system is suppressed (because of a disease such as cancer or HIV [human immunodeficiency virus] infection, or medication such as steroids) should be evaluated by a doctor before getting MMR vaccine.

- A child who has recently gotten a transfusion or other blood product might have to wait up to several months before getting MMR.

- A child who has a moderate or severe illness on the day an MMR (or any) vaccination is scheduled should probably delay the vaccination until he or she has recovered.

Your doctor or nurse can give you more details.

After getting MMR vaccine, if the child has any serious or unusual problems after getting this vaccine, call a doctor or get the child to a doctor right away.

Note: Additional information about the MMR vaccine can be found in Chapter 51—Measles.

Chapter 53

Rabies

What is rabies?

Rabies is an acute and deadly viral infection of the central nervous system. It is one of the most terrifying diseases known to man. Although rabies in humans is rare in the United States, as many as 18,000 Americans get rabies shots each year because they have been in contact with animals that may be rabid (rabies-infected). In 1998 according to the U.S. Centers for Disease Control and Prevention (CDC), only one person died of rabies in this country.

In other parts of the world, however, many people die of rabies each year. The World Health Organization (WHO) estimates that around the world more than 40,000 people die every year from rabies. WHO also estimates that 10 million people worldwide are treated after being exposed to animals that may have rabies.

Rabies is caused by a virus that is in the saliva of infected animals, and it is usually transmitted by bites from infected animals. All warm-blooded animals can get rabies, and some may serve as natural reservoirs of the virus.

Rabies is found in all of the United States, except Hawaii, and in many other countries around the world, including Canada and Mexico. The disease may be absent from large areas for many years, and then reappear suddenly or gradually by invasion from bordering countries or by the introduction of an infected animal.

National Institute of Allergy and Infectious Diseases (NIAID), National Institutes of Health (NIH), http://www.niaid.nih.gov/factsheets/rabies.htm, April 2002.

331

What animals usually get infected with rabies?

Rabies can affect wildlife such as raccoons, skunks, and bats, as well as household pets such as dogs and cats. Vaccination of pets and livestock is the most effective control measure to prevent the disease in these animals and subsequent human exposure. In fact, in the United States, such programs have largely eliminated canine (dog) rabies. In 1998, wild animals accounted for 93 percent of the 7,962 reported animal rabies cases in the United States and Puerto Rico. Rabies in raccoons accounted for 44 percent of cases, skunk rabies for 28.5 percent, bat rabies for 12.5 percent, and fox rabies for 5.5 percent of the cases. Only rarely, rabies is found in rabbits, squirrels, rats, and opossums.

Health officials are particularly concerned about rabies in raccoons because raccoons are often in close contact with household pets, especially dogs and cats. Increasingly, bats are being shown to be important transmitters of rabies to humans.

How can an animal with rabies infect a person?

Most people get rabies from being bitten by a rabid animal. Rarely, if a person has broken skin, like a scratch, which comes in contact with animal saliva full of rabies virus, that person may get infected. But rabies also can be spread in the air, as has occurred in caves where infected bats live.

What should I do if I think I've been in contact with rabies?

If you have been bitten or scratched by any animal, you should:

- Clean the wound immediately with soap and water to remove saliva from the area.
- Call a doctor right away.
- Notify the state or local health department.

If soap is not available, for example, when hiking, you can use water alone. But be sure to wash with soap and water as soon as possible. Allow the wound to bleed, which also will help to clean it.

There are situations in which it is possible that a person has had close contact with a bat and not known it, as when a sleeping person awakens to find a bat in the room. Therefore, CDC now recommends that people seek medical help even if they can't see a bat bite or scratch, or may have had mucous membrane exposure. Mucous membranes include the linings of the eyes, mouth, and nose.

The possibility of getting rabies from rodents, including squirrels, is small. If you have been bitten by one, however, you should still consult a doctor right away.

In fact, you should avoid contact with any wild animal.

How do doctors diagnose rabies?

If you think you may have been exposed to rabies, the doctor or other health care worker will ask you questions about when you possibly were in contact with an infected animal and if you have any symptoms. Laboratory tests to make sure that the diagnosis is correct involve looking for the rabies virus in your saliva or brain tissue. Unfortunately, this is usually not possible until late in the disease. The doctor must use sophisticated laboratory tests to show rabies or evidence of rabies virus.

What are the symptoms of rabies?

When symptoms do appear, it is usually 30 to 50 days following exposure. There is a direct relationship between how severe the bite is and where on the body the person was bitten and how long it takes for symptoms to appear. For example, if a person's head is severely bitten, symptoms may show up in as few as 14 days. Under rare conditions, a person may not have symptoms for a year or longer after exposure to the virus.

The doctor will suspect rabies if someone has symptoms such as:

- a short period of mental depression
- restlessness
- abnormal sensations such as itching around the site of the bite
- headache
- fever
- tiredness
- nausea
- sore throat
- loss of appetite

Other early symptoms include:

- stiff muscles

- dilation (enlargement) of pupils of the eye

- increased production of saliva

- unusual sensitivity to sound, light, and changes of temperature

If the disease has progressed, a person will have episodes of irrational excitement which alternate with periods of alert calm. Convulsions are common. Most dramatic of all are the severe and extremely painful throat spasms suffered by the person when trying to swallow—or even upon seeing—liquids. This reaction to water, sometimes seen as a fear of it, is typical in people with rabies and gives the disease its medical name, hydrophobia.

A person usually dies from cardiac or respiratory failure within a week after the appearance of rabies symptoms, while the excited state is most prominent. If the patient survives this stage, muscle spasms and agitation stop, only to be replaced by a growing paralysis leading to death.

In human rabies resulting from the bite of a rabid vampire bat, excitement and hydrophobia are usually not present and paralysis usually starts in the legs and moves upward.

Once symptoms appear, the only treatment is strong support to help the person feel more comfortable. This support includes controlling the symptoms in the respiratory, circulatory, and central nervous systems.

People do not recover and eventually die from the infection.

How is rabies treated?

If a doctor decides that you probably have been exposed to rabies, postexposure (after a being bitten) rabies shots should begin at once, preferably within 24 to 48 hours of exposure. In fact, many experts recommend that treatment should be started even if the delay is much longer than that.

The first treatment, sometimes called passive immunization, provides immediate but temporary protection by injecting antibodies (disease-fighting proteins or immunoglobulins) into the patient. Currently, CDC recommends treating a patient immediately with one dose of human rabies immunoglobulin (HRIG) shots.

After the first treatment, CDC recommends that patients be given a rabies shot, which starts the body producing its own antibodies. It takes some time for the body to produce the antibodies, but these antibodies provide longer-lasting protection. Because rabies has an unusually long incubation period, however, the body has time to respond to the vaccine and produce protective antibodies.

There are now three types of rabies vaccines, all of which are made from killed rabies virus:

- Human diploid cell vaccine (HDCV)

- Rabies vaccine adsorbed (RVA)

- Purified chick embryo cell culture (PCEC)

After possible exposure to the rabies virus, the doctor will give you five shots with one of these vaccines into your upper arm muscle over a four-week period. The vaccines can cause mild reactions such as swelling or redness at the vaccine site, headache, fever, nausea, muscle aches, and dizziness.

If you are a veterinarian, animal caretaker, laboratory worker, cave explorer, or forest ranger, or are often involved in other activities which put you in high risk of being bitten by an animal, health specialists recommend that you get pre-exposure shots with a rabies vaccine. You should get these shots in three injections over four weeks.

If you are traveling to areas where rabies is not well-controlled, such as parts of Africa, Asia, and Central and South America, and where the vaccine for postexposure treatment might not be readily available, you should also get the pre-exposure shots. Then, if you do come in contact with the rabies virus, then the postexposure regimen would require only two booster injections.

People with continuing risk of exposure should receive a booster about every two years.

How can I prevent getting rabies?

Control of rabies in animals and avoiding contact with possibly rabid animals are the best methods to prevent getting rabies.

- Make sure your pets and other domesticated animals, including dogs, cats, ferrets, sheep, cattle, and horses, regularly get animal rabies shots.

- Keep your dog on a leash when it's outside of the yard and do not chain it inside the yard.

- Avoid contact with wild or unfamiliar animals, and don't touch them even when they are dead.

- Seal basement, porch, and attic openings and cap chimneys to prevent animals from entering your home.

- Report strays or animals acting strangely or sick to your local animal control authorities.

What is rabies like in animals?

Early signs of rabies in animals include a change in behavior, fever, loss of appetite, and often, a change in phonation, such as a change in tone of a dog's bark. These signs are often slight, however, and people may not notice them. A few days after infection, the animal may be very restlessness and become very agitated and tremble. An affected dog may growl and bark constantly, and will viciously attack any moving object, person, or animal it comes across. This excited state usually lasts three to seven days, and is followed by convulsions and paralysis.

In some instances, signs of excitement and irritability are slight or absent, and paralysis develops within a few days of disease onset. In cases of this type, an early sign is often paralysis of the lower jaw, accompanied by increased drooling and foaming of saliva. The animal may appear to be choking on a foreign object. This is a dangerous trap for humans, who, in trying to help the animal, may expose themselves to infection without knowing it.

What research is going on?

Scientists supported by the National Institute of Allergy and Infectious Diseases (NIAID) are focusing their rabies research on basic research and vaccine development. These scientists showed that the current human diploid cell vaccine provides protection against all strains of rabies isolated from around the world. Scientists are trying to develop a lower-cost vaccine because it is too expensive for many countries to use it widely. One new vaccine approach supported by NIAID is attempting to develop a modern, DNA-based vaccine that would show broad protection against rabies and be less costly.

Chapter 54

Rocky Mountain Spotted Fever

What is Rocky Mountain spotted fever?

Rocky Mountain spotted fever is an acute infectious disease transmitted to humans by the bite of an infected tick. The disease is caused by *Rickettsia rickettsii*, which are some of the smallest known bacteria. The bacteria are parasites inside ticks' bodies, and spread to humans when the ticks bite. The disease occurs throughout the United States during months when ground temperatures reach 40° Fahrenheit or more and ticks are active.

Who gets Rocky Mountain spotted fever?

Both children and adults can be affected by Rocky Mountain spotted fever, but it is more common in children under 15 years old. Disease incidence is directly related to exposure to tick-infested habitats or to infested pets. It is most common between April and September. In spite of the disease's name, few cases have been reported from the Rocky Mountain region of the United States. However, it occurs in every U.S. state except Maine, Alaska, and Hawaii. It is most common in the Mid-Atlantic States: Virginia, West Virginia, and North and South Carolina.

"Rocky Mountain Spotted Fever," Illinois Department of Public Health, http://www.idph.state.il.us/public/hb/hbrmsf.htm. Updated in August 2001 by Dr. David A. Cooke, MD, Diplomate, American Board of Internal Medicine.

How is Rocky Mountain spotted fever spread?

Rocky Mountain spotted fever is spread by the bite of an infected tick (the American dog tick or the lone-star tick) or by contamination of the skin with tick blood or feces. Person-to-person transmission does not occur.

What are the symptoms of Rocky Mountain spotted fever?

Rocky Mountain spotted fever is characterized by a sudden onset of moderate to high fever (which can last for two or three weeks), severe headache, fatigue, deep muscle pain, chills, and rash. The rash consists of many small, flat, red-brown spots on the skin. Unlike most rashes, the spots do not briefly lighten in color (blanch) when you press on them with your finger. The rash begins on the legs or arms, may include the soles of the feet or palms of the hands, and may spread rapidly to the trunk or the rest of the body. Not every case of Rocky Mountain spotted fever will have the rash. People with Rocky Mountain spotted fever may become extremely ill, and it can be fatal if not diagnosed and treated appropriately.

How soon do symptoms appear?

Symptoms usually appear between three and 14 days after the bite of an infected tick. Any person experiencing illness with a fever following a tick bite should consult his or her physician and advise the physician of the tick bite.

How is Rocky Mountain spotted fever diagnosed?

Diagnosis of Rocky Mountain spotted fever is based largely on the patient's signs and symptom's of illness. Blood tests are important in confirming a diagnosis, but treatment should begin promptly if symptoms and exposure history support this diagnosis.

What is the treatment for Rocky Mountain spotted fever?

Treatment involves the use of certain antibiotics, such as tetracycline or chloramphenicol. Antibiotic treatment can be terminated two or three days after a person's temperature returns to normal for a full 24-hour period. Overall mortality hovers between 3 percent and 5 percent but ranges from 13 percent to 25 percent in untreated individuals. Death primarily occurs in patients in whom the diagnosis is not made until the second week of illness. The absence or delayed appearance of the typical rash contributes to a late diagnosis and thereby increases the incidence of fatality.

How can Rocky Mountain spotted fever be prevented?

Persons spending time outdoors in areas where ticks are commonly found—wooded areas, tall grass and brush—should take precautions against all tick-borne diseases:

- Check your clothing often for ticks climbing toward open skin. Wear white or light-colored long-sleeved shirts and long pants so the tiny ticks are easier to see. Tuck long pants into your socks and boots. Wear a head covering or hat for added protection.

- For those who may not tolerate wearing all of these clothes in hot, muggy weather, apply insect repellent containing DEET (n,n-diethyl-m toluamide) (30 percent or less) to exposed skin (except the face). Be sure to wash treated skin after coming indoors. If you do cover up, use repellents containing permethrin to treat clothes (especially pants, socks, and shoes) while in locations where ticks may be common. Follow label directions; do not misuse or overuse repellents. Always supervise children in the use of repellents.

- Walk in the center of trails so weeds do not brush against you.

- Check yourself, children, and other family members every two to three hours for ticks. Most ticks seldom attach quickly and rarely transmit tick-borne disease until they have been attached for four or more hours.

- If you let your pets outdoors, check them often for ticks. Infected ticks also can transmit some tick-borne diseases to them. Check with your veterinarian about preventive measures against tick-borne diseases. You are at risk from ticks that hitch a ride on your pets but fall off in your home before they feed.

- Make sure the property around your home is unattractive to ticks. Keep your grass mowed and keep weeds cut.

How should an attached tick be removed?

Remove any tick promptly. Do not try to burn the tick with a match or cover it with petroleum jelly or nail polish. Do not use bare hands.

The best way to remove a tick is to grasp it with fine-point tweezers as close to the skin as possible and gently, but firmly, pull it straight out. Do not twist or jerk the tick. If tweezers are not available, grasp the tick with a piece of cloth or whatever can be used as a barrier between your fingers and the tick. You may want to put the tick in a jar of rubbing alcohol labeled with the date and location of the bite in case you seek medical attention and your physician wishes to have the tick identified.

The mouthparts of a tick are shaped like tiny barbs and may remain embedded and lead to infection at the bite site if not removed properly.

Be sure to wash the bite area and your hands thoroughly with soap and water, and apply an antiseptic to the bite site.

Chapter 55

Rubella

The name rubella is derived from Latin, meaning "little red." It was initially considered to be a variant of measles or scarlet fever and was called third disease. It was not until 1814 that it was first described as a separate disease in the German medical literature.

Rubella is also called German measles or three-day measles. It is a very contagious disease caused by the rubella virus. The virus causes fever, swollen lymph nodes behind the ears, and a rash that starts on the face and spreads to the torso and then to the arms and legs. Rubella is no longer very common because most children are immunized beginning at 12 months of age. Rubella is not usually a serious disease in children, but can be very serious if a pregnant woman becomes infected. Infection with rubella in the first 3 months of pregnancy can cause serious injury to the fetus, resulting in heart damage, blindness, deafness, mental retardation, miscarriage, or stillbirth.

Rubella is spread person-to-person by breathing in droplets of respiratory secretions exhaled by an infected person. It may also be spread when someone touches his or her nose or mouth after their hands have been in contact with infected secretions (such as saliva) of an infected person. A person can spread the disease from as many as 5 days before the rash appears to 5 to 7 days after.

This chapter includes excerpts adapted from *Epidemiology and Prevention of Vaccine-Preventable Diseases, 7th Edition*, Centers for Disease Control and Prevention, April 2002; and "Rubella in the Child Care Setting," Centers for Disease Control and Prevention, January 1997, updated in June 2002 by Dr. David A. Cooke, MD, Diplomate, American Board of Internal Medicine.

Symptoms of Acquired Rubella

The incubation period of rubella is 14 days with a range of 12 to 23 days. Symptoms are often mild, and 20%–50% of cases may be subclinical or inapparent. In children, rash is usually the first manifestation. In older children and adults, there is often a 1–5 day period of symptoms before the appearance of the rash. These symptoms include low-grade fever, malaise, involvement of the lymph nodes, and upper respiratory symptoms. The rash of rubella usually occurs initially on the face and then progresses from head to foot. It lasts about 3 days and is occasionally itchy. The rash is fainter than the measles rash and does not coalesce.

Joint pain and arthritis occur so frequently in adults that they are considered by many to be an integral part of the illness rather than a complication. Other symptoms of rubella include conjunctivitis and pain or inflammation in the testes.

Complications of Rubella

Complications are uncommon, but tend to occur more often in adults than in children. Arthritis or joint pain may occur in up to 70% of adult women who contract rubella, but is rare in children and adult males. Fingers, wrists, and knees are often affected. Joint symptoms tend to occur about the same time or shortly after appearance of the rash and may last for up to one month; chronic arthritis is rare.

Encephalitis occurs in one in 5,000 cases, again more frequently in adults (especially in females) than in children. Mortality estimates vary from 0 to 50%.

Bleeding complications occur in approximately one per 3,000 cases, occurring more often in children than in adults. These manifestations may be secondary to low platelets and damage to blood vessels, with thrombocytopenic purpura being the most common manifestation. Gastrointestinal, cerebral, or intrarenal hemorrhage may occur. Effects may last from days to months, and most patients recover.

Additional complications include inflammation of the testes, nerve inflammation, and a rare late syndrome of progressive inflammation of the brain.

Rubella Vaccine

Rubella may be prevented by immunization. The rubella vaccine is part of the MMR (measles, mumps, rubella) vaccine series administered to children beginning at 12 months of age. Two doses are normally given, although immunity to rubella usually develops after the first. MMR is a live-virus vaccine, and should not be given to immunosuppressed children unless recommended by a specialist.

In recent years, a new formulation of the MMR vaccine has come into use. Older versions of the vaccine contained a preservative called thimerosal. Although thimerosal is considered safe, it does contain mercury. As a precaution, all new batches of the vaccine are thimerosal-free. This does not affect the effectiveness of the vaccine in any way.

Note: Additional information about the MMR vaccine can be found in Chapter 51—Measles.

Rubella in the Child Care Setting

All child care providers should be immune to rubella. People are considered immune only if they have received at least one dose of rubella vaccine on or after their first birthday or if they have laboratory evidence of rubella immunity.

If a child or adult in the child care facility develops rubella:

- Exclude the infected child or adult until 6 days after the onset of the rash.

- Notify the local health department immediately.

- Review all immunization records of the children in your care.

- Any children under 12 months who have not yet been vaccinated against rubella should be excluded until they have been immunized or until 3 weeks after the onset of rash in the last case.

- Refer any pregnant woman who has been exposed to rubella to her doctor.

- Follow good handwashing and hygiene procedures.

- Carefully observe other children, staff, or family members for symptoms.

Chapter 56

Streptococcal Infections: Strep Throat and Scarlet Fever

Few childhoods go by without the tell-tale fever and sore throat of a *Streptococcus*, or strep, infection. Although these throat infections are common and easily treated, the recent rise of particularly deadly or troublesome strains of Group A *Streptococcus* has pushed the bacterium into the medical limelight—again.

In the past, Group A strep has played a starring role in a number of deadly medical epidemics, particularly the scourges of rheumatic fever that swept across the nation in the first half of this century, killing or debilitating thousands of children each year.

After World War II, the number of cases of rheumatic fever dramatically declined until, during the 20 years between 1965 and 1985 alone, the yearly number of cases of rheumatic fever among school-age children dropped by more than 90 percent. The medical community had assumed that less crowded living conditions and the use of antibiotics were keeping the disease at bay. Some physicians even went so far as to call rheumatic fever a "vanishing disease in suburbia."

That complacency was shaken in the mid-1980s when outbreaks of rheumatic fever were reported among children and young adults in various cities scattered throughout the country. Those reports were followed by others of a new and deadly form of strep infection that was afflicting adults. This disease, which is called toxic streptococcal syndrome, made the headlines when public television's "Sesame

"Strep Demands Immediate Care," by Margie Patlak, *FDA Consumer*, October 1991, updated in April 2001 by Dr. David A. Cooke, MD, Diplomate, American Board of Internal Medicine.

Street" puppeteer Jim Henson was reported to have died from it in 1990. There's also evidence to suggest that blood infections caused by Group A strep are on the rise.

"Group A *Streptococcus* seems to have taken a little twist again," says Rosemary Roberts, MD, a medical officer with the Food and Drug Administration's (FDA) division of anti-infective drug products. "We're seeing manifestations like rheumatic fever that we haven't seen for awhile, as well as more invasive strains of Group A strep that are making people sicker much more quickly."

The jury isn't in yet on why Americans are experiencing such a boost in the severity of strep infections. Preliminary findings by researchers at the national Centers for Disease Control in Atlanta suggest that a population increase among previously rare strep types may be behind both the recent rheumatic fever outbreaks and cases of the new toxic streptococcal syndrome. Heightened production of disease-causing toxins by more common strep types may also be responsible for the latest strep casualties.

There are more than 80 known types of Group A *Streptococcus*, which can cause more than a dozen different illnesses. Group A *Streptococcus*, in turn, is part of a broader category of strep organisms that cause an even larger number of diseases.

Some of the more well-known Group A strep afflictions include upper respiratory diseases such as strep throat and scarlet fever, skin disorders such as impetigo, and inflammatory diseases such as rheumatic fever or kidney disease. In addition, blood infections due to Group A strep are a serious and frequent complication of wounds or surgery.

Group A strep infections are treatable with antibiotics, the drug of choice being penicillin. Other antibiotics, such as erythromycin and various cephalosporins, are effective alternatives for patients allergic to penicillin. FDA is responsible for ensuring the safety and effectiveness of these drugs.

Strep Throat

Strep throat (streptococcal pharyngitis) is probably the most well-known Group A strep infection. Although strep throat can occur at any age and at any time of the year, it mainly afflicts school-age children during the winter and spring. The many symptoms of strep throat include an extremely red and painful sore throat, ear pain, fever, enlarged and tender lymph nodes in the neck, white spots on the tonsils, or dark red spots on the soft palette. However, about 1 out of 5 people who has strep throat experiences no symptoms.

Because nearly all the symptoms of strep throat can also occur with viral infections, laboratory tests are used to confirm a doctor's suspicion that a patient's sore throat is caused by Group A strep. The traditional laboratory test to identify strep is a throat culture. To isolate and identify Group A strep from a throat swab takes from one to three days using the culture method. In recent years, a number of tests have become available that use antibodies to detect the presence of Group A strep directly on a throat swab, and these devices can provide test results in a matter of minutes. The different test kits available vary in their accuracy, and some do not detect as many positive results as the culture method. Therefore, if the rapid test is negative, a follow-up throat culture may be recommended.

Strep throat is highly contagious among children because they are in close contact with one another. In addition, they have not yet developed resistance to any of the strains, as adults have.

The incubation period for strep throat is two to five days. During epidemics, siblings of a strep throat patient have a fifty-fifty chance of also developing the disease, whereas only 20 percent of the parents of such patients will develop strep throat. Children with strep throat should not return to school until their fever returns to normal and they've had at least a day's worth of antibiotics.

Strep throat is easily treated with antibiotics in affected persons. However, there is no need to test or treat others who have been in contact with an infected person unless they develop symptoms themselves. Individuals who harbor the strep throat microbe but show no signs of an active infection are unlikely to spread infection to others, according to the American Academy of Pediatrics, or experience the complications of a strep infection.

Scarlet Fever

One of the more colorful variants of a strep infection is scarlet fever. The hallmarks of this disease include a bright red tongue, a brilliant scarlet rash (particularly on the trunk, arms and thighs), a flushed face, sore throat, and fever.

"Scarlet fever is simply strep throat with a rash," says Roberts. The red rash that typifies this disease is prompted by a toxin generated by the *Streptococcus* bacterium. At present, only a small minority of strains of strep produce this particular toxin, so Scarlet Fever remains rare. The striking symptoms of scarlet fever make it easy to diagnose, but most physicians confirm their clinical diagnosis with laboratory tests.

Like strep throat, scarlet fever primarily afflicts school-aged children during the winter and spring months. It is treated exactly the same way as ordinary strep throat. Left untreated, it carries the same risk of complications as other strep infections.

Skin Infection

When Group A *streptococci* literally get under the skin, they can foster a common skin disease known as impetigo. This contagious disease frequently afflicts mainly children during the summer, when insect bites, cuts, and scrapes are prevalent. These skin infringements serve as portals of entry for the *streptococci*.

Impetigo starts out as a rash of pinhead-sized blisters or pimples that rapidly run together to form yellow, flaky crusts. The impetigo rash may itch or burn, but rarely causes pain. The disease is diagnosed with the aid of cultures of the fluid lodged beneath the crusts. If large numbers of strep bacteria crop up in these cultures, their guilt in causing the disease is firmly established. Impetigo can also be caused by other bacteria, including *Staphylococcus*, or by mixtures of staphylococcal and streptococcal bacteria.

Impetigo is combated with the use of topical or oral antibiotics, depending on its severity and frequency within a given population. Doctors advise impetigo patients to remove the skin crusts and wash their rash with soap on a regular basis. Rarely, if not treated, streptococcal impetigo develops into a blood infection, and it can also foster kidney disease.

Rheumatic Fever

Probably the most serious and feared complication of strep infections is rheumatic fever. Although a relatively uncommon disease, the effects of rheumatic fever are serious enough to warrant concern. Signs of rheumatic fever include a red rash, pea-sized lumps under the skin, tender joints, fever, involuntary jerky movements, heart palpitations, chest pain, and, in severe cases, heart failure. Although most symptoms disappear within weeks to months, about half the time the disease leaves behind deformed heart valves that may limit patients' physical activities and foster premature death from heart failure.

Diagnosis of rheumatic fever is based on its symptoms in conjunction with a history of a recent strep infection, which can be confirmed by tests for strep antibodies in the blood.

Rheumatic fever is thought to be triggered by an overly active immune system, which inadvertently destroys body tissues in its zeal to rid the body of a strep infection. Most symptoms of rheumatic fever crop up one to four weeks after a strep infection, although involuntary jerky movements may not surface for as long as six months after infection. About half of the recent cases of rheumatic fever, however, developed with mild to no previous signs of a strep throat infection, such as a sore throat with fever.

It's these signs of a strep infection that physicians rely on to prevent rheumatic fever. As many as 3 percent of untreated cases of strep throat can develop into rheumatic fever. The good news, however, is that antibiotics can prevent rheumatic fever even if not started until several days after the onset of symptoms. Therefore, it is safe in most cases to wait for the results of a throat culture before starting antibiotics if the diagnosis is in question.

Once rheumatic fever occurs, doctors can do little to prevent its damage in the body. Anti-inflammatory drugs (such as aspirin or steroids) can ease many of the symptoms and possibly prevent some of rheumatic fever's more serious developments. Antibiotics are also used to treat any lingering strep infections. But even with such therapies, the disease often wreaks such damage on heart valves that they have to be surgically repaired or replaced with synthetic or animal implants.

Rheumatic fever usually recurs whenever its victims experience any new strep infections. To prevent such flare-ups, the American Heart Association recommends that anyone who has experienced rheumatic fever take prophylactic (preventive) doses of antibiotics. How long rheumatic fever patients require such a preventive drug regime depends on whether they experienced heart damage and whether they're likely to develop a future strep infection. Children who've had rheumatic fever, for example, generally take antibiotics on a daily or weekly basis until they reach adulthood, when the risk of a strep infection greatly diminishes.

Kidney Disease

The other dreaded complication of strep infections is post-streptococcal glomerulonephritis. This is a sudden, intense inflammation of the kidneys that can cause kidney failure. All kinds of strep infections can foster an inflammation of the kidneys (acute glomerulonephritis), but it most often follows impetigo. Less than 1 percent of all strep infections foster kidney disease, but because certain strains of strep are particularly prone to causing this complication, small epidemics of acute glomerulonephritis can crop up in private homes or in schools.

Symptoms of the disorder include a puffy face due to water retention, blood in the urine, pain in the loins, malaise, nausea, headache, and high blood pressure. These symptoms usually surface one to three weeks following a strep infection and subside within the same amount of time.

Diagnosis of acute post-streptococcal glomerulonephritis is based on symptoms, a history of a recent strep infection, and elevated levels of antibodies to strep in the blood. This form of kidney disease, like rheumatic fever, is thought to stem from an overactive immune response to strep.

Little can be done to prevent this heightened immune response once it's begun, although various drugs (such as diuretics) and dietary measures (such as restricted salt or protein intake) can ease many of its symptoms. Most patients recover without any permanent problems, although occasionally kidney damage inflicted by the disease may require dialysis or a kidney transplant.

Patients rarely experience a recurrence of acute glomerulonephritis following additional strep infections because of the immunity they develop to the specific type of strep bacterium that caused their disorder. (Only a handful of strep types can cause glomerulonephritis, and most cases of the disorder can be traced to a specific Group A streptococcal strain known as Type 12.)

Blood Infection

Although the number of bloodstream infections (septicemia) of Group A strep appears to be on the rise, they are still extremely rare. Only about 4 to 5 people out of 100,000 develop these infections each year, according to the national Centers for Disease Control in Atlanta. But nearly one-third of all patients with *Streptococcus* blood infections will die from them.

Septicemia usually gets its start when streptococcal bacteria on the skin delve into an opening as large as a surgical or battle wound or as small as a minor cut or scrape. Normally, the body's immune system checks these bloodstream invaders before they wreak havoc in the body. In those individuals whose resistance is lowered, however, *Streptococcus* travels far and wide, causing such symptoms as fever, low blood pressure, chills, confusion, diarrhea, vomiting, or a red skin rash. Septicemia usually afflicts people over 60 who have an underlying disease such as diabetes or renal failure that compromises their immune defenses.

In addition to relying on clinical signs to diagnose septicemia, physicians use laboratory findings, including positive blood cultures, positive antibody tests, and extremely high numbers of white blood cells in the blood.

Toxic Streptococcal Syndrome

The new toxic streptococcal syndrome, first described in 1987 in this country, is similar to septicemia. Patients with this disorder have many of the same symptoms as those of septicemia, but because of the disease's rapid progression, by the time they seek treatment they are often gravely ill. Toxic streptococcal syndrome patients frequently go into shock and experience multi-organ failure, as well as complications such as the pneumonia that reportedly killed Jim Henson.

Only 1 or 2 people out of 100,000 fall prey to toxic streptococcal syndrome each year. Unlike septicemics, most of these patients don't have any underlying diseases hampering their immune defenses. Of 21 cases studied extensively by researchers, most patients were in their 30s and the youngest was 25 years old.

"The individuals who are getting strep septicemia and toxic strep syndrome," points out Centers for Disease Control (CDC) epidemiologist Walter Straus, "are not the same ones who are getting strep throat."

Patients with toxic streptococcal syndrome are treated with antibiotics as well as with medical measures aimed at curbing the severe complications of the disease. The sooner patients are treated with antibiotics, the more likely they will recover from the syndrome, which kills about one-third of its victims.

Whether Group A *Streptococcus* infects the skin, blood, internal organs, or the throat, it is usually checked by prompt and appropriate antibiotic therapy. This is why, though recent outbreaks of serious strep infections are cause for some concern, they are not likely to prompt the extensive death or debilitation once tied to them.

Signs of a Group A Strep Infection

- sore throat accompanied by fever
- chest pain
- shortness of breath
- shock
- red rash accompanied by fever

351

- tender joints
- involuntary jerky movements
- blood in urine
- yellow flaky crusts on the skin
- puffy face and malaise

Persons developing any of these symptoms should seek immediate medical care.

The Streptococci *Family*

The streptococcal bacteria are extremely versatile and common. Able to invade almost any part of the body, *streptococci* cause a host of diseases. These microbes are divided into more than a dozen different groups, based on the proteins they harbor in their cell walls and their performance on various laboratory tests. Here's a list of some of the more troublesome categories or species of *Streptococcus* and the diseases for which they are well known:

- Group A: strep throat, scarlet fever, rheumatic fever, impetigo, toxic streptococcal syndrome, streptococcal kidney disease, blood infections
- Group B: blood infections in newborns, meningitis, childbed fever
- Groups C, D, G, H, K: urinary tract infections, heart infections, meningitis, upper and lower respiratory tract infections
- *Streptococcus* mutans: dental caries (cavities)
- *Streptococcus* pneumoniae: pneumonia, ear infections, meningitis, sinus infections.

—by Margie Patlak

Margie Patlak is a freelance writer in Elkins Park, Pennsylvania.

Chapter 57

Tetanus

Bacteria Causes Tetanus

Tetanus is an acute, often fatal, disease caused by an toxic substance produced by bacteria *Clostridium tetani* (*C. tetani*). It is characterized by generalized rigidity and convulsive spasms of skeletal muscles. The muscle stiffness usually involves the jaw (lockjaw) and neck and then becomes generalized.

C. tetani is a slender, gram-positive, anaerobic rod that may develop a terminal spore, giving it a drumstick appearance. The spores are widely distributed in soil and in the intestine and feces of horses, sheep, cattle, dogs, cats, rats, guinea pigs, and chickens. Manure-treated soil may contain large numbers of spores. In agricultural areas, a significant number of human adults may harbor the organism. The spores can also be found on skin surfaces and in contaminated heroin.

C. tetani usually enters the body through a wound. In the presence of anaerobic (low oxygen) conditions, the spores germinate. Toxins are produced, and disseminated via blood and lymphatics. Toxins act at several sites within the central nervous system, including peripheral motor end plates, spinal cord, brain, and sympathetic nervous system. The typical clinical manifestations of tetanus are caused when tetanus toxin interferes with release of neurotransmitters, blocking inhibitor impulses. This leads to unopposed muscle contraction and spasm.

Excerpted from *Epidemiology and Prevention of Vaccine-Preventable Diseases, 7th Edition*, Centers for Disease Control and Prevention, April 2002.

353

Seizures may occur, and the autonomic nervous system may also be affected.

Clinical Features

The incubation period varies from 3 to 21 days, usually about 8 days. In general the further the injury site is from the central nervous system, the longer the incubation period. The shorter the incubation period, the higher the chance of death. In neonatal tetanus, symptoms usually appear from 4 to 14 days after birth, averaging about 7 days.

The most common type (about 80 percent) of reported tetanus is generalized tetanus. The disease usually presents with a descending pattern. The first sign is trismus or lockjaw, followed by stiffness of the neck, difficulty in swallowing, and rigidity of abdominal muscles. Other symptoms include a temperature rise of 2 to 4 degrees centigrade above normal, sweating, elevated blood pressure, and episodic rapid heart rate. Spasms may occur frequently and last for several minutes. Spasms continue for 3 to 4 weeks. Complete recovery may take months.

Neonatal tetanus is a form of generalized tetanus that occurs in newborn infants. Neonatal tetanus occurs in infants born without protective passive immunity, because the mother is not immune. It usually occurs through infection of the unhealed umbilical stump, particularly when the stump is cut with an unsterile instrument. Neonatal tetanus is common in some developing countries (estimated over 270,000 deaths worldwide per year), but very rare in the United States.

Medical Management

All wounds should be cleaned; necrotic tissue and foreign material should be removed. If tetanic spasms are occurring, supportive therapy and maintenance of an adequate airway are critical.

Tetanus immune globulin (TIG) is recommended for persons with tetanus. TIG can only help remove unbound tetanus toxin. It cannot effect toxin bound to nerve endings. A single intramuscular dose of 3000 to 5000 units is generally recommended for children and adults, with part of the dose infiltrated around the wound if it can be identified. Intravenous immune globulin (IVIG) contains tetanus antitoxin and may be used if TIG is not available.

Due to the extreme potency of the toxin, tetanus disease does not result in tetanus immunity. Active immunization with tetanus toxoid should begin or continue as soon as the person's condition has stabilized.

How Is Tetanus Transmitted?

Tetanus is primarily transmitted by contaminated wounds (apparent and inapparent). The wound may be major or minor. In recent years, however, a higher proportion of cases had minor wounds, probably because severe wounds are more likely to be properly managed. Tetanus may follow elective surgery, burns, deep puncture wounds, crush wounds, otitis media (ear infections), dental infection, animal bites, abortion, and pregnancy.

During 1995–1997 (the most recent years data are available), acute injuries such as punctures, lacerations and abrasions accounted for 64 percent of reported cases of tetanus. Thirteen of those with acute injuries reported stepping on a nail. Other acute injuries included self-performed body piercing and tattooing, animal bites, and splinters. Twenty-two (18 percent) of cases reported injection drug use (IDU). Three cases were reported after surgical procedures (hemorrhoid banding, spine implant, knee surgery). Eight cases had various chronic wounds. Three had diabetes mellitus without a known injury or wound. The type of injury or condition was unknown for 8 reported cases.

Tetanus is not contagious from person to person. It is the only vaccine-preventable disease that is infectious, but not contagious.

Preventing Tetanus

A marked decrease in mortality occurred from the early 1900s to the late 1940s. In the late 1940s, tetanus toxoid was introduced into routine childhood immunization and tetanus became nationally notifiable. At that time, there were 500–600 cases reported per year (approximately 0.4 cases per 100,000 population).

After the 1940s, reported tetanus incidence rates fell steadily. Since the mid-1970s, 50–100 cases have been reported annually (about 0.05 cases per 100,000). The death-to-case ratio has declined from 30 percent to approximately 10 percent in recent years. A provisional all-time low of 27 cases (0.02 cases per 100,000) were reported in 2001. Almost all reported cases of tetanus are in persons who have either never been vaccinated, or who completed a primary series, but have not had a booster in the preceding 10 years.

Tetanus toxoid used for immunization is available as a single antigen preparation, combined with diphtheria as pediatric DT or adult

Td, and with both diphtheria toxoid and acellular pertussis vaccine as DTaP. Pediatric formulations (DT and DTaP) contain a similar amount of tetanus toxoid as adult Td, but contain 3–4 times as much diphtheria toxoid. Children younger than 7 years of age should receive either DTaP or pediatric DT. Persons 7 years of age or older should receive the adult formulation (adult Td), even if they have not completed a series of DTaP or pediatric DT. There is virtually no reason to use single antigen tetanus toxoid. Tetanus toxoid should be given in combination with diphtheria toxoid, since periodic boosting is needed for both antigens.

After a primary series of three properly spaced doses of tetanus toxoid in persons 7 years of age and older and four doses in children under 7 years of age, essentially all recipients achieve antitoxin levels considerably greater than the minimal protective level of 0.01 IU/ml.

Following a properly administered primary series, virtually all persons develop a protective level of antitoxin. Antitoxin levels fall over time. While some persons may be protected for life, most persons have antitoxin levels that approach the minimal protective level by 10 years after the last dose. As a result, routine boosters are recommended every 10 years. Cases of tetanus occurring in fully immunized persons whose last dose was within the last 10 years are extremely rare.

Chapter 58

Toxocariasis

What is toxocariasis?

Toxocariasis is an infection caused by the parasitic roundworms commonly found in the intestines of dogs (*Toxocara canis*) and cats (*T. cati*). In the United States, an estimated 10,000 cases of *Toxocara* infections occur yearly in humans.

What are symptoms of toxocariasis?

There are two forms of toxocariasis:

Ocular larva migrans (OLM). *Toxocara* infections can cause OLM, an eye disease that can cause blindness. OLM occurs when a microscopic worm enters the eye; it may cause inflammation and formation of a scar on the retina. Each year more than 700 people infected with *Toxocara* experience permanent partial loss of vision.

Visceral larva migrans (VLM). Heavier, or repeated *Toxocara* infections, while rare, can cause VLM, a disease that causes swelling of the body's organs or central nervous system. Symptoms of VLM, which are caused by the movement of the worms through the body, include fever, coughing, asthma, or pneumonia.

Centers for Disease Control and Prevention (CDC), Division of Parasitic Diseases (DPD), http://www.cdc.gov/ncidod/dpd/parasites/toxocara/factsht_ toxocara.htm, reviewed March 2002.

How serious is infection with Toxocara?

In most cases, *Toxocara* infections are not serious, and many people, especially adults infected by a small number of larvae (immature worms), may not notice any symptoms. The most severe cases are rare, but are more likely to occur in young children, who often play in dirt, or eat dirt (pica) contaminated by dog or cat stool.

How is toxocariasis spread?

The most common *Toxocara* parasite of concern to humans is *T. canis*, which puppies usually contract from the mother before birth or from her milk. The larvae mature rapidly in the puppy's intestines; when the pup is 3 or 4 weeks old, they begin to produce large numbers of eggs that contaminate the environment through the animal's stool. The eggs soon develop into infective larvae.

How can I get toxocariasis?

You or your children can become infected after accidentally ingesting (swallowing) infective *Toxocara* eggs from larvae in soil or other contaminated surfaces.

What should I do if I think I have toxocariasis?

See your health care provider to discuss the possibility of infection and, if necessary, to be examined. A blood test is available for diagnosis.

What is the treatment for toxocariasis?

VLM is treated with antiparasitic drugs, usually in combination with anti-inflammatory medications. Treatment of OLM is more difficult and usually consists of measures to prevent progressive damage to the eye.

Who is at risk for toxocariasis?

Young children; owners of dogs and cats.

How can you prevent toxocariasis?

- Have your veterinarian treat your dogs and cats, especially young animals, regularly for worms.

- Wash your hands well with soap and water after playing with your pets and after outdoor activities, especially before you eat. Teach children to always wash their hands after playing with dogs and cats and after playing outdoors.

- Do not allow children to play in areas that are soiled with pet or other animal stool.

- Clean your pet's living area at least once a week. Feces should be either buried or bagged and disposed of in the trash.

- Teach children that it is dangerous to eat dirt or soil.

Part Seven

Chronic Conditions

Chapter 59

Caring for a Seriously Ill Child

Taking care of a chronically ill child is one of the most draining and difficult tasks a parent can face. A prolonged childhood illness affects all family members emotionally and physically and changes relationships within the family. Luckily, this tough balancing act doesn't have to be accomplished alone: support groups, social workers, and family friends often can lend a helping hand.

Explaining Long-Term Illness

Experts once believed that the less a sick child knew about his medical condition, the better. But this protective posture is no longer the norm.

"Honest communication is the most important element in helping a child adjust to a long-term medical condition," says Donna Copeland, PhD. "Children should know that they have a serious illness and that they will have lots of medicine, but that the end goal is to get them well."

Communicating medical information clearly and honestly to your child means addressing his needs in an age-appropriate manner. "Even the smallest baby can be reassured," Dr. Copeland notes. "An

This information was provided by KidsHealth, one of the largest resources online for medically reviewed health information written for parents, kids, and teens. For more articles like this one, visit www.KidsHealth.org, or www. TeensHealth.org. © 2001 The Nemours Center for Children's Health Media, a division of The Nemours Foundation. Reprinted with permission.

extra calming touch or soothing tone of voice lets the child know you're there."

When dealing with an older, verbal child, you should use correct medical terminology. The aim is not to frighten your child, but to give him the words to communicate information and concerns to medical professionals and others. "The words malignant or cancer don't have the same implications for a 3-year-old child that they do for adults," says Dale Perkel, an oncology social worker.

To maintain your child's trust, treatments and their possible discomfort also should be accurately explained to sick children. "Don't say, 'This won't hurt,'" Perkel advises if the procedure is likely to be painful. Instead, tell your child that a procedure may cause some discomfort, but then reassure him that you'll be there to support him.

Although some parents may prefer to discuss the medical facts with their child alone, others invite a doctor to answer specific questions a child may have about treatment or care issues. Many hospitals offer parents the choice of talking to their child about a long-term diagnosis alone, addressing the child with the doctor present, or including the entire medical team made up of doctors, social workers, and nurses. Perkel prefers the team approach, which allows the child to see that everyone (including his parents) is working together and that he can ask questions and get immediate and accurate answers.

Tackling Tough Emotions

Dr. Copeland urges children to regularly express their fears and feelings about changes to their bodies throughout a long-term illness. You can also ask your child what he is experiencing and listen to everything he has to say before bringing up your own feelings and explanations.

"You can't always promise everything is going to be fine," she warns. "Children need to acknowledge the reality of the situation." This kind of communication doesn't always have to be verbal. Dr. Copeland points out that music, drawing, or writing can often help a child living with a life-threatening disease to express his emotions and to escape through a fantasy world of his own design.

Your child may also need reminders that he is not responsible for his illness. "Sometimes children lapse into magical thinking, and they may connect their own behavior with their disease. Reassure them that neither they nor anyone else has caused their illness," Perkel says.

Childhood Behavior

Although kids with chronic long-term illnesses certainly require extra TLC (tender loving care), Perkel notes that special medical requirements don't eliminate the routine needs of childhood. The foremost—and perhaps trickiest—task for worried parents is to treat a sick child as normally as possible. Despite the circumstances, this means setting limits on unacceptable behavior, sticking to a regular routine, and avoiding overindulgence. Although this may seem impossible to a guilt-ridden or overprotective parent, spoiling or coddling your child can make it harder for him to readjust when he becomes well.

When your child leaves the hospital for home, normalcy remains the goal. All children need to visit with friends, go to school or receive homebound instruction, and have private time alone. As much as possible, it helps for parents to respect these aspects of childhood.

Siblings

Family dynamics can be severely tested by the demands of a sick child. Clinic visits, checkups, and changes in physical appearance can prove demanding and at times, overwhelming. To ease these pressures, experts encourage families to try to maintain as normal a family routine as possible. Siblings should continue to attend school and their usual recreational activities; the family should attempt to provide some predictability and time for everyone to be together.

Flexibility is key. "The old 'normal' may have been the entire family around the table for a home cooked meal at 5, while the new 'normal' may be take-out pizza on clinic nights," Perkel says.

Ask school personnel to note any changes in behavior among the siblings of a sick child. Reactions to a brother's or sister's illness can take many different forms. Siblings of the chronically ill child may show the signs of stress by becoming angry, sullen, resentful, fearful, or withdrawn. They may pick fights or fall behind in schoolwork. Conversely, such children may also become too good, taking on an overly mature role in an attempt to protect their parents from further harm. In all cases, parents should pay close attention. Siblings who feel shunted aside by the demands of a sick child have been shown to be prime candidates for future emotional difficulties.

To keep siblings from feeling excluded, brothers and sisters of a sick child can and should be included in the treatment process. Depending on their ages and interest, visiting the hospital, meeting the nursing and physician staff, or accompanying their sick sibling to the clinic for treatments can also help make the situation less frightening and more understandable.

"What they imagine about the illness and hospital visits are often a lot worse than the reality," Perkel notes. "When they come to the hospital, hopefully they'll develop a more realistic picture and see that, while unpleasant things may be part of the treatment, there are also people who care about their sibling and try to minimize discomfort."

Stress Busters

Although no magic potion exists to reduce the stress involved in caring for a child with a long-term illness, there are ways to ease the strain. They include:

- Break problems into manageable parts. If your child's treatment is expected to be given over an extended time, Perkel suggests viewing it in more manageable time blocks. Planning a week or a month at a time may be less overwhelming.

- Attend to your own needs. Get appropriate rest and food. To the extent possible, pay attention to your relationship with your spouse, hobbies, and friendships.

- Depend on friends. Let them car pool siblings to soccer or theater practice. Permit others—relatives, friends—to share responsibilities of caring for your child. Remember that you can't do it all.

- Ask for help in managing the financial implications of your child's illness.

- Recognize that everyone handles stress differently. If you and your spouse have distinct worrying styles, talk about them and try to accommodate them. Don't pretend that they don't exist.

- Develop collaborative working relationships with health care professionals. Realize you are all part of the team. Ask questions and learn all you can about your child's illness.

- Consult other parents in support groups at your care center or hospital. They can offer information and understanding.

Chapter 60

Children with Cancer

Chapter Contents

Section 60.1

Basic Information about Cancer in Children

Excerpted from "Young People with Cancer, A Handbook for Parents," Chapters 1–3, National Cancer Institute (NCI), originally published in January 1993. Updated in January, 2001 by Dr. David A. Cooke, MD, Diplomate, American Board of Internal Medicine.

Introduction

Cancer is actually a group of diseases, each with its own name, its own treatment, and its own chances of control or cure. It occurs when a particular cell or group of cells begins to multiply and grow uncontrollably, crowding out the normal cells. Cancer may take the form of leukemia, which develops from the white blood cells, or solid tumors, found in any part of the body.

Despite considerable and continuing research, no one knows why children get cancer. Some common misconceptions about cancer are addressed below:

1. So far as scientists have been able to determine, nothing you or your child did or didn't do caused the disease. Cancer in children is still a largely unexplained disease, and there is no evidence that you could have prevented it.

2. Few cases of childhood cancer are due to genetic (inherited) factors.

3. In almost all cases of childhood cancer, its appearance in one child does not mean that a brother or sister is more likely to develop it.

4. Cancer is not contagious. It cannot be spread from person to person like a cold, or from an animal to a person.

5. No food or food additive has been implicated as a cause of any childhood cancer.

Leukemia

Leukemia is a cancer of the blood and develops in the bone marrow, the body tissue that produces blood cells. The bone marrow is a jelly-like substance that fills the inside of the bones.

Solid Tumors

The word tumor does not always imply cancer. Some tumors (collections of abnormally growing cells) are benign (not cancerous). In discussing tumors that are malignant (cancerous), however, the term solid tumor is used to distinguish between a localized mass of tissue and leukemia. (Leukemia is actually a type of tumor that takes on the fluid properties of the organ it affects—the blood.)

Treatment

Your child's treatment will be based on medical advances learned from treating many other young people. For some types of cancer, treatment programs may be well established. However, research for effective treatments is constantly under way, and your child may be treated under a research protocol (or regimen), which is a general treatment plan that several hospitals use for treatment of one type of cancer. The protocol is carefully designed to establish the ideal type, frequency, and duration of treatment.

Still, because children's reactions to therapy vary, the treatments may need to be modified to allow for individual differences. If a child is unable to tolerate a treatment plan or protocol, and minor adjustments do not correct this, another treatment plan may be begun or a specially designed program created. Before any therapy begins, the doctor should discuss the treatment program with you, including benefits and risks, and obtain your consent. Depending on the hospital's policy on the age at which a patient's agreement is necessary to undertake therapy, your child may also be required to approve it.

The treatment plan may look complicated at first, but each of the steps will be carefully explained, and you will soon become familiar with the routine.

At the treatment center, your child may be seen by different physicians from time to time, all of whom will follow the basic treatment plan. Your child may also be examined by resident physicians, fellows, and medical students who are working in the center as part of the educational program in cancer medicine and pediatrics. All residents and fellows are experienced physicians who are near the end of their training period, and their work is supervised by a senior physician.

In addition to these physicians at the treatment center, your family physician or pediatrician may continue to play an active role in the care of your child. With current information on the therapy prescribed for your child, your doctor can remain a source of advice and treatment for routine medical care and problems. Especially if distance between your home and the treatment center is a factor, your local physician may be called on to do blood tests or administer chemotherapy prescribed by the center physicians; thus, the number of visits to the center may be reduced. If that is the case, your child's initial hospitalization or outpatient treatment will usually take place at the center, and you will return there for periodic checkups.

The exact type of treatment your child will receive depends on the type of cancer. Most patients receive surgery, radiation therapy, chemotherapy, or a combination of these. These treatments aim at bringing about a remission, the decrease or disappearance of symptoms of the cancer. There are two major phases of treatment: remission induction and remission maintenance. Remission induction attempts to establish a "clinical" remission, in which detectable cancer has been eliminated. If this phase is successful, maintenance therapy aims at reaching undetectable cancer cells, which experience has shown may remain in the body. Remission induction may be accomplished through surgery, radiation, or chemotherapy. Maintenance therapy involves the use of chemotherapy and may last only a few months or go on for several years.

Hospitalization

Hospitalization can be a traumatic experience for any child. Experiencing difficult medical procedures and continually meeting new people who do all sorts of things to the child build up tension. The young patient may become nervous, anxious, and unruly. For the hospitalized child, some form of outlet in play is essential.

Most hospitals have playrooms for patients. These offer children an opportunity to interact with one another in a way similar to their play with friends at home. In hospital playrooms, children may relax and become less fearful and better able to cope with their feelings about hospital equipment, medical procedures, and medical personnel. They may act out their concerns in play and thus deal with them in their own way.

Playrooms may also be equipped to provide outlets for the energies of older children and adolescents who may enjoy taking part in crafts of playing games appropriate to their ages. Video games and tape players for use in the playroom or their own rooms are popular with teens.

Hospitalization threatens the growing sense of independence in older children. The young person is taken to the doctor, taken to the hospital, given treatment. This role is passive rather than active. The lack of independence resulting from hospitalization and cancer treatment is particularly displeasing to the adolescent, who may frequently and loudly protest the forced dependence. It is not uncommon for adolescents to refuse treatment, break hospital rules, miss outpatient appointments, or undertake activities against the doctor's orders. Besides rebelling against the feelings of dependence, teenagers may be acting on the normal adolescent resistance to authority figures and reluctance to appear different from peers outside the hospital. Parents can help by allowing the adolescent a share of the responsibility for his or her own care and by respecting the need for independence and privacy, hard as that may be under the circumstances. But more than anything else, your teenager needs to know that you are there if you are needed and that you can be relied on for honest, dependable answers.

Surgery

For many solid tumors, surgery is the primary and most effective treatment. For very large tumors, radiation or chemotherapy is often used before surgery to reduce the size of the tumor, make surgery safer for the patient, and lessen any physical or functional defects.

The young person facing surgery is likely to be afraid. To counter some of that fear, many hospitals prepare patients for surgery by letting them visit the operating and recovery rooms, where they can meet and talk with the people who will be present during the operation. These people explain what they will be doing and how they will look. They might, for instance, bring along a surgical mask and put it on for the younger child. This advance preparation can at least ease the shock and accompanying fear of the sterile operating room, strange equipment, and uniformed, masked personnel.

Your child will have questions about the surgery, and these must be answered as honestly as possible, because the child may feel betrayed if what you said does not match up with what actually happened.

Chemotherapy

Chemotherapy is treatment with anticancer drugs. These drugs can be given orally (pills or liquids) or by injection. There are several types of injections: into a muscle (intramuscular, or IM), into a vein (intravenous, or IV), into an artery (intra-arterial), or into a cavity (intracavitary). Doctors also inject anticancer drugs into the spinal fluid (intrathecal, or IT) to treat brain tumors and to prevent central nervous system disease in leukemia. Often, special devices, such as catheters and pumps, are used to help deliver the drugs.

Insertion of the IV needle may be painful and, once in the vein, the drugs may cause an uncomfortable burning sensation. If the drug leaks from the vein, it may severely burn the skin, so care must be taken to make sure the IV line is securely in place, and the nurse or doctor must act immediately if the needle comes out of the vein.

Injections are generally given by physicians or nurses, but pills may be given at home. Taking chemotherapy pills can sometimes be a problem with younger children, but the tablets can be broken into smaller pieces for swallowing or powdered and mixed with apple sauce, jam, or custard. Older children, particularly adolescents, may wish to be responsible for taking and keeping track of their oral medication(s). However, it is still important for parents to be familiar with the medications and check to be sure they are being taken correctly.

Whether you or your child is responsible, you may want to develop a system for keeping track of when medications are taken. Marking a special calendar is one way of doing this.

Chemotherapy and Its Side Effects

Anticancer drugs can affect not only cancer cells but also other rapidly dividing normal cells such as those in the gastrointestinal tract, bone marrow, hair follicles, and reproductive system. Because of this, unwanted side effects of the treatment can and often do occur. Most side effects, however, are temporary.

Many side effects from anticancer drugs are possible, and the following points are good to keep in mind:

1. Most side effects can be lessened by taking appropriate measures before, during, and after chemotherapy.

2. Side effects vary in severity and type from person to person and treatment to treatment. Your child will not necessarily have the same reactions as another child, but it is important

for you to be aware of those problems that occur commonly so you can recognize them early.

3. Most side effects are reversible and will improve after the drug is stopped. Some, such as hair loss and bone marrow depression, may lessen or disappear even without discontinuing chemotherapy.

4. Side effects of chemotherapy may be classified as common or uncommon and as acute (immediate) or delayed (days to weeks after chemotherapy).

Common side effects:

*   nausea and vomiting
*   pain and burning at injection site
*   hair loss
*   mouth soreness and ulcers
*   constipation (especially with the drug vincristine)
*   bone marrow depression (low blood counts)

Less common side effects:

*   allergic reactions (hives; rash; swelling of eyelids, hands, and feet; shortness of breath)
*   drug extravasation (leaking of drug out of vein into skin)
*   jaundice (yellow tint to skin and eyes due to liver problems)
*   hemorrhagic cystitis (bloody urine due to bladder irritation especially with the drug cyclophosphamide)
*   mental or nervous system changes (lethargy, tiredness, lack of coordination)

Finally, it is helpful to discuss with your physician any of the listed side effects and any other changes that you observe in your child.

Radiation Therapy

Radiation therapy is treatment with high-energy x-rays. High levels of radiation can kill cells or keep them from growing and dividing. Radiation therapy is used to treat cancer because cancer cells are growing and dividing more rapidly than many of the normal cells around them. In addition, most normal cells appear to recover more fully from radiation effects than cancer cells.

Radiation may be used alone, in combination with surgery or chemotherapy, or both. There is no pain or discomfort during the treatment. It is much like having an ordinary x-ray taken, except that the child needs to hold still for a few minutes longer.

Before therapy is started, a physician specializing in radiation therapy will talk with you and explain the details of the treatment. The physician will also use dye to mark the area to be irradiated. Once in place, this dye should not be washed off for the duration of the treatments, because it will be used as a guide for aiming the radiation. While radiation therapy is being received, soap or lotion should not be used on these lines or within the radiation field, where the skin will become tender. The area should also be kept dry.

Areas of the body not being treated are often protected from radiation by special shields made of lead.

Side Effects of Radiation Therapy and Controlling Them

Your child will not be radioactive during or after radiation therapy. Neither you nor anyone else need fear contact with the child. Among the real side effects of treatment, which vary according to the site receiving the radiation, are:

1. Skin damage. The skin in the treated area may be somewhat sensitive and therefore should be protected against exposure to sunlight and irritation. During treatment, it should not be exposed to sunlight. After treatment is completed, the skin will still be sensitive, and a sun-blocking lotion containing PABA should be used to prevent burning. If the head is affected, soft hats and scarves may be worn. Your physician may also prescribe baby powder or cornstarch, an antibiotic ointment, or steroid cream to relieve itching and pain and to speed healing. Nothing, however, should be applied to the treatment area without the recommendation of the person in charge of the treatment.

2. Sore mouth (if the head and neck are within the irradiated area). Your physician may prescribe a mouth rinse.

3. Hair loss. Hair is frequently lost from the area receiving the radiation therapy. This loss is usually temporary, with hair

growth beginning about 3 months after the completion of treatment. Initial adjustment to even temporary hair loss can be difficult, but after a time, children are able to play, work, and go to school without undue embarrassment. Some will want to wear a wig, cap, or scarf.

4.   Nausea, vomiting, and headaches. A few children have these symptoms following radiation therapy to specific sites, such as the head or abdomen. These problems may last for about 4 or 5 hours and can be relieved by medicines prescribed by your doctor. In terms of diet, small, frequent meals are recommended. You may want to see that your child eats 3 to 4 hours before treatment.

5.   Diarrhea after radiation to the abdomen (or pelvic area). This condition usually responds to simple measures such as non-prescription drugs or medications prescribed by your doctor. A low-residue diet avoiding fresh fruits, vegetables, and fried foods may also help. Occasionally, treatment will have to be suspended until the symptoms subside.

6.   Late effects. Following irradiation to the brain and/or central nervous system, some children seem to be drowsy and need more sleep. This symptom may begin at various times, even as late as 5 to 7 weeks after therapy has been completed. It usually lasts about 5 to 10 days. Several days before the drowsiness occurs, the child may lose his appetite, have fever or headache, have nausea and vomiting, and be irritable in general. This is a temporary condition; nevertheless, it is important to report such symptoms to your physician. Other post therapy symptoms your doctor will want to evaluate are dizziness, sight disturbances, increased appetite, and stiff neck. None of these may occur, but if they do, you should contact the physician.

7.   Long-term effects. Research suggests that radiation therapy to the head may affect intelligence and/or coordination, depending on several factors, including the age of the child at the time of exposure. In some cases, growth may be affected. Research also points to the increased possibility of developing a second tumor in an area treated with radiation. Your child's physician or radiation therapist can tell you more about these long-term effects in relation to your child and the treatment.

New Treatments

The search for new and more effective drugs to treat cancer is a continuing one. Each year, thousands of drugs are tested in experimental animals for activity against cancer. The most promising of these are further studied to determine whether they might be safe and effective for human use and to establish the proper dosage.

Some parents are concerned that if a cure for cancer is found in one hospital, it will not be known in another. Actually, the medical world is relatively small, and in this age of rapid communications, the discovery of a successful new treatment method will become generally known almost immediately.

Unconventional Methods of Cancer Treatment

Unusual remedies and approaches to cancer treatment often achieve public notoriety. As the parent of a child with cancer, inevitably you will hear of these yourself or have them brought to your attention by others. Patients, particularly older ones, may also hear of such treatments.

These treatments may involve unusual forms of therapy or strict dietary regimens that are reported to cure cancer. Despite many claims, no dietary or vitamin therapy has ever been shown to cure or improve cancer, and many patients suffer more from these regimens than from conventional treatment. As a group, these treatment techniques have not been tested in the same strict method as have treatments employed by your physician. Reports of unconventional cures seldom provide enough information to compare their effectiveness with that of more conventional therapies. Be very suspicious of therapies that rely heavily on testimonials to prove themselves; they frequently are frauds. Also keep in mind that some of these therapies are not necessarily safe, and can even cause injuries or death.

The guarantee of cure these treatments offer may seem attractive when judged against the difficult treatment course of conventional therapies and the fact that your physician cannot absolutely predict the results of that treatment. If you develop an interest in an unconventional treatment or have any questions, discuss it with your physician, who should be able to provide or direct you to relevant information. The treatment team's primary concern is that your child receive the most effective treatment possible. If some magical, easy cure for cancer existed, caregivers would be the first to make it available.

Because many people have heard of these alternative methods of cancer treatment, you, or occasionally the older patient, may find yourself in the position of defending your decision to follow conventional treatment methods. This can be a frustrating situation and place a burden on you during an already stressful time. It is important to remember that suggestions are usually well intentioned and that they come from those who are not well informed about treatment advances. The best way to deal with this may be to provide these people with more information and make it clear that you appreciate their interest but that you feel your child is already receiving the best treatment available.

Section 60.2

Talking with Your Child about Cancer

Excerpted from "Talking with Your Child about Cancer," National Cancer Institute (NCI), originally published in January 1993. Reviewed in January 2001 by Dr. David A. Cooke, MD, Diplomate, American Board of Internal Medicine.

Introduction

Learning that your child has cancer is perhaps the hardest news you ever have had to face. As a parent, you must now decide how to tell your child.

The questions that many parents ask are: "What should my child be told?" "Who should tell my child?" and "When should my child be told?" This text was written to help you answer these questions.

You probably already are asking, "Should I tell my child about the cancer at all?" In the past, children were often shielded from the diagnosis. But, studies show that most children know they have a serious illness despite attempts of parents and health care workers to protect them.

Most likely, your child already suspects that something is wrong. He or she may not feel well, is seeing the doctor more often, and has had some uncomfortable and frightening tests. Your child also may sense the anxiety and fears of family members and close friends.

Children who are not told about their illness often depend on their imagination and fears to explain their symptoms. Many children with cancer believe their illness is punishment for something they have done; as a result, they may feel unnecessary anxiety and guilt. Health professionals generally agree that telling children the truth about their illness decreases stress and guilt. Knowing the truth also increases a child's cooperation with treatment. In addition, talking about cancer often helps bring the family closer together and makes dealing with illness a little easier for everyone.

Who Should Tell My Child?

The answer to this question is personal. It depends on the relationship you have with your child and on your own feelings and attitudes. You may want to tell your child yourself, or you may want your child's doctor to help explain the illness. Either way, you or someone close to your child should offer support, encouragement, and love.

If you choose to tell your child yourself, talking to others might help you decide what to say. Health professionals such as your child's doctor, nurse, or social worker can offer ideas. Talk with parents of other children with cancer. Contact members of support groups such as the Candlelighters Childhood Cancer Foundation for advice (to find the Candlelighters chapter nearest you, contact the Candlelighters Childhood Cancer Foundation, P.O. Box 498, Kensington, MD 20895-0498, Toll-Free: 800-366-CCCF, Phone: 301-962-3520, Fax: 301-962-3521; Website: www.candlelighters.org; E-mail: info@candlelighters.org). Thinking about what you want to say, talking it over with other concerned adults, and rehearsing it with someone close to you will help you feel more at ease.

When Should My Child Be Told?

Because you are the best judge of your child's personality and moods, you are probably the best person to decide when your child should be told about the illness. There is no "right" moment to tell a child he or she has cancer. Try to choose a quiet time and place where you and your child can be alone. This will create a calm and supportive atmosphere. It is probably best to talk with your child soon after diagnosis. Waiting days or weeks gives children more time to use their imagination and develop fears that may be hard to get rid of later.

What Should My Child Be Told?

Before you speak with your child, you need to understand the type of cancer he or she has and the treatment that will be given. This way, you will be prepared for questions. Your child will feel more secure if you can provide the correct information.

The amount of information and the way it should be told depend on the child's age and intellectual maturity. As a rule, a gentle, open, and honest approach is best. The following describes general stages in child development and what children are likely to understand about a serious illness at different ages. Please keep in mind that these are only general guidelines. Your child may fit into more than one or none of these categories.

Newborn to 2-Year-Olds

Children this young can't understand an illness such as cancer. They can't see it or touch it. They are more concerned with what's happening to them. Separation from their parents is a major worry. Children more than a year old are concerned with how things feel and how to control things around them. Very young children are most afraid of medical procedures and tests. Many cry, run away, or squirm to try to control what's happening.

After 18 months, children begin to think about what is going on around them. That's why an honest approach is best. Be truthful about trips to the hospital and procedures that may hurt. You can tell your child that needle-sticks will hurt for a minute and that it is okay to cry. This lets your child know that you understand and accept his or her feelings. Your honesty also helps build trust.

Being able to make choices, as long as they do not interfere with treatment or harm health, can increase your child's confidence and sense of control. For example, if a medicine is taken by mouth, your child could choose to have it mixed in apple juice, grape juice, or apple-sauce.

2- to 7-Year-Olds

Children ages 2 to 7 are better able to understand illness. They tend to look at things from one point of view—their own—and believe that the world revolves around them. They link events to one thing. For example, they usually tie illness to a specific event such as staying in bed or eating Jell-O or popsicles. Children at this age often think their illness is caused by a specific action. Therefore, getting better will happen automatically if they follow a set of rules.

Younger children, in particular, need to be reassured often that they did nothing to cause their illness and that their cancer treatment is not punishment for something they have done, said, or thought. Children in this age group also need to have medical procedures explained honestly and realistically. It helps to remind children that all of the tests and treatments are done to help them feel better.

Simple explanations about cancer are also important. Stories that relate cancer to familiar ideas will help in explaining the diagnosis. These comparisons may be tailored to the child's specific cancer type. The 2- to 7-year-old, for example, understands good and bad. Try explaining cancer and treatments in terms of a battle between "good guy cells" and "bad guy cells." Taking medicine will help the good guys become stronger so they can beat the bad guys.

7- to 12-Year-Olds

Children ages 7 to 12 years are still limited by their own experiences but are starting to understand relationships among several events. Thus, they see their illness as a set of symptoms. They are less likely to believe that their illness resulted from something they did. They understand that getting better comes from taking medicines and doing what the doctor says. Children at this age are able to cooperate with treatment.

An explanation of cancer to this child can be more detailed but should still include familiar situations. Comparisons also are useful in explaining cancer to children in this age group. You might say that there are different kinds of cells in the body, and these cells have different jobs to perform. Like people, these cells must work together to get their jobs done. Cancer cells can be described as "troublemakers," that disrupt the work of the good cells. Treatment helps to get rid of the "troublemakers" so the other cells can work together once again.

Although the understanding of death varies among 7- to 12-year olds, many children in this age group think or worry about dying. However, they often are afraid to say anything to you. Be open and honest with your child. Tell your child that you, the doctors, nurses, and others are doing everything they can to make the cancer cells go away. Reassure your child that a lot of children with cancer get better, but no matter what happens, you'll be there. If you are not sure what to say, ask the doctor, nurse, social worker, or chaplain for help.

Keeping Lines of Communication Open

Throughout treatment and followup care, you should continue to talk openly with your child. Like many other children, your child may, with time, ask more complex questions. Setting up patterns of open communication early will support your child now and strengthen your relationship for years to come.

At times, you may feel strong emotions when you are with your child. You do not want to burden your child with your fear, anger, or sadness. But children often are aware of how you feel. In fact, children may hide their own feelings to protect their parents. You may want to discuss your feelings with your child if you think they interfere with your relationship. You can tell your child why you are sad. This reassures your child that you are not angry with him or her and also lets your child express feelings. Let your child know that it is okay to cry and be sad. This gives him or her permission to show feelings.

During treatment, it is important to remember that you, your child, and the health care team are partners. Children who truly feel like a member of this team are more likely to cooperate and to accept treatment. You can help your child by explaining what will happen and allowing him or her to make simple, safe decisions about care.

Questions Your Child May Ask

Children often are curious and may have many questions about their illness and treatment. Your child knows and trusts you and will expect you to respond to questions. Some children will ask questions right away, while others will ask them later. Here are some ideas to help you answer some of the questions your child is likely to ask.

"Why Me?"

Children, like adults, wonder why they have cancer. They may feel strongly that their cancer was caused by something they did. A child with cancer should be told honestly that no one—not even the experts—knows why a person develops cancer. Children need to be reassured that nothing they did, or didn't do, caused their disease. Children also need to know that their illness is not contagious—they did not "catch" cancer from someone else.

"Will I Get Well?"

Often, children know about family members or friends who have died from cancer. As a result, many children are afraid to ask if they will get well; they fear the answer will be "no." You should tell your child that cancer is a serious disease but that the medicine, x-rays, and/or an operation will help to get rid of the cancer. You should also tell your child that the doctors, nurses, and family are trying their best to cure the cancer. By using this approach, you are giving your child an honest, hopeful answer. Knowing there are caring people such as doctors, nurses, counselors, and others also may help your child feel more secure.

"What Will Happen to Me?"

When children are first diagnosed with cancer, many new and frightening things happen to them. While at the doctor's office, clinic, or hospital, they may see other children with cancer who are not feeling well, are bald, or have had amputations. A child may be too afraid to ask questions and may develop unrealistic fears about what will happen. For this reason, children should be told in advance about their treatment and possible side effects. They should know what will be done to help if side effects occur. Children also should know that there are many types of cancer and that what happens to another child will not necessarily happen to them, even if they have the same type of cancer or the same type of treatment.

Children should know about their treatment schedule. They also should be told about any changes in their schedule or in the type of treatment they receive. Having your child keep a calendar that shows the days for doctor's visits, treatments, or special tests will help prepare for these visits.

"Why Must I Take Medicines When I Feel Okay?"

Most of us link taking medicine to feeling sick. It's confusing to children to take medicines when they feel well. Answers to this question may relate back to the original explanation of the cancer. For example, children could be told that even though they are feeling well and have no signs of disease, the "bad-guy cells" are hiding. They must take the medicine for a while longer to help find the bad guys and stop them from coming back.

"What Should I Tell the Kids at School?"

Children with cancer are concerned about how their friends and schoolmates will react. This is especially true when they have missed a lot of school or return with obvious physical changes such as weight loss, weight gain, or hair loss. Encourage your child to keep in touch with close friends and classmates. Friends often want to know what happens when a child is away from school. Encourage your child to talk honestly about the disease and the kind of treatment being given. Suggest that your child reassure friends that they cannot "catch" cancer from anyone. You or one of the teachers at school also may be able to talk to other students.

Try to help your child understand that not all people, including some adults, know about cancer. People who don't understand cancer often act differently or may give your child incorrect information.

Such talks with others may cause your child to have doubts and fears despite all your reassurance. Ask your child about conversations with others so that you can correct any misunderstandings.

You may want to ask your child's doctor, nurse, or social worker about a school conference, classroom presentations, or a school assembly that includes a question and answer session to help other students better understand cancer and what is happening to your child. Your child's teachers or the school counselor can help.

Your child will learn two important lessons about how people react to illness. First, some people, no matter what they are told, may act different because they do not know much about cancer. Second, good friends will remain friends. They know your child is still the same friend as before.

"Will I Be Able to Do the Things I Did before I Got Cancer?"

The answer to this question is individual and depends on the child's type of cancer and treatment. Most likely, your child will need some restrictions at different times during treatment. Tell your child why the doctors or nurses think it's best to restrict certain activities and how long this will last. Help your child substitute one kind of activity for another. For example, you could suggest that friends come over to paint, have a snack, or play video games if the doctor feels that your child should not ride a bike because the chance of injury is high.

Section 60.3

Coping with Cancer

Excerpted from "Young People with Cancer, A Handbook for Parents,"
Chapter 4, National Cancer Institute (NCI), originally published in January 1993. Updated in January 2001 by Dr. David A. Cooke, MD, Diplomate,
American Board of Internal Medicine.

Dealing with the Diagnosis

Even though many parents suspect what the outcome of their child's diagnostic tests will be, the diagnosis confirming these fears comes as a shock. Initial explanations of the disease and treatment may be lost as parents try to come to grips with the reality that their child has cancer. This initial confusion is common, and repeated explanations of the diagnosis, treatment, and possible outcome of the disease may be necessary. Because this is a time when many important decisions must be made, as a parent, you should not be hesitant or embarrassed about asking and re-asking questions about your child's disease and its treatment. Treatment centers often provide printed materials that give further explanations about cancer and its treatment and allow parents to absorb details at their own pace. Many materials are available from the National Cancer Institute (see Chapter 84—Resources for Information about Childhood Diseases" for contact information).

Parents' Initial Reactions

Parents may experience many feelings upon hearing that their child has cancer. Common reactions are denial, anger, guilt, grief, fear, and confusion. These reactions are natural and may be a way of helping you cope with the necessity of accepting a situation that you want to change but cannot. It is important to remember, however, that this is a time when your child needs your support and is particularly sensitive to your moods and feelings.

Although the diagnosis is usually definite once the test results have been examined, parents often ask for a second opinion from another physician. Your physician or treatment center can recommend someone to you, or you may wish to get a recommendation from another source. Second opinions are useful for confirming the diagnosis and reassuring parents about its accuracy and for confirming recommended treatment or exploration of another approach to treatment. However, once the diagnosis and treatment have been agreed upon by two physicians, seeking a third opinion may in fact reflect a parent's need to find another, more acceptable diagnosis. This puts an unfair burden on the sick child and delays treatment.

Accepting the Diagnosis

Gradually, parents realize that their child has cancer and nothing can change it. At this point they begin to cope with the diagnosis and their feelings about it. Some parents become angry. Targets for this anger may vary and can include God, themselves, the physician, or even the sick child for becoming ill. Because it is difficult to express anger toward the sick child, spouses and healthy children can become the scapegoats for unresolved feelings. Parents sometimes lose their tempers. Letting the anger out may occasionally be helpful. It is important to remember, however, that other members of the family experience similar feelings. Realizing that some reactions stem from this anger and talking things through with family members, treatment staff, or others who can give support may help in dealing with these feelings.

Reassuring Your Child

Whatever you tell your child about the illness, he or she may bring up the issue of death and the fears it creates. Be prepared to cope with questions about death, even if they are painful. Refusing to discuss death may deny your child an outlet for some strong and possibly frightening feelings, and it will deny you the opportunity to offer comfort or reassurance. In addition to discussing the child's feelings and fears, it is important to stress to all young people with cancer the fact that cancer can be treated, that research for better methods is ongoing, and that treatments are improving all the time.

Finally, young people of all ages tend to feel guilt and anger at the time of a severe illness. Guilt feelings may stem from the often subconscious feeling that disease is a punishment for being bad. Your child, therefore, needs frequent reassurances that he or she has done nothing wrong and is loved. The child may direct anger inward or at you for letting the illness happen. It is important for you to remember that even when your child is angry with you, your child loves you.

Telling the Brothers and Sisters

The diagnosis of cancer affects the entire family. For the siblings, the initial period can be a time of confusion and fear. Children, even young ones, are sensitive to what is happening. They are aware of a brother's or sister's hospitalization and of trips to the doctor and clinic. They notice their parents crying and trying to comfort one another. They may overhear parts of conversations that are difficult to understand. Children often conspire to figure out what is going on. Pieces of information are gathered, pooled, and analyzed. Because of this, it is important to take time early in the diagnosis and treatment process to have an honest discussion of the situation with the siblings. Explain the facts about cancer, keeping in mind the age and maturity of each child, and update the information periodically as the siblings and patient get older and are able to understand more.

All of the children need to know that cancer is not contagious and that they will not become sick from contact with the patient. They need to be reassured that they are healthy themselves and that the possibility of cancer running in the family is highly unlikely.

Siblings also need to be told emphatically that they are in no way responsible for the illness. Angry outbursts, such as "Drop dead!" or "I hate you," which are said by all normal children at one time or another, frequently haunt a child after learning about a sibling's illness. Feelings of guilt or wrongdoing need to be dealt with immediately. Failure to do so may result in problems later on.

Continuing Life

One of the challenges facing the family of a child with cancer is maintaining a normal life. This is not always an easy task, particularly during moments of high stress such as at the time of diagnosis and during the hospitalizations and relapses. Even when treatment is going successfully, the lives of the patient and family members are influenced by the disease and its treatment and side effects. Schedules are rearranged to accommodate hospitalization or clinic visits, family members may be separated, siblings may feel neglected. Everyone may be worried or tense.

Despite all this, the continued development of family members demands that life continue as normally as possible under the circumstances.

To see that this happens, the sick child should be treated as normally as possible, the needs and feelings of the patient's siblings attended to, and prediagnosis sources of support kept open for both the parents and the child. In addition, new sources of support such as other parents of children with cancer and treatment team members, can help parents cope.

The Parents

To cope with the child's illness and the changes this brings in your own life, you may want to consider the following suggestions:

- Make a special effort to find private times to communicate with your spouse, or if you are a single parent, with others close to you. Don't allow all your discussions to revolve around the sick child. Make time to do things you enjoyed doing together before your child became sick.

- Find ways to reduce the frustration you may feel when clinic visits require waiting for procedures, test results, or consultations with physicians. Bring something to read or do while the child is sleeping or doesn't need your individual attention.

- If work schedules permit and the distance between hospital and home is close enough, you and your spouse may alternate staying with the hospitalized child. This allows both parents to become familiar with the child's life in the hospital and various aspects of treatment. It reduces the gap that may grow between parents when one becomes much more actively involved in the treatment than the other. If you are a single parent, other family members or friends who are close to the child may be able to stay at the hospital occasionally so you can rest.

- Don't hesitate to turn to treatment staff for support. Most treatment centers have psychologists, social workers, nurse clinicians, or chaplains available to talk about special concerns.

- You may want to look for other sources of support. Talk to other parents of children with cancer informally in the hospital or clinic. Your treatment center may have a parents' group supervised by a staff member for more formal discussions. In addition, organizations outside the center may also exist. One national group, the Candlelighters Childhood Cancer Foundation, has local chapters. Treatment center staff may be able to help you locate such a group.

The Patient

Although the diagnosis of cancer will change your child's life for a time, the child still has the same needs as other young people for friends, school, and the activities enjoyed before the illness. You can help by encouraging your child to continue a "normal" life as much as possible.

Friendships may be maintained during hospitalization or when your child is sick at home through visits, letters, or telephone calls.

School

For the school-aged child, continuing with school is vital. School is the major activity of children the same age, and continuing to attend school will reinforce the child's sense of well-being. Furthermore, it prevents the child from falling behind others the same age in learning and in the emotional development that comes from participating in school and school activities. When your child is hospitalized, a special hospital school program may be available. If your child is receiving frequent treatments or is too ill to attend school while at home, a home tutor may be available through the school system (the treatment center may be able to help you arrange for this). But home tutoring should be undertaken with the understanding that it is directed toward easing the eventual return to school.

Discipline

Discipline is important to the normal development of all children. This is no less true when they have cancer. However, the special circumstances of these children's lives may make maintaining discipline more difficult. Having seen their child ill and in pain, parents may attempt to make up for this by giving extra presents or allowing behavior they would not tolerate in another child. They may find it difficult to discipline the child with cancer because of the uncertainty of the future. Although it is true that for many of these young people the future is uncertain, and some will die, discipline is an important part of seeing that the quality of life is maintained.

It may also be tempting to overprotect your child, to keep the child with you and away from situations you cannot control. This may deny your child the opportunity to participate in normal activities necessary for growth and development.

Siblings

Siblings of cancer patients may have many different feelings about the patient, the illness, and the attention the patient receives. While sympathizing with their brother or sister who is ill, they may still feel some resentment and believe that they are being neglected. In many cases, this is true. During times of hospitalization or when the patient is not feeling well, attention may focus on the sick child. As parents, you may not be able to pay as much attention to the siblings as you did before. You may have to miss school functions or ball games in which the siblings are participating. You may have little emotional reserve left after dealing with your sick child to talk with siblings about their concerns, to play with them, or help with their homework.

When you do have the energy, try to make special time for the siblings. Encourage them to become involved in outside activities and make a point of recognizing their achievements. When you can, make plans to spend time alone with them and do things that interest them.

One way to help them to understand their brother's or sister's illness is by involving them in the treatment. Older children in particular welcome the opportunity to be taken into their parents' confidence and will often respond in helpful ways. Finding things for them to do for their sick brother or sister, or their worried parents, gives many young people a sense of belonging and usefulness that might otherwise be lacking in the family's focus on cancer.

Remember, the patient's brothers and sisters may be asked questions about the illness by schoolmates or others in the community. They should have enough information to answer these questions. In fact, you might want to help them anticipate questions or comments and discuss possible answers.

Family and Friends

A diagnosis of cancer affects not only the patient's parents and siblings but also the grandparents, other relatives, and family friends. Ideally, these people can provide support and assistance. They can babysit and spend time with the siblings, stay with the sick child to relieve you, or assist in the many practical problems that arise when a household must continue to function under stress.

Unfortunately, they are not always able to do this. Grandparents may feel particularly lost and helpless, because they are concerned about their grandchild and at the same time cannot stop the suffering of their own child. If grandparents do not understand and accept the situation, you may find yourself in the difficult position of dealing with your own emotional difficulties while attempting to support the grand parents. Treatment team members may be helpful; they can explain the child's condition to the grandparents. Being allowed to participate in meetings of parents' groups may also help grandparents deal with their feelings about the child's illness.

Each family has its own way of relating to relatives, friends, and neighbors. Above all, initial honesty is of real value in the long-term handling of any problems. People want and need to help, but they may need assistance from you to do so. They will need information about the disease and its treatment. Some may have to be told such basics as the fact that cancer is not contagious.

Your employers may also need to be told about your child's sickness so they can understand the reason for requests for time off from work. If you feel it is necessary, the child's doctor may write your employer and explain the situation.

Finally, in their efforts to help, people will give all sorts of advice. If their comments are confusing or upsetting, make a point of discussing them with medical personnel.

Finances

The cost of your child's treatment may cause additional pressure in an already tense situation. The desire to have the best in care may be offset by fear about the costs and how they will be met. As soon as financial questions arise, ask your doctor or the social worker for help.

Because health and life insurance questions can influence major health decisions, you'll need a clear understanding of the coverage your policies offer. Caregivers, particularly medical social workers, can clarify individual policies and help you fill out forms.

You should also keep complete records; store your bills and insurance forms together for easy reference at tax time. Keeping track of bills, your payments, and insurance payments by date and type of charge will simplify this further.

Treatment center staff may also be able to help you with other costs associated with cancer treatment. Check with them to see if you are eligible for special rates for parking or food at the hospital. If your child is hospitalized or needs daily treatment away from home, lodging costs for parents may be substantially reduced if special arrangements have been made. Medical social workers may be familiar with other programs such as those of voluntary cancer related organizations or state or local programs, that may be able to assist you.

Section 60.4

Managing Your Child's Eating Problems during Cancer Treatment

Excerpted from "Managing Your Child's Eating Problems during Cancer Treatment," National Cancer Institute (NCI), originally published in March 1994. Updated in January 2001 by Dr. David A. Cooke, MD, Diplomate, American Board of Internal Medicine.

This section offers practical hints for coping with treatment side effects that may affect your child's appetite.

These suggestions have helped other parents manage eating problems that can be frustrating to handle. Try all the ideas to find what works best for your child.

Loss of Appetite

- Make mealtimes calm and relaxed. Don't hurry meals.

- Encourage normal activities, but don't force them.

- Try changing the time, place, and surroundings of meals, once in a while. A picnic, even if it is in the house, can make mealtime more fun. Watching a favorite TV show or inviting a special friend to join your child at meal or snack time also can enhance willingness to eat.

- Let your child eat whenever hungry. A child does not need to eat just three main meals a day. Several smaller meals throughout the day may be even better. Sometimes having a regular schedule can help the body adjust to a new eating pattern. See what works best for your child.

- Praise good eating. Try using small rewards such as a favorite dessert or new toy, to encourage good eating.

- Avoid arguing, nagging, or punishing. Forcing a child to eat may make the situation worse.

- Offer food often during the day, even at bedtime. Have healthy snacks handy. Taking just a few bites of the right foods or sips of the right liquids every hour or so can help increase protein and calories.

- Ask your child's doctor about medicines that can improve appetite if the problem becomes serious.

Sore Mouth or Throat

- Try soft foods that are easy to chew and swallow such as: ice cream; milkshakes; bananas, applesauce, and other soft fruits; peach, pear, and apricot nectars; watermelon; cottage cheese; mashed potatoes or macaroni and cheese; custards, puddings, and gelatin; scrambled eggs; oatmeal or other cooked cereals; pureed or mashed vegetables such as peas and carrot; pureed meats; liquids.

- Avoid serving your child foods that can irritate the mouth: citrus fruit or juices such as orange, grapefruit, or tangerine; spicy or salty foods such as potato chips; rough, coarse, or dry foods such as raw vegetables, crackers, or toast.

- Cook foods until they are soft and tender.

- Cut foods into small pieces.

- Mix food with butter, thin gravies, and sauces to make it easier to swallow.

- Use a blender or food processor to puree food.

- Give your child a straw for drinking liquids.

- Try serving foods cold or at room temperature. Hot and warm foods can irritate a tender mouth and throat.

- To make swallowing easier, have your child try tilting his or her head back or moving it forward.

- If teeth and gums are sore, the dentist may be able to recommend a special product for teeth cleaning.

- Have your child rinse his or her mouth often with water to help remove food and bacteria and to promote healing.

- Ask the doctor about anesthetic lozenges and sprays that can numb your child's mouth and throat during meals.

Changed Sense of Taste

- Choose and prepare foods that look and smell good.

- If red meat such as beef tastes unpleasant, replace with chicken, turkey, eggs, dairy products, or fish without a strong odor.

- Help the flavor of meat, chicken, or fish by marinating it in sweet fruit juices, Italian dressing, or sweet-and-sour sauce.

- Try using small amounts of flavorful seasonings such as basil, oregano, or rosemary.

- Try tart foods such as oranges or lemonade that may have more taste. A tart lemon custard might taste good and also will provide needed protein and calories. Do not try this if your child also has a sore mouth, throat, or gums.

- Try using bacon, ham, or onion to add flavor to vegetables.

- Stop serving problem foods.

- Try serving foods at different temperatures (cold, unheated, warm, or hot) to see which preparation your child likes best. Warm or hot foods may have more flavor and taste than cold foods. However, do not serve warm or hot foods if your child has a sore throat, mouth, or gums; feels nauseated; or is vomiting.

Talk to your child 's doctor or registered dietitian if a sore throat, mouth, or gums makes eating difficult for your child. They can suggest ways to improve the taste of food without hurting the sore area.

Dry Mouth

- Try very sweet or tart foods and beverages such as lemonade; these foods may help the mouth produce more saliva. Do not try this if your child also has a tender mouth or sore throat.

- Have your child suck on sugar-free hard candy or popsicles or chew sugar-free gum, which also can help produce more saliva. Because some cancer treatments such as radiation therapy can increase the chance of tooth decay, sugar-free candies and gum usually are better than those with sugar.

- Fix soft and pureed foods, which may be easier to swallow.

- Keep your child's lips moist with lip salves.

- Serve foods with sauces, gravies, and salad dressings to make them moist and easier to swallow.

393

- Offer a sip of water every few minutes to help make it easier to swallow and talk.

- To lessen dry mouth, have your child try to breathe through his or her nose rather than through the mouth. If this is too difficult ask the doctor, nurse, or dentist for suggestions.

- If the dry mouth problem is severe, ask your doctor or dentist about products that coat and protect the mouth and throat.

Nausea

- Ask your doctor about medicine to help control nausea. Medicines used to control nausea and vomiting are called antiemetics. Very effective antiemetics have been developed in recent years, and can help immensely.

- Try foods such as: toast and crackers, yogurt, sherbet, pretzels, angel food cake, oatmeal, skinned chicken (baked or broiled, not fried), fruits and vegetables that are soft or bland such as canned peaches, clear liquids sipped slowly, sugar-free hard candies, popsicles, or ice chips.

- Avoid foods such as: fatty, greasy, or fried foods; very sweet foods; spicy, hot foods; and foods with strong odors.

- Have your child eat small amounts of food frequently and slowly.

- Avoid serving meals in a room that is stuffy, too warm, or has cooking odors or scents that might be disagreeable.

- Offer liquids throughout the day, except at meal times. Liquids are filling and may reduce the appetite for solid foods. Some good choices include cooled, liquid, fruit-flavored gelatin and flat soda. Stir the soda until the fizz is gone before serving the drink to your child. Give your child a straw to make drinking easier.

- Serve beverages cool or chilled. Try freezing favorite beverages in ice cube trays.

- Serve foods at room temperature or cooler; hot foods may add to nausea.

- Don't force favorite foods during nausea attacks. It may cause a permanent dislike of those foods.

- Let your child rest after meals because activity may slow digestion. It's best to rest sitting up for about an hour after meals.

- If nausea is a problem in the morning, try serving dry toast or crackers while the child remains in bed.

- Make loose-fitting clothes available; they are more comfortable.

- Avoid giving food for 1 or 2 hours before treatment if nausea occurs during radiation therapy or chemotherapy.

- Try to keep track of the time when the nausea occurs and the causes of it (specific foods, events, surroundings). If possible, make appropriate changes in your menus or schedule. Share the information with your doctor or nurse.

Vomiting

- Ask your doctor about medicine to control nausea.

- Do not give your child anything to drink or eat until the vomiting is under control.

- Once you have controlled vomiting, offer small amounts of clear liquids (e.g., water, broth, milk-free ices and gelatin desserts, fruit drinks). Begin with 1 teaspoonful every 10 minutes; gradually increase the amount to 1 tablespoonful every 20 minutes; and finally, try 2 tablespoonfuls every 30 minutes.

Your child's doctor or nurse may suggest oral rehydration therapy to replace the water and important electrolytes lost as a result of vomiting. Solutions that contain sodium, potassium, chloride, and sugars may be used.

When your child is able to keep down clear liquids, try a full-liquid diet (e.g., strained cereal, pudding, yogurt, milkshakes, cream soups). Continue offering small amounts as often as your child can keep them down. If your child feels okay on a full-liquid diet, gradually work up to a regular diet.

Diarrhea

When diarrhea occurs, food passes quickly through the bowel before the body gets enough vitamins, minerals, and water. This may cause dehydration and increase the risk of infection. Contact your doctor if the diarrhea is severe. Here are some ideas for coping with diarrhea:

- Try foods that are high in protein and calories, but low in fiber: plain or vanilla yogurt without fruits; rice with broth; noodles;

Farina or cream of wheat; eggs (cooked until the whites are solid; not fried); ripe bananas; canned or cooked fruit without skins; cottage cheese, cream cheese; chicken or turkey, skinned; tender or ground beef; or fish that is baked or broiled, not fried.

- Eliminate foods such as: greasy, fatty, or fried foods; raw vegetables and fruits; high-fiber vegetables such as broccoli, corn, beans, cabbage, peas, and cauliflower; strong spices such as hot pepper, curry, and Cajun spice mix; high-sugar foods such as fruit-flavored gelatin desserts; caffeine-containing beverages such as coffee or cocoa; carbonated beverages.

- Offer small amounts of food and liquids throughout the day instead of three large meals.

- Serve plenty of liquids during the day, except at mealtimes because liquids are filling and may reduce the appetite for solid foods. Drinking fluids is important. The body needs water and fluids, and your child may lose a lot of fluids from diarrhea.

- Offer liquids at room temperature. Avoid serving very hot or very cold foods.

- Serve plenty of foods and liquids that contain sodium (salt) and potassium. These minerals often are lost during diarrhea. Good liquid choices include bouillon or fat-free broth. Foods high in potassium that don't cause diarrhea include bananas, peach and apricot nectar, and boiled or mashed potatoes.

- Do not give your child any antidiarrheal medicines without the doctor's okay—some of these products can actually make the diarrhea last longer.

- After sudden, short-term attacks of diarrhea (acute diarrhea), a clear-liquid diet may be helpful for the first 12 to 14 hours. This lets the bowel rest while replacing the important body fluids lost during diarrhea. Rehydrating solutions may be given to replace the water and important minerals lost as a result of diarrhea, especially if the diarrhea is severe or lasts for a few days or more. Ask your child's doctor or registered dietitian for guidelines.

- Be careful when using milk and milk products. Diarrhea may be caused by lactose intolerance. Ask the doctor or dietitian for advice if you think your child has this problem.

Constipation

Keep track of changes in your child's bowel movements; if there are no bowel movements for 48 hours, talk with the doctor or nurse.

- Serve plenty of liquids, except at mealtime. (Liquids are filling and may reduce the appetite for solid foods.) This will help to keep stools soft.

- Constipation may be more easily avoided or relieved if your child has a usual time for a bowel movement. The morning and the hour after meals are best. Offering a hot drink about 30 minutes before these times may help.

- Serve high-fiber foods such as whole-grain breads and cereals; brown rice; dried fruits such as raisins and prunes; and raw fresh vegetables and fruits such as cauliflower, potatoes with skin, peas, apples, pears, oranges, and berries.

- Keeping the skins on vegetables and fruits, whether raw or cooked, also will increase the amount of fiber in the diet.

- Add wheat bran to foods such as casseroles and homemade breads.

- When possible, encourage exercise. Talk to the doctor or a physical therapist about the amount and type of exercise that is right for your child.

If none of these suggestions work for your child, ask your doctor about medicine to ease constipation. Be sure to check with your doctor before giving your child any laxatives or stool softeners.

Weight Gain

Sometimes children gain excess weight during treatment without eating extra calories. For example, certain anticancer drugs such as prednisone, can cause the body to hold fluid and, thus, to gain weight. This buildup of excess fluids is called edema. The weight is in the form of water buildup and does not mean the child is eating too much.

It is important not to put your child on a diet if you notice weight gain. Instead, tell your doctor, so you can find out what may be causing this change. If anticancer drugs cause weight gain, the doctor may recommend limiting salt because salt causes the body to hold on to water. The doctor also may prescribe drugs called diuretics to get rid of extra fluid.

Lactose Intolerance

Lactose intolerance means that the body cannot digest or absorb the milk sugar called lactose. Milk, other dairy products, and foods to which milk has been added contain lactose.

Cells in the intestine normally produce an enzyme that breaks down the lactose in dairy products. However, most types of cancer treatment affect the cells in the intestine and the rest of the digestive tract. As a result, many people who had no problem digesting milk and dairy products before being treated for cancer, find it difficult to eat or drink these foods during, and sometimes after, their treatment. Usually, this will resolve once cancer treatment has been completed, but it may take several weeks to several months for digestion to return to normal.

Chapter 61

Children and Acquired Immune Deficiency Syndrome (AIDS)

Section 61.1

Children and the
Human Immunodeficiency Virus
(HIV)

"Children and HIV," Fact Sheet Number 612, revised September 9, 2002, © 2002 University of New Mexico, New Mexico AIDS InfoNet (www. aids infonet.org). New Mexico AIDS InfoNet is partially funded by the National Library of Medicine and the New Mexico Department of Health. Fact Sheets are regularly updated. The most recent information can be obtained from the website at http://www.aidsinfonet.org. Reprinted with permission.

How Serious is HIV for Children?

Most children with HIV were born to mothers with HIV or got a transfusion of infected blood. These infections are rare in the developed world. Blood for transfusions is screened. Pregnant women are taking antiviral medications. However, where antiviral medications are not available, or where blood is not routinely screened, children still get infected.

Anyone age 13 or younger is counted as a child in U.S. health statistics. Fewer children in the U.S. are infected with HIV each year. In 1992, almost 1,000 children were infected. By 2000, there were just over 100 new infections.

How Are Children Different?

Children's immune systems are still developing. They have a different response to HIV infection. T-cell and viral load counts are higher than in adults. An infant's viral load usually declines until age 4 or 5. Then it stabilizes.

Children also respond differently to anti-HIV medications. They have larger increases in T-cell counts and more diverse T-cells. They seem to recover more of their immune response than adults.

Infants have more fat and water in their bodies. This affects the amount of medication available. Children have a very high rate of metabolism. This gradually slows as they mature.

The liver processes drugs and removes them from the body. It takes several years to mature. As it matures, drug levels in children can change significantly.

Bones develop quickly during the early years of life. Antiviral medications seem to weaken bones in adults. This could be a serious problem for children. It has not yet been carefully studied.

Research on Children

The U.S. government supported the Pediatric AIDS Clinical Trials Group to study AIDS in children. In Europe, the Pediatric European Network for Treatment of AIDS does similar work.

It is very difficult to recruit children into HIV clinical trials. Many children with HIV have already been studied more than once. With falling infection rates, there are very few new cases of pediatric HIV. The U.S. might end support for its pediatric trials network. Important research questions may be studied in adults.

Treatment for Children

HIV-infected children should be treated by a pediatrician with experience treating HIV.

Anti-HIV therapy works very well for children. The death rate from AIDS has dropped as much as for adults. However, there are not very many HIV-infected children to study in the developed world. Manufacturers were not required to study their products in children until very recently in the U.S. As a result, very few antiviral medications have been studied in children.

The correct doses are not always known. Children's doses are sometimes based on their weight. Another method is body surface area. This formula considers both height and weight. As mentioned above, several factors affect drug levels in children. Medications may have to be adjusted several times as a child develops.

The most convenient medications for infants and very young children allow for individualized dosing. They come in liquid or powder form. Others come in a granular form. Some pills can be crushed and added to food or liquids. Some clinics teach children how to swallow pills. If children can swallow pills, they may be able to use a broader range of medications.

It is difficult to know when to start treatment for children. Immediate treatment might prevent immune system damage. Delayed treatment may provide better quality of life for several years. However,

HIV-related diseases show up much faster in untreated children than in adults. Without treatment, about 20% of children die or develop AIDS within one year. A recent study showed that most HIV-infected children in the U.S. start antiviral treatment before they are 3 months old.

Children and Adherence

Adherence is a major challenge for children and infants. Both the child and the parents may need extra psychological and logistic support. Many children do not understand why they should put up with medication side effects.

Parents are usually HIV-positive. They may have their own difficulties with adherence. Their children may be on a different schedule, and probably take different medications. Many antiviral medications taste bad or have a strange texture. A feeding tube directly into the stomach may be necessary if an infant refuses to swallow medications.

The Bottom Line

Where antiviral medications are available, new infections of children are rare. Antiviral medications are very effective in preventing HIV-related complications and death.

Treatment of HIV-infected children is complicated. Not all anti-HIV medications are approved for use by children. The correct dosing is not always known. Children may have a difficult time tolerating medications and taking every dose as scheduled.

However, because children's immune systems are still developing, they might have a better chance of fully recovering from damage caused by HIV.

Treatment of HIV-infected children should be provided by a pediatrician with experience in HIV.

Section 61.2

Pediatric AIDS

Excerpted from "Backgrounder: HIV Infection in Infants and Children," National Institute of Allergy and Infectious Disease (NIAID), updated July 31, 2000; available online at http://www.niaid.nih.gov/newsroom/simple/background.htm.

HIV infection is often difficult to diagnose in very young children. Infected babies, especially in the first few months of life, often appear normal and may exhibit no telltale signs that would allow a definitive diagnosis of HIV infection. Moreover, all children born to infected mothers have antibodies to HIV, made by the mother's immune system, that cross the placenta to the baby's bloodstream before birth and persist for up to 18 months. Because these maternal antibodies reflect the mother's but not the infant's infection status, the test is not useful in newborns or young infants.

In recent years, investigators have demonstrated the utility of highly accurate blood tests in diagnosing HIV infection in children 6 months of age and younger. One laboratory technique called polymerase chain reaction (PCR) can detect minute quantities of the virus in an infant's blood. Another procedure allows physicians to culture a sample of an infant's blood and test it for the presence of HIV.

Currently, PCR assays or HIV culture techniques can identify at birth about one-third of infants who are truly HIV-infected. With these techniques, approximately 90 percent of HIV-infected infants are identifiable by 2 months of age, and 95 percent by 3 months of age. One innovative new approach to both RNA and DNA PCR testing uses dried blood spot specimens, which should make it much simpler to gather and store specimens in field settings.

Progression of HIV Disease in Children

Researchers have observed two general patterns of illness in HIV-infected children. About 20 percent of children develop serious disease in the first year of life; most of these children die by age 4 years.

The remaining 80 percent of infected children have a slower rate of disease progression, many not developing the most serious symptoms of AIDS until school entry or even adolescence. A recent report from a large European registry of HIV-infected children indicated that half of the children with perinatally acquired HIV disease were alive at age 9. Another study, of 42 perinatally HIV-infected children who survived beyond 9 years of age, found about one-quarter of the children to be asymptomatic with relatively intact immune systems.

The factors responsible for the wide variation observed in the rate of disease progression in HIV-infected children are a major focus of the NIAID pediatric AIDS research effort. The Women and Infants Transmission Study, a multisite perinatal HIV study funded by NIH, has found that maternal factors including Vitamin A level and CD4 counts during pregnancy, as well as infant viral load and CD4 counts in the first several months of life, can help identify those infants at risk for rapid disease progression who may benefit from early aggressive therapy.

Signs and Symptoms of Pediatric HIV Disease

Many children with HIV infection do not gain weight or grow normally. HIV-infected children frequently are slow to reach important milestones in motor skills and mental development such as crawling, walking and speaking. As the disease progresses, many children develop neurologic problems such as difficulty walking, poor school performance, seizures, and other symptoms of HIV encephalopathy.

Like adults with HIV infection, children with HIV develop life-threatening opportunistic infections (OIs), although the incidence of various OIs differs in adults and children. For example, toxoplasmosis is seen less frequently in HIV-infected children than in HIV-infected adults, while serious bacterial infections occur more commonly in children than in adults. Also, as children with HIV become sicker, they may suffer from chronic diarrhea due to opportunistic pathogens.

Pneumocystis carinii pneumonia (PCP) is the leading cause of death in HIV-infected children with AIDS. PCP, as well as cytomegalovirus (CMV) disease, usually are primary infections in children, whereas in adults these diseases result from the reactivation of latent infections.

A lung disease called lymphocytic interstitial pneumonitis (LIP), rarely seen in adults, also occurs frequently in HIV-infected children. This condition, like PCP, can make breathing progressively more difficult and often results in hospitalization.

Children with HIV suffer the usual childhood bacterial infections—only more frequently and more severely than uninfected children. These bacterial infections can cause seizures, fever, pneumonia, recurrent colds, diarrhea, dehydration and other problems that often result in extended hospital stays and nutritional problems.

HIV-infected children frequently have severe candidiasis, a yeast infection that can cause unrelenting diaper rash and infections in the mouth and throat that make eating difficult.

Section 61.3

Pediatric Antiretroviral Drug Information

This section includes excerpts from "Guidelines for the Use of Antiretroviral Agents in Pediatric HIV Infection," National Institutes of Health, December 14, 2001, available online at http://www.aidsinfo.nih.gov/guidelines/pediatric/html; and "Pediatric Antiretroviral Drug Information," National Institutes of Health, December 14, 2001, available online at http://www.aidsinfo.nih.gov.

As of February 2001, there were 15 antiretroviral drugs approved for use in HIV-infected adults and adolescents; 11 of these have an approved pediatric treatment indication. These drugs fall into three major classes, nucleoside analogue reverse transcriptase inhibitors (NRTIs), non-nucleoside analogue reverse transcriptase inhibitors (NNRTIs), and protease inhibitors (PIs). The most recent information is available on the HIV/AIDS Treatment Information Service Website (http://aidsinfo.nih.gov).

Nucleoside Analogue Reverse Transcriptase Inhibitors

Abacavir (ABC, Ziagen®)

In December of 1998, abacavir (ABC) was approved by the FDA for combination therapy in adults and children age 3 months or older, based on controlled trials in adults and children.

Didanosine (ddI, Videx®)

Didanosine (ddI) received FDA approval in 1991 for adults and pediatric patients older than 6 months of age with advanced HIV infection who were intolerant to or deteriorating on ZDV. Since that time the indications have been broadened and dosage recommendations reduced. In October 2000 a new delayed-release formulation of enteric-coated beadlets was approved for use in adults allowing for once-daily ddI administration in selected patients.

Lamivudine (3TC, Epivir®)

Lamivudine (3TC) was approved in November 1995 for use in infants greater than 3 months of age and children based on efficacy studies in adults in conjunction with safety and pharmacokinetic studies in children. In September 1997, it was approved as a fixed combination of 3TC/ZDV for adults and adolescents greater than 12 years old. In November 2000, it was approved as a fixed-dose combination of 3TC/ZDV/abacavir for adolescents and adults weighing greater than 40 kg.

Stavudine (d4T, Zerit®)

Stavudine (d4T) was approved in September 1996 for use in infants and children greater than six months of age based on evidence from controlled trials in adults and on safety and pharmacokinetic data from children.

Zalcitabine (ddC, Hivid®)

In August 1994 zalcitabine (ddC) was approved for use in adults and adolescents older than 13 years of age. It is not FDA-approved for use in pediatric patients.

Zidovudine (ZDV, AZT, Retrovir®)

Zidovudine (ZDV) was the first NRTI studied in adult and pediatric clinical trials and the first antiretroviral agent approved for therapy of HIV infection. ZDV first received FDA approval for the treatment of HIV infection in adults in 1987. It was approved for use in children ages 3 months to 12 years in May 1990. Perinatal trial PACTG 076 established that a ZDV prophylactic regimen given during pregnancy, labor and to the newborn reduced the risk of perinatal

HIV transmission by nearly 70%. Zidovudine received FDA approval for that indication in August 1994.

Non-Nucleoside Analogue Reverse Transcriptase Inhibitors

Delavirdine (DLV, Rescriptor®)

Delavirdine (DLV) was approved in April 1997 for use in adolescents 16 years and older and adults in combination with other antiretroviral agents. This agent, similar to others in its class has no activity against HIV-2 but is specific for HIV-1. This NNRTI has had very limited study in pediatric patients under age 13 years.

Efavirenz (DMP-266, EFV, Sustiva™)

Efavirenz (EFV) was approved in September 1998 for children older than 3 years of age, adolescents and adults.

Nevirapine (NVP, Viramune®)

Nevirapine (NVP) is approved for use in children greater than 2 months old. NVP is a dipyridodiazepinone derivative and is specific for HIV-1. It does not inhibit any of the human cellular DNA polymerases.

Protease Inhibitors

Amprenavir (APV, Agenerase®)

The Food and Drug Administration in April 1999 approved amprenavir (APV) for use in combination with other antiretrovirals in adults and children over 4 years of age. This approval was based upon the results of controlled trials of up to 24 weeks duration in treatment naive and experienced adults. Pediatric approval was based upon analysis of two open label trials in treatment experienced children, one after 8 weeks of therapy and one after 4 weeks of therapy. APV is available in both liquid and solid formulations.

Indinavir (IDV, Crixivan®)

Indinavir (IDV) was approved in 1996 for use in adolescents and adults older than 18 years of age. Like the other PIs, IDV is prone to multiple drug interactions due to its interaction with the cytochrome

P450 system (see product label). A liquid formulation is not yet available. Administration of IDV with a meal high in calories, fat and protein results in a reduction in plasma IDV concentrations; administration with lighter meals (e.g. dry toast with jelly, apple juice and coffee with skim milk and sugar) results in little to no change in IDV pharmacokinetics.

Lopinavir/Ritonavir (LPV/RTV, ABT-378/r, Kaletra™)

Lopinavir/Ritonavir (LPV/RTV) is a fixed combination of these two protease inhibitors (133.3 mg of lopinavir plus 33.3 mg of ritonavir). LPV/RTV received FDA approval in 2000 for combination with other antiretroviral agents for the treatment of HIV-1 infection in adults and pediatric patients age six months and older. It is available in both liquid and solid formulations.

Nelfinavir (NFV, Viracept®)

Nelfinavir (NFV) is approved for use in children over two years of age in combination with NRTIs and NNRTIs. It is available in both oral powder and tablet formulations. Like other agents in this class it is an inhibitor of the HIV-1 protease enzyme, which results in preventing cleavage of the gag-pol polyprotein. This inhibits viral replication by producing and releasing immature, non-infectious virions. NFV is active against HIV-1 and HIV-2 strains. Oral bioavailability of NFV has been reported to be 70-80% when administered with food; bioavailability is significantly reduced when the drug is taken in a fasting state. Like other PIs, NFV is metabolized by the cytochrome P450 enzyme system in the liver, inhibits CYP3A4 and is associated with a number of clinically significant pharmacologic drug interactions (see product label).

Ritonavir (RTV, Norvir®)

Ritonavir (RTV) is approved for use in children over the age of 2 years in combination with other antiretroviral agents. It was the first PI approved for use in children and is available as liquid and capsule formulations. It has specific activity for HIV-1, and to a lesser extent, HIV-2.

Saquinavir (SQV, hard gel capsule, Invirase®; soft gel capsule, Fortovase®)

In 1995, saquinavir (SQV) became the first protease inhibitor approved for use in adolescents and adults older then 16 years, in combination therapy with NRTIs. In its original formulation, as a hard gel capsule (Invirase), it had very limited bioavailability (~ 4%) following oral administration. In 1997, the FDA approved a soft gel capsule preparation (Fortovase) with significantly enhanced oral bioavailability. SQV has not been formally approved for use in children and is not yet available in a liquid preparation. Absorption of SQV soft gel capsule is enhanced by food.

Chapter 62

Iron Deficiency Anemia

Introduction

Iron deficiency anemia (IDA) is a condition where one has inadequate amounts of iron to meet body demands such as during periods of rapid growth and pregnancy. IDA is usually due to a diet insufficient in iron or from blood loss. Blood loss can be acute as in hemorrhage or trauma or long term as in heavy menstruation.

Risk Groups

Most at risk are young children whose growth demands are great, the elderly whose diets are many times lacking, and women who are pregnant or of childbearing age.

Symptoms

Fatigue is the most common complaint, along with malaise (vague feeling of physical discomfort or uneasiness), sensitivity to cold, shortness of breath, dizziness, and restless legs syndrome (uncomfortable feeling in legs, sensations of pulling, tingling, crawling, accompanied by a need to move the legs).

Excerpted from "Disorders: Iron Deficiency Anemia," © 2000 Iron Disorders Institute; reprinted with permission. The full text is available online at http://www.irondisorders.org/disorders/ida/index.htm.

Detection

Hemoglobin and serum ferritin are the most common ways to test for anemia. A new test called serum transferrin receptor is a good way to determine iron deficiency anemia because this test is not affected by inflammation.

Your physician may determine you are iron deficient if your hemoglobin is low.

Note: One can be anemic as reflected in a low hemoglobin but have an elevated ferritin.

Treatments

IDA can be the result of inadequate daily intake of iron, pregnancy, growth spurts, or blood loss due to heavy period or internal bleeding. If IDA is related to inadequate iron in diet, usually adding three portions of lean red meat (heme iron sources) per week, along with all other essential vitamins and minerals will correct anemia.

If anemia is due to increased demand for iron such as a growth spurt (toddlers, adolescents) or pregnancy, oral supplementation may be necessary. Short term supplementation with moderate doses (30–60 mg daily) of oral iron, combined with increased consumption of heme-rich sources of iron may be sufficient to address iron demands. Much will depend upon the patient's general health, established hemoglobin pattern, ferritin levels, symptoms, family history and current diet.

Large doses of supplemental oral iron have not been proven beneficial. Studies conducted by Dr. Janet Hunt, Grand Forks Nutritional Center, U.S. Department of Agriculture, indicate that our body's natural regulation mechanism will adjust for the amount of iron absorption during periods of growth and pregnancy. Increased supplementation in normal individuals can cause additional and possibly unnecessary iron to go into burial as reflected by ferritin elevation.

If hemoglobin does not respond within 30–45 days, perhaps anemia is due to another cause and should be further investigated. Among other causes of anemia are disorders such as problems of iron utilization, absorption, red blood cell production, vitamin B_{12} deficiency or other mineral deficiencies, kidney function, bone marrow production, and hemoglobinopathies such as thalassemia. Also, potentially serious infection or inflammation may be present.

When hemoglobin levels are seriously low, the heart is particularly vulnerable. Whole blood transfusion or IV iron may needed to stabilize hemoglobin levels. Parenteral or IV iron can be administered by injection or infusion. Again, this type therapy is usually reserved for cases of trauma where blood loss is life-threatening and not used for insufficiency due to inadequate dietary iron intake.

Chapter 63

Thalassemia

A Basic Description

Thalassemia is the name of a group of genetic blood disorders. To understand how thalassemia affects the human body, you must first understand a little about how blood is made.

Hemoglobin is the oxygen-carrying component of the red blood cells. It consists of two different proteins, an alpha and a beta. If the body doesn't produce enough of either of these two proteins, the red blood cells do not form properly and cannot carry sufficient oxygen. The result is anemia that begins in early childhood and lasts throughout life.

Since thalassemia is not a single disorder but a group of related disorders that affect the human body in similar ways, it is important to understand the differences between the various types of thalassemia.

Alpha Thalassemia

People whose hemoglobin does not produce enough alpha protein have alpha thalassemia. It is commonly found in Africa, the Middle East, India, Southeast Asia, southern China, and occasionally the Mediterranean region. Types of alpha thalassemia range from mild to severe in their effect on the body.

Silent Carrier State: This condition generally causes no health problems because the lack of alpha protein is so small that the hemoglobin functions normally. It is called "silent carrier" because of how difficult it is to detect. Silent carrier state is "diagnosed" by deduction when an apparently normal individual has a child with hemoglobin H disease or alpha thalassemia trait.

Hemoglobin Constant Spring: This is an unusual form of Silent Carrier state that is caused by a mutation of the alpha globin. It is called Constant Spring after the region of Jamaica in which it was discovered. As in silent carrier state, an individual with this condition usually experiences no related health problems.

Alpha Thalassemia Trait or **Mild Alpha Thalassemia:** In this condition, the lack of alpha protein is somewhat greater. Patients with this condition have smaller red blood cells and a mild anemia, although many patients do not experience symptoms. However, physicians often mistake mild alpha thalassemia for iron deficiency anemia and prescribe iron supplements that have no effect on the anemia.

Hemoglobin H Disease: In this condition, the lack of alpha protein is great enough to cause severe anemia and serious health problems such as an enlarged spleen, bone deformities, and fatigue. It is named for the abnormal hemoglobin H (created by the remaining beta globin) that destroys red blood cells.

Hemoglobin H-Constant Spring: This condition is more severe than hemoglobin H disease. Individuals with this condition tend to have a more severe anemia and suffer more frequently from enlargement of the spleen and viral infections.

Homozygous Constant Spring: This condition is a variation of hemoglobin H-Constant Spring that occurs when two Constant Spring carriers pass their genes on to their child (as opposed to hemoglobin H Constant Spring, in which one parent is a Constant Spring Carrier and the other a carrier of alpha thalassemia trait). This condition is generally less severe than hemoglobin H Constant Spring and more similar to hemoglobin H disease.

Hydrops Fetalis or **Alpha Thalassemia Major:** In this condition, there are no alpha genes in the individual's DNA, which causes the gamma globins produced by the fetus to form an abnormal hemoglobin called hemoglobin Barts. Most individuals with this condition die before or shortly after birth. In some extremely rare cases where the condition is discovered before birth, in utero blood transfusions have allowed the birth of children with hydrops fetalis who then require lifelong blood transfusions and medical care.

Beta Thalassemia

People whose hemoglobin does not produce enough beta protein have beta thalassemia. It is found in people of Mediterranean descent, such as Italians and Greeks, and is also found in the Arabian Peninsula, Iran, Africa, Southeast Asia and southern China.

There are three types of beta thalassemia that also range from mild to severe in their effect on the body.

Thalassemia Minor or **Thalassemia Trait:** In this condition, the lack of beta protein is not great enough to cause problems in the normal functioning of the hemoglobin. A person with this condition simply carries the genetic trait for thalassemia and will usually experience no health problems other than a possible mild anemia. As in mild alpha thalassemia, physicians often mistake the small red blood cells of the person with beta thalassemia minor as a sign of iron-deficiency anemia and incorrectly prescribe iron supplements.

Thalassemia Intermedia: In this condition the lack of beta protein in the hemoglobin is great enough to cause a moderately severe anemia and significant health problems, including bone deformities and enlargement of the spleen. However, there is a wide range in the clinical severity of this condition, and the borderline between thalassemia intermedia and the most severe form, thalassemia major, can be confusing. The deciding factor seems to be the amount of blood transfusions required by the patient. The more dependent the patient is on blood transfusions, the more likely he or she is to be classified as thalassemia major. Generally speaking, patients with thalassemia intermedia need blood transfusions to improve their quality of life, but not in order to survive.

Thalassemia Major or **Cooley's Anemia:** This is the most severe form of beta thalassemia in which the complete lack of beta protein in the hemoglobin causes a life-threatening anemia that requires regular blood transfusions and extensive ongoing medical care. These extensive, lifelong blood transfusions lead to iron-overload which must be treated with chelation therapy to prevent early death from organ failure.

Other Forms of Thalassemia

In addition to the alpha and beta thalassemias, there are other related disorders that occur when the gene for alpha or beta thalassemia combines with an abnormal or mutant gene.

E Beta Thalassemia: Hemoglobin E is one of the most common abnormal hemoglobins. It is usually found in people of Southeast Asian ancestry, such as Cambodians, Vietnamese, and Thai. When combined with beta thalassemia, hemoglobin E produces E beta thalassemia, a moderately severe anemia which is similar in symptoms to beta thalassemia intermedia.

Sickle Beta Thalassemia: This condition is caused by a combination of beta thalassemia and hemoglobin S, the abnormal hemoglobin found in people with sickle cell disease. It is commonly found in people of Mediterranean ancestry, such as Italians, Greeks, and Turks. The condition varies according to the amount of normal beta globin produced by the beta gene. When no beta globin is produced by the beta gene, the condition is almost identical with sickle cell disease. The more beta globin produced by the beta gene, the less severe the condition.

Treatment of Thalassemia

Blood Transfusions

The most common treatment for all major forms of thalassemia is red blood cell transfusions. These transfusions are necessary to provide the patient with a temporary supply of healthy red blood cells with normal hemoglobin capable of carrying the oxygen that the patient's body needs.

While thalassemia patients were given infrequent transfusions in the past, clinical research led to a more frequent program of regular blood cell transfusions that has greatly improved the patients' quality of life. Today, most patients with a major form of thalassemia receive red blood cell transfusions every two to three weeks, amounting to as much as 52 pints of blood a year.

Iron Overload

Because there is no natural way for the body to eliminate iron, the iron in the transfused blood cells builds up in a condition known as "iron overload" and becomes toxic to tissues and organs, particularly the liver and heart. Iron overload typically results in the patient's early death from organ failure.

Chelation Therapy

To help remove excess iron, patients undergo the difficult and painful infusion of a drug, Desferal. A needle is attached to a small battery-operated infusion pump and worn under the skin of the stomach or legs five to seven times a week for up to twelve hours. Desferal binds iron in a process called "chelation." Chelated iron is later eliminated, reducing the amount of stored iron.

The Compliance Problem

Compliance with Desferal is vital to the thalassemia patient's long term survival. However, many patients find the treatment so difficult that they do not keep up with it or abandon treatment altogether. Lack of compliance with chelation therapy leads to accelerated health problems and early death. To combat the compliance problem, researchers are at work on less stressful new chelators that can improve patient compliance.

Chapter 64

Sickle Cell Disease

Facts about Sickle Cell Anemia

What Is Sickle Cell Anemia?

Sickle cell anemia is an inherited blood disorder, characterized primarily by chronic anemia (low blood count) and periodic episodes of pain. The underlying problem involves hemoglobin, a component of the red cells in the blood. The hemoglobin molecules in each red blood cell carry oxygen from the lungs to the body organs and tissues and bring back carbon dioxide to the lungs. In sickle cell anemia, the hemoglobin is defective. After the hemoglobin molecules give up their oxygen, some of them may cluster together and form long, rod-like structures. These structures cause the red blood cells to become stiff and to assume a sickle shape. Unlike normal red cells, which are usually smooth and donut-shaped, the sickled red cells cannot squeeze through small blood vessels. Instead, they stack up and cause blockages that deprive the organs and tissue of oxygen-carrying blood. This process produces the periodic episodes of pain and ultimately can damage the tissues and vital organs and lead to other serious medical

This chapter contains text from "Facts about Sickle Cell Anemia," National Heart, Lung, and Blood Institute (NHLBI), NIH Pub. No. 96-4057, November 1996, and "Management and Therapy of Sickle Cell Disease," NHLBI, NIH Pub. No. 95-2117, revised December 1995 (Third Edition). The combined text was updated in May 2001 by Dr. David A. Cooke, MD, Diplomate, American Board of Internal Medicine.

problems. Unlike normal red blood cells, which last about 120 days in the bloodstream, sickled red cells die after only about 10 to 20 days. Because they cannot be replaced fast enough, the blood is chronically short of red blood cells, a condition called anemia.

What Causes Sickle Cell Anemia?

Sickle cell anemia is caused by an error in the gene that tells the body how to make hemoglobin. The defective gene tells the body to make abnormal hemoglobin that results in deformed red blood cells. Children who inherit copies of the defective gene from both parents will have sickle cell anemia. Children who inherit the defective sickle hemoglobin gene from only one parent will not have the disease, but will carry the sickle cell trait. Individuals with sickle cell trait generally have no symptoms, but they can pass the sickle hemoglobin gene on to their children.

How Common Is Sickle Cell Anemia?

Sickle cell anemia affects millions of people throughout the world. It is particularly common among people whose ancestors come from sub-Saharan Africa; Spanish-speaking regions (South America, Cuba, Central America); Saudi Arabia; India; and Mediterranean countries, such as Turkey, Greece, and Italy. However, sickle cell anemia can occur among people of any race.

In this country, it affects approximately 72,000 people, most of whose ancestors come from Africa. The disease occurs in approximately 1 in every 500 African-American births and 1 in every 1,000–1,400 Hispanic-American births. Approximately 2 million Americans, or 1 in 12 African Americans, carry the sickle cell trait.

What Are the Signs and Symptoms of Sickle Cell Anemia?

The clinical course of sickle cell anemia does not follow a single pattern; some patients have mild symptoms, and some have very severe symptoms. However, the basic problem is the same—the sickle-shaped red blood cells tend to get stuck in narrow blood vessels, blocking the flow of blood.

The presence of two defective genes is needed for sickle cell anemia. If each parent carries one sickle hemoglobin gene and one normal gene, with each pregnancy, there is a 25 percent chance of the child's inheriting two defective genes and having sickle cell anemia; a 25 percent chance of inheriting two normal genes and not having the disease; and a 50 percent chance of being an unaffected carrier like the parents.

Sickle cell anemia can result in the following conditions:

- Hand-foot syndrome. When the small blood vessels in the hands or feet are blocked, pain and swelling can result, along with fever. This may be the first symptom of sickle cell anemia in infants.

- Fatigue, paleness, and shortness of breath—all symptoms of anemia, or a shortage of red blood cells.

- Pain that occurs unpredictably in any body organ or joint, wherever the sickled blood cells block oxygen flow to the tissues. The frequency and amount of pain varies. Some patients have painful episodes (also called crises) less than once a year, and some have as many as 15 or even more episodes in a year. Sometimes the pain lasts only a few hours; sometimes it lasts several weeks. For especially severe, ongoing pain, the patient may have to be hospitalized and treated with painkillers and intravenous fluids. Pain is the principal symptom of sickle cell anemia in both children and adults.

- Eye problems. When the retina, the film at the back of the eye that receives and processes visual images, does not get enough nourishment from circulating red blood cells, it can deteriorate. Damage to the retina can be serious enough to cause blindness.

- Yellowing of the skin and eyes. These are signs of jaundice, resulting from the rapid breakdown of red blood cells.

- Delayed growth and puberty in children and often a slight build in adults. The slow rate of growth is caused by a shortage of red blood cells.

- Infections. In general, both children and adults with sickle cell anemia are more vulnerable to infections and have a harder time fighting them off once they start. This is the result of damage to the spleen from the sickled red cells which prevents the spleen from destroying bacteria in the blood. Infants and young children, especially, are susceptible to bacterial infections that can kill them in as little as 9 hours from onset of fever. Pneumococcal infections used to be the principal cause of death in young children with sickle cell anemia until physicians began routinely giving penicillin on a preventive basis to infants who are identified at birth or in early infancy as having sickle cell anemia.

- Stroke. The defective hemoglobin damages the walls of the red blood cells, causing them to stick to blood vessel walls. This can result in the development of narrowed, or blocked, small blood vessels in the brain, causing a serious, life-threatening stroke. This type of stroke occurs primarily in children.

- Acute chest syndrome—a life-threatening complication of sickle cell anemia, similar to pneumonia, that is caused by infection or trapped sickled cells in the lung. This is characterized by chest pain, fever, and an abnormal chest x-ray.

How Is Sickle Cell Anemia Detected?

Early diagnosis of sickle cell anemia is critical so that children who have the disease can receive proper treatment. More than 40 states now perform a simple, inexpensive blood test for sickle cell disease on all newborn infants. This test is performed at the same time and from the same blood samples as other routine newborn screening tests. Hemoglobin electrophoresis is the most widely used diagnostic test. If the test shows the presence of sickle hemoglobin, a second blood test is performed to confirm the diagnosis. These tests also tell whether the child carries the sickle cell trait.

Management and Therapy of Sickle Cell Disease

Child and Adolescent Health Care Maintenance

Health care maintenance services for children and adolescents with sickle cell disease include those services provided to healthy children and services specifically provided for sickle cell disease. Routine services include immunizations and dietary counseling as well as education about preventive health measures. The frequency of visits should depend on the needs of the child and family. During the first 2 years of life, health care maintenance visits should be scheduled concurrently with needed immunizations. Older patients who are doing well can be seen semi-annually. Children also should be seen within a short time after a hospitalization or emergency room visit so the physician can review the situations that may have precipitated the event and make any necessary changes in the treatment plan.

Immunizations should be administered according to schedules recommended by either the American Academy of Pediatrics or the American Academy of Family Practice. In addition, all children with sickle cell disease should be immunized against hepatitis B virus and

Haemophilus influenza b (Hib). Vaccination against pneumococcus is very important, but there is currently some uncertainly about how it should be done. An older pneumococcal vaccine (Pneumovax) has been recommended at age 2 years, with a booster at age 5 years for some time. Recently, a newer form designed for young children called Prevnar was introduced. It is not yet clear whether children with sickle cell anemia should receive just one or both vaccines. Check with your physician, as recommendations are evolving. Seasonal influenza vaccines are recommended.

Dietary counseling is an important part of routine health care. Mothers should be encouraged to breast-feed their infants, although iron-fortified formulas are an alternative.

Sickle Cell-Specific Issues

In addition to the general health maintenance issues, there are health maintenance issues specific for sickle cell disease. These include the need for parents to learn specific physical assessment skills, to administer prophylactic antibiotics, to implement measures that minimize the risk of vaso-occlusive complications, and to use analgesics and comfort measures to minimize pain. During health maintenance visits, providers also should carefully review the history and physical examination for evidence of organ dysfunction. When performing the physical examination, providers should pay attention to growth parameters and physical development. Physical growth and sexual maturation are delayed in sickle cell anemia patients compared with normal children, but the child eventually will catch up during the late teenage years. Common physical findings in children with sickle cell disease include mild generalized lymphadenopathy, functional systolic murmurs, and slight hepatic enlargement.

Because limitation of motion and pain are common signs of aseptic necrosis, the range of motion of the hips of older children and adolescents should be assessed. Scleral icterus is another common physical finding. Because children and adolescents are often teased about their yellow eyes, they should be taught the nature of this characteristic and reassured that it will not affect their visual acuity and does not necessarily reflect liver disease.

Blood counts should be done frequently during the first year of life to establish the patient's baseline, but after 12 months of age, the hemoglobin and hematocrit are relatively stable and need to be checked only once or twice a year in uncomplicated patients. For patients who are doing well, an annual urinalysis and measurement of blood urea nitrogen (BUN), serum creatinine, and liver enzymes are adequate for monitoring the patient for evidence of organ damage. Before the administration of the first transfusion, the patient's red blood cell antigens should be determined and recorded in the patient's permanent medical record.

Specific physical assessment skills that should be taught to parents include taking the body temperature and assessing respiratory effort, degree of pallor, and spleen size. Parents of children who have an enlarged spleen should be taught to palpate the spleen and may be given a tongue depressor that indicates the level at which the spleen extends below the left costal margin in the mid-clavicular line. The parent can use this spleen stick to determine if the spleen size has changed and can provide the stick to other health care providers who assess the child. The skin around the ankles of adolescents should be examined carefully for ulcers, and patients should be reminded to avoid trauma to the lower extremities because this may precipitate ulcerations. Parents should also be told that the child may have repeated episodes of enuresis or nocturia as a result of the renal concentrating defect and should be provided with suggestions on how to manage this rather difficult problem. Parents should remind school officials that their child will need access to fluids while at school and will also need to be excused periodically from class to use lavatory facilities.

Parents and patients should be instructed in the proper use of analgesia. Fear of addiction may prevent parents from administering adequate analgesics to their children. Similarly, older patients may under-medicate themselves for fear of becoming addicted to the analgesic.

Hydroxyurea is a new medication therapy for sickle cell anemia which has emerged in recent years. It can help increase production of normal hemoglobin in children and adolescents with sickle cell disease. While it is not a cure for the condition, it can reduce the frequency of crises, and is also helpful in patients with leg ulcers. It is helpful, but also requires monitoring during treatment. Parents should discuss with their specialist whether hydroxyurea is appropriate for their child.

There is often a need to provide counseling in the area of recreation and physical activities. Patients should be encouraged to get regular exercise. School-age children should participate in physical education classes, but they should be allowed to rest if they tire, and they should be encouraged to drink fluids after exercise. The potential risks of recreational activities that involve strenuous exertion should be discussed with the patient. Patients with sickle cell disease should dress warmly for cold weather and should avoid direct exposure to cold temperatures, including swimming in cold water. Children and adolescents should engage in competitive athletics with caution because it is difficult to heed the signs of fatigue in the heat of competition, and the team may find it difficult to replace an athlete sidelined by illness. Children with sickle cell disease may benefit from a summer camping experience, either in an appropriate regular camp or through participation in a special camp for children with sickle cell disease. If the camp staff members are knowledgeable about the disease and comfortable with the care of these children, the camper can learn self-reliance and share experiences with other children about sickle cell disease while having fun. Health care providers and others who attend camp with sickle cell children typically find this a rewarding experience.

Chapter 65

Diabetes in Children and Adolescents

Diabetes is one of the most serious health problems facing the world today. In the United States each year, more than 13,000 children are diagnosed with type 1 diabetes. Increasingly, health care providers are finding more and more children and teens with type 2 diabetes, a disease usually seen in people over age 40. Although there are no national data, some clinics report that one-third to one-half of all new cases of childhood diabetes are now type 2. African American, Hispanic/Latino and American Indian children who are obese and have a family history of type 2 diabetes are at especially high risk for this type of diabetes.

What Is Diabetes?

Diabetes is a chronic disease in which the body does not make or properly use insulin, a hormone that is needed to convert sugar, starches, and other food into energy. People with diabetes have increased blood glucose (sugar) levels due to a lack of insulin, insufficient insulin, or resistance to insulin's effects. High levels of glucose build up in the blood, and spill into the urine and out of the body. As a result, the body loses its main source of fuel.

Taking care of diabetes is important. If not treated, diabetes can lead to serious problems. Diabetes can affect the eyes, kidneys, nerves, gums,

"Diabetes in Children and Adolescent," a fact sheet produced by the National Diabetes Education Program (NDEP), National Institute of Diabetes and Digestive and Kidney Diseases (NIDDK), February 2002. For more information about diabetes visit NDEP online at http://ndep.nih.gov or NIDDK online at http://www.niddk.nih.gov.

teeth, and blood vessels. Diabetes is the leading cause of adult blindness, lower limb amputations, and kidney failure. It can cause heart disease and stroke, and even death if untreated. Some of these problems can occur in teens and young adults who develop diabetes during childhood. Research in adults shows that these problems can be greatly reduced or delayed by keeping blood glucose levels near normal.

What Are Special Concerns for Children and Adolescents with Diabetes?

Diabetes presents unique issues for children and teens with the disease. Simple things—like going to a birthday party, playing sports, or staying overnight with friends—need careful planning. Every day, children with diabetes may need to take insulin or oral medication. They also need to check their blood glucose several times during the day and remember to make correct food choices. For school-age children, these tasks can make them feel "different" from their classmates. These tasks can be particularly bothersome for teens.

For any child or teen with diabetes, learning to cope with the disease is a big job. Dealing with a chronic illness such as diabetes may cause emotional and behavioral challenges. Talking to a social worker or psychologist may help a child or teen and his or her family learn to adjust to lifestyle changes needed to stay healthy.

What Can Families and Others Do?

Managing diabetes in children and adolescents is most effective when the entire family makes a team effort. Families can share concerns with physicians, diabetes educators, dietitians, and other health care providers to get their help in the day-to-day management of diabetes. Extended family members, teachers, school nurses, counselors, coaches, day care providers, or other resources in the community can provide information, support, guidance, and help with coping skills. These individuals also may help with resources for health education, financial services, social services, mental health counseling, transportation, and home visiting.

Diabetes is stressful for both the children and their families. Parents should be alert for signs of depression or eating disorders and seek appropriate treatment. While all parents should talk to their children about avoiding tobacco, alcohol, and other drugs, this is particularly important for children with diabetes. Smoking and diabetes each increase the risk of cardiovascular disease and people with diabetes who smoke have a greatly increased risk of heart disease and circulatory problems. Binge drinking can increase the risk of hypoglycemia (low blood sugar) and symptoms of hypoglycemia can be mistaken for those of intoxication and not properly treated. Local peer groups for children and teens with diabetes can provide positive role models and group activities.

What Are the Types of Diabetes?

There are two main types of diabetes. Type 1 and type 2 diabetes are described below. A third type—gestational diabetes—occurs only during pregnancy and often resolves after pregnancy. Women who have had gestational diabetes are more likely to develop type 2 diabetes later in life.

Type 1 Diabetes

Type 1 diabetes is a disease of the immune system, which is the body's system for fighting infection. In people with type 1 diabetes, the immune system attacks the beta cells, the insulin-producing cells of the pancreas, and destroys them. The pancreas can no longer produce insulin, so people with type 1 diabetes need to take insulin daily to live. Type 1 diabetes can occur at any age, but the disease occurs most often in children and young adults.

Symptoms: The symptoms of type 1 diabetes usually develop over a short period of time. They include increased thirst and urination, constant hunger, weight loss, and blurred vision. Children may also feel very tired all the time. If not diagnosed and treated with insulin, the child or teen with type 1 diabetes can lapse into a life-threatening diabetic coma, known as diabetic ketoacidosis or DKA.

Risk Factors: Though scientists have made much progress in predicting who is at risk for developing type 1 diabetes, they do not know exactly what triggers the immune system's attack on beta cells. They believe that type 1 diabetes is due to a combination of genetic and environmental factors. Researchers are working to identify these factors and stop the auto-immune process that leads to type 1 diabetes.

Type 2 Diabetes

The first step in the development of type 2 diabetes is often a problem with the body's response to insulin, called insulin resistance. For reasons scientists do not completely understand, the body cannot use the insulin very well. This means that the body needs increasing amounts of insulin to control blood glucose. The pancreas tries to make more insulin, but after several years, insulin production may drop off.

Type 2 diabetes used to be found mainly in adults who were overweight and age 40 or older. Now, as more children and adolescents in the United States become overweight and inactive, type 2 diabetes occurs more often in young people. Type 2 diabetes is also more common in certain racial and ethnic groups, such as African Americans, American Indians, Hispanic/Latinos, and some Asian and Pacific Islander Americans. To control their diabetes, children with type 2 diabetes may need to take oral medication, insulin, or both.

Symptoms: Type 2 diabetes develops slowly in some children, but quickly in others. Symptoms may be similar to those of type 1 diabetes. A child or teen can feel very tired, thirsty, or nauseated (sick to the stomach), and have to urinate often. Other symptoms may include weight loss, blurred vision, frequent infections, and slow healing of wounds or sores. Some children or adolescents with type 2 diabetes may show no symptoms at all when they are diagnosed. For that reason, it is important for parents and caregivers to talk to a health care provider about testing children or teens who are at high risk for the disease.

Risk Factors: Being overweight, being older than 10 years of age, experiencing puberty, and having a family member who has type 2 diabetes are risk factors for the disease. Certain populations, as noted above, are at higher risk. In addition, physical signs of insulin resistance, such as acanthosis nigricans, may appear: the skin around the neck or in the armpits appears dark, thick, and velvety. High blood pressure also may be a sign of insulin resistance. For children and teens at risk, health care providers can encourage, support, and educate the entire family to make lifestyle changes that may delay—or prevent—the onset of type 2 diabetes. Such lifestyle changes include keeping at a healthy weight and staying active.

What Should a Child or Teen with Diabetes Do Every Day?

To control diabetes and prevent complications, blood glucose levels must be as close to a "normal" range as safely possible. Families should work with a health care provider to help set a child's or teen's targets for blood glucose levels. The provider can help develop a personal diabetes plan for the child and discuss ways to manage hypoglycemia (low blood glucose) and hyperglycemia (high blood glucose).

A Personal Diabetes Plan

A personal diabetes plan ensures that a daily schedule is in place to keep a child's diabetes under control. A health care provider develops this plan in partnership with a child or teen and his or her family. The plan shows the child or teen how to follow a healthy meal plan, get regular physical activity, check blood glucose levels, and take insulin or oral medication as prescribed.

Follow a Healthy Meal Plan: A child or teen needs to follow a meal plan developed by a physician, diabetes educator, or a registered dietitian. A meal plan outlines proper nutrition for growth. A meal plan also helps keep blood glucose levels in the target range. Children or adolescents and their families can learn how different types of food—especially carbohydrates such as breads, pasta, and rice—can affect blood glucose levels. Portion size, the right amount of calories for the child's age, and ideas for healthy food choices at meal and snack time also should be discussed. Family support for following the meal plan and setting up regular meal times is a key to success, especially if the child or teen is taking insulin.

Get Regular Physical Activity: A child or teen with diabetes needs regular physical activity. Exercise helps to lower blood glucose levels, especially in children and adolescents with type 2 diabetes. Exercise is also a good way to help children control their weight. If possible, a child or teen should check blood glucose levels before beginning a game or sport. A child or teen should not exercise if blood glucose levels are too low.

Check blood glucose levels regularly: A child or teen should check blood glucose levels regularly with a blood glucose meter, preferably a meter with a built-in memory. A health care professional can teach a child how to use a blood glucose meter properly and how often to use it. Blood glucose meter results show if blood glucose levels are in the target range, too high, or too low. A child should keep a journal or other records of blood glucose results to discuss with his or her health care provider. This information helps the provider make any needed changes to the child's or teen's personal diabetes plan.

Take all diabetes medication as prescribed: A child or teen should take all diabetes medication as prescribed. Parents, caregivers, school nurses, and others can help a child or teen learn how to take medications properly. For type 1 diabetes, a child or teen takes insulin shots at regular times each day. Some children and teens use an insulin pump, which delivers insulin. Some children or teens with type 2 diabetes need oral medication or insulin shots or both. In any case, all medication should be balanced with food and activity every day.

Hypoglycemia and Hyperglycemia

Keeping blood glucose levels within the target range is the goal of diabetes control. However, extremes in blood glucose levels can occur for several reasons. The parent or caregiver should talk with a health care provider about how to deal with these potential problems related to a child's or teen's diabetes.

Blood glucose levels can sometimes drop too low—a condition called hypoglycemia. Taking too much diabetes medicine, missing a meal or snack, or exercising too much may cause hypoglycemia. A child or teen can become nervous, shaky, and confused. When blood glucose levels fall very low, the person can lose consciousness or develop seizures. Talk to the child's or teen's health care provider about how to deal with this serious but manageable condition.

Blood glucose levels can sometimes rise too high—a condition known as hyperglycemia. Forgetting to take medicines on time, eating too much, and getting too little exercise may cause hyperglycemia. Being ill also can raise blood glucose levels. Over time, hyperglycemia can lead to serious health problems and cause damage to the eyes, kidneys, nerves, blood vessels, gums, and teeth.

Are There Legal Considerations for Children and Teens with Diabetes?

Several Federal and state laws provide protections to children with disabilities, including children or teens with diabetes. These children must have full access to public programs, including public schools, and to most private schools as well. Students with diabetes are entitled to accommodations and modifications necessary for them to stay healthy at school and have the same access to an education as other students do.

A child's or teen's school should prepare a plan that outlines how the child's special health care needs will be met. The plan should identify school staff responsible for making sure the plan is followed. The parents should be present during development of the plan. Any changes to the plan should be made only with the parents' consent. Ideally, the plan should be updated every year. For information or questions about the Americans With Disabilities Act (ADA), call 800-514-0301 or 800-514-0383 (TDD), or go to U.S. Department of Justice's ADA website online at www.usdoj.gov/crt/ada/adahome1.htm.

Are Researchers Studying Diabetes in Children and Adolescents?

As the lead Federal Government agency for diabetes research, the National Institute of Diabetes and Digestive and Kidney Diseases (NIDDK) conducts and supports a wide range of research aimed at finding ways to prevent and treat diabetes and its health complications. The Institute's research on type 1 diabetes focuses on understanding its causes, improving treatment, and developing new therapies that could prevent or cure diabetes. In addition, NIDDK recently created Trialnet, a clinical trials network to test new ways to prevent type 1 diabetes and to preserve beta cell function in people who already have diabetes.

NIDDK is also setting up clinical centers to study the prevention and treatment of type 2 diabetes in children and adolescents. Treatment trials will look at lifestyle changes and drug therapy. Prevention trials will develop programs that can be used in schools and communities to lower risk factors for the disease. Other NIDDK-supported research on type 2 diabetes seeks to understand the causes of the disease, improve diagnosis, and develop new treatments. For more information about NIDDK research on children and adolescents with diabetes, visit the website www.niddk.nih.gov/research.

In 2000, the Centers for Disease Control and Prevention (CDC) began funding a 5-year multi-center study of childhood diabetes. Participating centers are located in California, Colorado, Hawaii, Ohio, South Carolina, and Washington. The goals of the program are to 1) develop population-based registries of childhood diabetes, 2) characterize the types of diabetes, 3) develop case definitions and study the prevalence and incidence of the different types of childhood diabetes, and 4) describe the natural history and the quality of care received during follow-up. For more information, call 877-232-3422 or visit the website http://www.cdc.gov/diabetes/projects/cda2.htm.

NIDDK and CDC are joint sponsors of the National Diabetes Education Program (NDEP). The goal of this program is to reduce illness and death associated with diabetes and its complications. The NDEP

435

has developed an initiative to help health care providers identify, diagnose, and treat children and teens with type 2 diabetes. In addition, the NDEP will launch an initiative to increase awareness in the school setting about the importance of helping children and teens with diabetes manage their disease.

Resources

American Diabetes Association
1701 N. Beauregard Street
Alexandria, VA 22311
Toll-Free: 800-DIABETES or
800-342-2383
Phone: 703-549-1500
Website: http://www.diabetes.org
E-mail: customerservice@
diabetes.org

CDC Division of Diabetes Translation
Public Inquiries/Publications
P.O. Box 8728
Silver Spring, MD 20910
Toll-Free: 877-CDC-DIAB or
877-232-3422
Fax: 301-562-1050
Website: www.cdc.gov/diabetes
E-mail: diabetes@cdc.gov

CDC's National Center for Chronic Disease Prevention and Health Promotion
1600 Clifton Road
Atlanta, GA 30333
Toll-Free: 800-311-3435
Phone: 404-639-3311
Fax: 770-448-5195
Website: www.cdc.gov/nccdphp/
index.htm

Juvenile Diabetes Foundation International
120 Wall Street, 19th Floor
New York, NY 10005
Toll-Free: 800-223-1138
Phone: 212-785-9500
Website: http://www.jdf.org

National Diabetes Education Program (NDEP)
1 Diabetes Way
Bethesda, MD 20892-3600
Toll-Free: 800-438-5383
Website: http://www.ndep.nih.gov

National Diabetes Information Clearinghouse
1 Information Way
Bethesda, MD 20892-3560
Toll-Free: 800-860-8747
Phone: 301-654-3327
Fax: 301-907-8906
Website: www.niddk.nih.gov/
health/diabetes/diabetes.htm
E-mail: ndic@info.niddk.nih.gov

Chapter 66

Pituitary Tumors in Children

Introduction

The pituitary gland is a peanut-shaped gland in the brain, behind and between the eyes.

Childhood pituitary tumors, although rare, do occur. Such tumors are usually benign, that is, non-cancerous. However, because the pituitary gland is very important in helping to regulate the hormones of the body, even a small disruption can have serious effects on mood, on the ability to focus and concentrate, as well as on growth and overall maturation. Pituitary tumors can also cause symptoms due to pressure on other parts of the brain and may cause headaches, dizziness, or problems with vision.

New diagnostic techniques and chemical assays or tests for specific hormones, as well as computerized imaging tools such as magnetic resonance tomography (MR) and computerized tomography (CT) are used to locate and diagnose pituitary tumors. Then microsurgery, radiation therapy, hormones, and/or drugs are used to treat pituitary tumors in children. The effects of some tumors can also often be improved by hormone replacement therapies. Scientists at the National Institutes of Health and others around the world are improving the diagnosis and therapy of pituitary tumors and learning about the molecular mechanisms that cause these tumors. There is also a constant

National Institute of Child Health and Human Development (NICHD), 1997; updated September 2002. Available online at http://www.nichd.nih.gov/publications/pubs/pit.htm.

search for genetic patterns and an on-going effort to develop new gene-based therapies to prevent or treat pituitary tumors.

The Pituitary Gland

The pituitary gland is called a master gland, one that coordinates signals for hormone production from the brain, the hypothalamus, and from other parts of the body. This gland secretes a number of hormones that help control and respond to stress, affect brain functions, such as the ability to focus and pay attention, and go govern growth and sexual development, energy metabolism, and the body's ability to defend itself.

Classification of Pituitary Tumors

Pituitary tumors that secrete hormones take the name of the hormone they secrete and the ending -oma. For instance, a tumor that secretes prolactin is called prolactinoma. Other pituitary tumors secreting corticotropin are termed corticotropinomas, and so on. Each of these tumors produces a characteristic syndrome in patients because of excessive hormone secretion. Tumors that do not secrete hormones can cause problems by interfering with the functioning of the pituitary gland and by causing pressure on other parts of the brain.

Symptoms

In general, the symptoms seen with pituitary tumors are related to a disturbance in production of a specific hormone or group of hormones and relate to the role the hormones play in maintaining health and development. The symptoms of pituitary tumors vary depending on the size and location of the tumor and whether the tumor presses on other organs or affects the secretion of hormones. For instance, pituitary tumors may press on the optic nerve, causing problems with vision.

The symptoms of a pituitary tumor can range from simple common complaints such as listlessness or restlessness to more severe symptoms such as headaches, vomiting or dizziness. One problem in determining whether or not a tumor is present is that every child has minor and relatively unimportant symptoms such as restlessness or headaches from time to time. Of course, when more distressing signs or multiple symptoms are seen, parents and doctors search for an explanation and more precise tests are recommended.

In older children or adolescents, other signs may be seen including problems with normal growth and development. For instance, sometimes young girls or boys, under age 9, experience a very early puberty, referred to as precocious puberty. This is caused by tumors that secrete luteinizing hormone (LH). Girls may develop breasts, have pubic hair, and begin menstruation. Boys may find their genitals enlarging and facial and pubic hair beginning to grow. Tumors that secrete follicle stimulating hormone (FSH), in contrast, can retard sexual development in both sexes and stunt growth.

If the tumor limits the secretion of gonadotropin, it can affect the development and functioning of the ovaries and testes. Adolescent boys may fail to enter puberty or may lose facial or pubic hair and notice an effect on their genital size. Adolescent girls may also fail to enter puberty or may find their breasts smaller, some loss of pubic hair, and perhaps an interruption of menstruation.

Where secretion of adrenocorticotropic hormone (ACTH) is low, the child can experience low blood sugar, fatigue, and low blood pressure, which can cause dizziness when standing. On the other hand, with pituitary tumors that secrete ACTH, a variety of problems can result. These include stunted growth, delayed or stopped puberty, weight gain, acne, purple streaks in the skin, a round red face, and a bulge of fat on the back of or below the neck. These tumors can also cause weakness, depression, or forgetfulness and trigger a sudden complete or partial loss of vision.

Some pituitary tumors can disrupt the function of the thyroid gland by secreting thyroid stimulating hormone (TSH). This in turn enlarges the thyroid, causing a visibly large lump in the neck known as a goiter. These tumors also cause nervousness, a rapid pulse, weight loss, excess eating and sweating, and a sensitivity to heat.

Pituitary tumors that limit the secretion of TSH can also affect a child in many ways, including making it harder to concentrate, tiredness, constipation, dry skin, and a sensitivity to cold. It may also cause girls to have irregular periods or not to menstruate at all.

Some pituitary tumors decrease the secretion of vasopressin, the hormone that triggers the kidney's reabsorption of water from urine. A lack of vasopressin can cause a great thirst, excess urination, voracious appetite accompanied by emaciation, loss of strength, and fainting.

Other pituitary tumors secrete an excess of the hormone prolactin. In girls who have gone through puberty, tumors that secrete the hormone prolactin can cause the production of breast milk and stop menstruation, while in post-pubertal boys they can cause impotence. An excess of prolactin can also delay or stop puberty in both sexes.

A pituitary tumor that limits the secretion of growth hormone (GH) can stunt the growth of children and cause low blood sugar, which can induce fainting, dizziness, anxiety, and intense hunger. Growth hormone secreting tumors in growing children can boost growth excessively so that, if not treated, the children can grow unusually tall.

In adolescent children who have gone through puberty, and whose bones have stopped growing, excess GH can cause enlargement of their feet, hands, lips, nose, and jaw, a condition referred to as acromegaly It also can foster excess perspiration and fatigue, a widening of the spaces between the teeth, furrows in the forehead and weakness in the hands.

The most common type of pituitary tumor in children is due to growth of embryonic remnants in the area of the pituitary gland and is called craniopharyngioma. This tumor often disrupts vision by pressing on the optic nerve. Craniopharyngiomas also cause a lack of most pituitary hormones, prompting a combination of some of the symptoms previously described for tumors that induce a deficiency of single pituitary hormones.

Diagnosis and Testing

Doctors can detect larger pituitary tumors on an x-ray, computerized tomography scan or magnetic resonance scan. Many pituitary tumors, however, are too small to be seen on these images of the pituitary region of the brain. To diagnose these tumors, doctors try to detect the hormonal abnormalities with various tests. Often blood or urine levels of specific hormones are measured within a few hours of giving the patient compounds known to stimulate or suppress production of the hormones.

For instance, sometimes patients are given a glucose tolerance test. After fasting overnight, the patient drinks a sugar solution, then has blood samples taken in which sugar or growth hormone levels are measured. Sometimes, in order to locate a very small tumor in the pituitary gland, an invasive procedure is required. This procedure is called inferior petrosal sinus sampling. A radiologist inserts special catheters from the groin veins into the vessels that drain the pituitary gland at the top of the neck and draws blood for measurement of the hormone that the tumor secretes.

Treatment

Doctors can successfully treat most pituitary tumors with microsurgery performed under the magnification of a surgical microscope, radiation therapy, surgery, drugs, or a combination of these treatments. Surgery is the treatment of choice for tumors that enlarge rapidly and threaten vision. The treatment plan for other pituitary tumors varies according to the type and size of the tumor.

Depending on each individual diagnosis, a physician can prescribe a wide variety of treatments. Sometimes treatments stimulate or compensate for missing hormones, others reduce the production of hormones. In some cases, drugs must be taken on a daily basis.

Chapter 67

Klinefelter Syndrome: XXY Males

What Is Klinefelter Syndrome?

In 1942, Dr. Harry Klinefelter and his coworkers at the Massachusetts General Hospital in Boston published a report about nine men who had enlarged breasts, sparse facial and body hair, small testes, and an inability to produce sperm.

By the late 1950s, researchers discovered that men with Klinefelter syndrome, as this group of symptoms came to be called, had an extra sex chromosome, XXY instead of the usual male arrangement, XY.

In the early 1970s, researchers around the world sought to identify males having the extra chromosome by screening large numbers of newborn babies. One of the largest of these studies, sponsored by the National Institute of Child Health and Human Development (NICHD), checked the chromosomes of more than 40,000 infants.

Based on these studies, the XXY chromosome arrangement appears to be one of the most common genetic abnormalities known, occurring as frequently as 1 in 500 to 1 in 1,000 male births. Although the syndrome's cause, an extra sex chromosome, is widespread, the syndrome itself—the set of symptoms and characteristics that may result from having the extra chromosome—is uncommon. Many men live

Excerpted from "A Guide for XXY Males and Their Families," by Robert Bock, National Institute of Child Health and Human Development (NICHD), NIH Pub. No. 93-3202, updated September 2002. The full text is available online at http://www.nichd.nih.gov/publications/pubs/klinefelter.htm.

out their lives without ever even suspecting that they have an additional chromosome.

"I never refer to newborn babies as having Klinefelter's, because they don't have a syndrome," said Arthur Robinson, MD, a pediatrician at the University of Colorado Medical School in Denver and the director of the NICHD-sponsored study of XXY males. "Presumably, some of them will grow up to develop the syndrome Dr. Klinefelter described, but a lot of them won't."

For this reason, the term "Klinefelter syndrome" has fallen out of favor with medical researchers. Most prefer to describe men and boys having the extra chromosome as "XXY males."

In addition to occasional breast enlargement, lack of facial and body hair, and a rounded body type, XXY males are more likely than other males to be overweight, and tend to be taller than their fathers and brothers.

Although they are not mentally retarded, most XXY males have some degree of language impairment. As children, they often learn to speak much later than do other children and may have difficulty learning to read and write. And while they eventually do learn to speak and converse normally, the majority tend to have some degree of difficulty with language throughout their lives. If untreated, this language impairment can lead to school failure and its attendant loss of self esteem.

Fortunately, however, this language disability usually can be compensated for. Chances for success are greatest if begun in early childhood. Sections that follow describe possible strategies for meeting the special educational needs of many XXY males.

Causes

No one knows what puts a couple at risk for conceiving an XXY child. Advanced maternal age increases the risk for the XXY chromosome count, but only slightly. Furthermore, recent studies conducted by NICHD grantee Terry Hassold, a geneticist at Case Western Reserve University in Cleveland, OH, show that half the time, the extra chromosome comes from the father.

Diagnosis

Because they often don't appear any different from anyone else, many XXY males probably never learn of their extra chromosome. However, if they are to be diagnosed, chances are greatest at one of the following times in life: before or shortly after birth, early childhood, adolescence, and in adulthood (as a result of testing for infertility).

In recent years, many XXY males have been diagnosed before birth, through amniocentesis or chorionic villus sampling (CVS). In amniocentesis, a sample of the fluid surrounding the fetus is withdrawn. Fetal cells in the fluid are then examined for chromosomal abnormalities. CVS is similar to amniocentesis, except that the procedure is done in the first trimester, and the fetal cells needed for examination are taken from the placenta. Neither procedure is used routinely, except when there is a family history of genetic defects, the pregnant woman is older than 35, or when other medical indications are present.

The next most likely opportunity for diagnosis is when the child begins school. A physician may suspect a boy is an XXY male if he is delayed in learning to talk and has difficulty with reading and writing. XXY boys may also be tall and thin and somewhat passive and shy. Again, however, there are no guarantees. Some of the boys who fit this description will have the XXY chromosome count, but many others will not.

A few XXY males are diagnosed at adolescence, when excessive breast development forces them to seek medical attention. Like some chromosomally normal males, many XXY males undergo slight breast enlargement at puberty. Of these, only about a third—10 percent of XXY males in all—will develop breasts large enough to embarrass them.

The final chance for diagnosis is at adulthood, as a result of testing for infertility. At this time, an examining physician may note the undersized testes characteristic of an XXY male. In addition to infertility tests, the physician may order tests to detect increased levels of hormones known as gonadotropins, common in XXY males.

A karyotype is used to confirm the diagnosis. In this procedure, a small blood sample is drawn. White blood cells are then separated from the sample, mixed with tissue culture medium, incubated, and checked for chromosomal abnormalities, such as an extra X chromosome.

Childhood

According to Dr. Robinson, the director of the NICHD-funded study, XXY babies differ little from other children their age. They tend to start life as what many parents call "good" babies—quiet, undemanding, and perhaps even a little passive. As toddlers, they may be somewhat shy

445

and reserved. They usually learn to walk later than most other children, and may have similar delays in learning to speak.

In some, the language delays may be more severe, with the child not fully learning to talk until about age 5. Others may learn to speak at a normal rate, and not meet with any problems until they begin school, where they may experience reading difficulties. A few may not have any problems at all—in learning to speak or in learning to read.

XXY males usually have difficulty with expressive language—the ability to put thoughts, ideas, and emotions into words. In contrast, their faculty for receptive language—understanding what is said—is close to normal.

Guidelines for Detecting Language Problems

Shortly after the first birthday, children should be able to make their wishes known with simple one word utterances. For example, a child may say "milk" to mean "I want more milk." Gradually, children begin to combine words to produce two-word sentences, such as "More milk." By age three, most children use an average of about four words per sentence.

If a child is not communicating effectively with single words by 18 to 24 months, then parents should seek a consultation with a speech and language pathologist.

The XXY Boy in the Classroom

Although there are exceptions, XXY boys are usually well behaved in the classroom. Most are shy, quiet, and eager to please the teacher. But when faced with material they find difficult, they tend to withdraw into quiet daydreaming. Teachers sometimes fail to realize they have a language problem, and dismiss them as lazy, saying they could do the work if they would only try. Many become so quiet that teachers forget they're even in the room. As a result, they fall farther and farther behind, and eventually may be held back a grade.

Help under the Law

According to Dr. Robinson, XXY boys do best in small, uncrowded classrooms where teachers can give them a lot of individual attention. He suggests that parents who can meet the expense consider sending their sons to a private school offering special educational services.

Parents who cannot afford private schools should become familiar with Public Law 94-142, the Education of the Handicapped Act—now called the Individuals with Disabilities Education Act. This law, adopted by Congress in 1975, states that all children with disabilities have a right to a free, appropriate public education. The law cannot ensure that every child who needs special educational services will automatically get them. But the law does allow parents to take action when they suspect their child has a learning disability.

Testosterone Treatment

Ideally, XXY males should begin testosterone treatment as they enter puberty. XXY males diagnosed in adulthood are also likely to benefit from the hormone. A regular schedule of testosterone injections will increase strength and muscle size, and promote the growth of facial and body hair.

Side effects of the injections are few. Some individuals may develop a minor allergic reaction at the injection site, resulting in an itchy welt resembling a mosquito bite. Applying a non-prescription hydrocortisone cream to the area will reduce swelling and itching.

In addition, testosterone injections may result in a condition known as benign prostatic hyperplasia (BPH). This condition is common in chromosomally normal males as well, affecting more than 50 percent of men in their sixties, and as many as 90 percent in their seventies and eighties. In XXY males receiving testosterone injections, this condition may begin sometime after age 40.

Health Considerations

Compared with other males, XXY males have a slightly increased risk of autoimmune disorders. In this group of diseases, the immune system, for unknown reasons, attacks the body's organs or tissues. The most well known of these diseases are type 1 (insulin dependent) diabetes, autoimmune thyroiditis, and lupus erythematosus. Most of these conditions can be treated with medication.

XXY males with enlarged breasts have the same risk of breast cancer as do women—roughly 50 times the risk XY males have. For this reason, these XXY adolescents and men need to practice regular breast self examination. The free booklet "Breast Exams: What You Should Know" is available from the National Cancer Institute, listed in the Resources section of this *Sourcebook*. The last page of the booklet is a pullout chart listing the instructions for breast self examination.

Although the booklet was written primarily for women, the breast self examination technique also can be used by XXY males. XXY males may also wish to consult their physicians about the need for more thorough breast examinations by medical professionals.

In addition, XXY males who do not receive testosterone injections may have an increased risk of developing osteoporosis in later life. In this condition, which usually afflicts women after the age of menopause, the bones lose calcium, becoming brittle and more likely to break.

Chapter 68

Fragile X Syndrome

Introduction

Fragile X syndrome is the most common genetically-inherited form of mental retardation currently known. In addition to intellectual disability, some individuals with Fragile X display common physical traits and characteristic facial features, such as prominent ears. Children with Fragile X often appear normal in infancy but develop typical physical characteristics during their lifetime. Mental impairment may range from mild learning disability and hyperactivity to severe mental retardation and autism. This genetic syndrome is caused by a defect on the X chromosome. Because of scientific advances, improvements in genetic testing, and increased awareness, the number of children diagnosed with Fragile X has increased significantly over the last decade.

A substantial research effort led to the 1991 discovery of FMR-1 (Fragile X mental retardation), the gene that when damaged causes Fragile X. Although the normal function of the FMR-1 gene is not fully understood, it appears to be important early in development. The mechanism by which the normal FMR-1 gene is converted into an altered, or mutant, gene capable of causing disease symptoms involves

Excerpted from "Facts about Fragile X Syndrome," National Institute of Child Health and Human Development (NICHD), National Institutes of Health (NIH). This publication was reviewed in August 2000 by NIH researchers. Although the publication does not include the newest research available, it has been determined to still be scientifically valid. The full text is available online at http://www.nichd.nih.gov/publications/pubs/fragilextoc.htm.

an increase in the length of the gene. A small region of the gene, CGG, undergoes repeated duplications, forming deoxyribonucleic acid (DNA) and repeats that result in a longer gene. The lengthened DNA region is susceptible to a chemical modification process called DNA methylation. When the number of repeats is small (less than 200) the individual often has no signs of the disorder. However, in individuals with a larger number of repeats, the characteristics that are typical of Fragile X are observed. In families that exhibit Fragile X, both the number of repeats and the length of the chromosome increase with succeeding generations. The severity of the symptoms increases with the increasing length of the repeated region.

Fragile X exhibits X-linkage. The effect of X-linkage is that the frequency of the syndrome is greater in males than in females. To understand the mechanism of X-linkage some background information on the organization of human chromosomes is needed. Human females typically have two X chromosomes, and human males have one X and one Y chromosome. A female who inherits a chromosome carrying the Fragile X gene from either parent is likely to inherit a normal X chromosome from the other parent. The normal X chromosome could provide the normal gene function and mask the presence of the Fragile X gene in a female. In that case, the female would still possess the Fragile X gene and be capable of passing it on to her offspring, but she would not exhibit symptoms. She would be a "carrier." On the other hand, a male who inherits the Fragile X gene from his mother would inherit a Y chromosome and not a normal X chromosome from his father, and therefore a male with one copy of the gene is likely to show symptoms. We do not yet have a complete understanding of the mechanism of genetic transmission of Fragile X. For example, it is not known why approximately one-fifth of males who carry mutated forms of FMR-1 are either unaffected or only mildly affected. In some cases, a single copy of the Fragile X gene is sufficient to cause the syndrome in females. The situation is made more complex by the fact that the intensity of the symptoms increases with succeeding generations. The observable characteristics of Fragile X occur in approximately 1 in 1,000 male births and 1 in 2,500 female births.

On a normal X chromosome, the FMR-1 region of the chromosome contains 50 or fewer copies of the CGG repeat. This same region may be repeated hundreds or even thousands of times in individuals with Fragile X. Researchers have made a surprising correlation between the number of DNA repeats and the degree of clinical impairment. Individuals with between 50 and 200 repeats are often carriers of Fragile X who have mild symptoms or no symptoms at all. When the number of repeats increases, the chemical modification process called DNA methylation is more likely to occur. It is this chemical modification that appears to inactivate the FMR-1 gene, leading to deficits in cognitive processing. Why methylation of this region of DNA leads to the symptoms of Fragile X is not understood. Mental impairment in Fragile X appears to correlate with DNA containing more than 200 repeats. In that case, most males are impaired and 50 percent of females show some learning disabilities. However, there are exceptions, including individuals with enormous numbers of repeats who have no apparent impairment.

Inheritance

In normal individuals the FMR-1 gene is passed on, in stable fashion, from the parent to the offspring. In Fragile X individuals, the repeated sequences not only expand abnormally, but are unstable and the degree of impairment in offspring may vary. The Fragile X mutation appears to increase in length as it is inherited by succeeding generations. This phenomenon is known as "genetic anticipation." Eventually, the mutation reaches a critical number of repeats and causes Fragile X syndrome. For example, a male may have normal IQ, no Fragile X symptoms, and a short region of DNA repeats at the Fragile X region of his X chromosome. This individual, called a "transmitting" male, may have a daughter with 50 to 200 repeats. At that stage the condition is considered a "premutation," as there still may be no apparent symptoms. This daughter, a "carrier," might have a son with 1,000 repeats and the full blown Fragile X syndrome. If a woman is a carrier, each of her children has a 50 percent chance of inheriting her Fragile X gene. Each time her Fragile X gene is inherited, it is likely to have expanded in length. A daughter who inherits the gene will be a carrier with some chance of impairment; a son who inherits the gene has an 80 percent likelihood of developing Fragile X syndrome.

Testing for Fragile X Carrier

A simple test is now available that can determine if a woman is a carrier of the Fragile X gene. A drop of blood can be taken from the woman's finger and analyzed quickly and inexpensively. If a woman who is found to be a carrier is pregnant, she can arrange for testing of the fetus, as described below. For a woman with a family history of retardation, testing before pregnancy will help determine if she is at risk.

Prenatal Testing

Three prenatal tests can determine if Fragile X is present in the fetus. Chorionic villi sampling (CVS) involves extracting a tiny amount of fetal tissue at 9 to 11 weeks of pregnancy. CVS is not widely used and carries a 1–2 percent risk of miscarriage following the procedure.

Amniocentesis is the removal and analysis of a small sample of fetal cells from the amniotic fluid. Amniocentesis is widely available and involves a lower risk of miscarriage. However, amniocentesis cannot be done until the 15th to 18th week of pregnancy and it usually takes an additional 2 to 4 weeks for the cells to grow and be analyzed. So a woman may have to wait until the 17th to 22nd week of her pregnancy to have the results of this test.

The third method, percutaneous umbilical blood sampling (PUBS), is the most accurate method and can be used to confirm the results of CVS or amniocentesis. However, PUBS is not widely available, PUBS is not done until the 18th to 22nd week and carries the greatest risk of miscarriage.

Diagnosing and Treating Fragile X Syndrome

Individuals with Fragile X may have a cluster of physical, behavioral, mental, and other characteristics. These symptoms may vary in number and degree among affected children. In the best of circumstances, early identification of a child with Fragile X and subsequent treatment involves a team of professionals. These might include a speech and language pathologist, an occupational therapist (perhaps even a specialist in sensory integration), a physical therapist, a special education teacher, a genetics counselor, and a psychologist.

Physical Characteristics

Males with Fragile X have some common physical characteristics: a long narrow face; large or prominent ears; and macroorchidism (enlarged testicles). More than 80 percent of males with Fragile X develop at least one of these features, but often not until after puberty. Other physical characteristics of males with Fragile X are double-jointed fingers, flat feet, puffy eyelids, and "hollow chest." These physical features may indicate an underlying abnormality of the connective tissue, although no specific connective tissue defect has been detected.

Females with Fragile X syndrome do not exhibit most of the physical characteristics found in males with Fragile X, although they often have large or prominent ears.

Behavioral Characteristics

The most prevalent behavioral characteristics of children with Fragile X are attention problems and hyperactivity, known as attention-deficit hyperactivity disorder (ADHD). ADHD is frequently treated with medication, generally central nervous system stimulants such as methylphenidate (Ritalin), pemoline (Cylert) and dextroamphetamine (Dexedrine). Because these drugs have side effects that include irritability and poor appetite, alternatives such as amantadine and clonidine may be appropriate. Amantadine has been used with surprising success to treat hyperactivity and attention difficulties in children with low IQs, for whom stimulants are generally less effective.

Fragile X children with ADHD may benefit from the addition of tricyclic antidepressants or a major tranquilizer such as thioridazine (Mellaril). Because mood swings and temper tantrums present major difficulties for children with Fragile X, psychotherapeutic medications such as Lithium and more recently fluoxetine (Prozac) have helped control aggression and outbursts. Anticonvulsants such as carbamazepine or valproate, used if seizures are present, can also help treat behavior problems, including aggression in males with Fragile X.

Children with Fragile X have strong reactions to changes in their environment, and their heightened anxiety can compound their behavioral difficulties. They appear to have an underlying disability related to processing external stimuli, called sensory integration. Extreme hypersensitivity to their environment makes is difficult for them to screen out stimuli such as noise, lights, or odors. This, in turn, often provokes emotional outbursts or tantrums.

Some of the other behaviors associated with Fragile X are similar to those of autism, including hand flapping, hand biting, poor eye contact, and tactile defensiveness (responding negatively to being touched). However, one strength of males with Fragile X is their great sociability and friendliness, in contrast to autistic children, who appear unable to relate to others. Researchers recommend that autistic children be screened for Fragile X.

Mental Impairment

Mental retardation associated with Fragile X is similar to that of Down syndrome in that most of those affected fall somewhere in the middle range of impairment. There are differences between males and females with Fragile X with respect to their mental impairment. There are differences between males and females with Fragile X with respect to their mental impairment.

Many females with Fragile X syndrome are learning disabled in math, but perform exceptionally well in reading and spelling. In addition, one-third of females with Fragile X have metal disabilities similar to those associated with schizophrenia, such as dependence on odd forms of communication and preference for social isolation. Males with Fragile X appear to differ in mental development from both females with Fragile X and children with other kinds of developmental delays who exhibit learning disabilities. Males with Fragile X may actually achieve more than some other developmentally disabled children with higher IQ scores. It is important for educators to understand the particular difficulties of males with Fragile X. They appear to process information in simultaneous fashion; this causes difficulty when they are taught skills that require sequential processing of information, such as reading. For males with Fragile X, learning often involves seeing the whole in order to understand the parts.

Speech, Language, and Learning Disabilities

Speech and language present special difficulties. Children with Fragile X often speak in rapid bursts or repeat words (called echolalia). For males with Fragile X, the primary language difficulty is perseveration. Perseveration is the inability to complete a sentence because of continuous repetition of words at the end of a phrase. Another language-based behavior displayed by males with Fragile X is talking inappropriately and incessantly about one topic. This particular difficulty distinguishes males with Fragile X from individuals with other forms of mental retardation or autism. Speech problems are made worse in situations where the child must have eye contact with another person or when the child becomes anxious, leading researchers to suspect some underlying relationship between difficulties with language and difficulties with sensory processing.

Medical Problems

Although most children with Fragile X do not have serious physical problems, they are at greater risk for certain types of moderate medical problems than are normal children. For example, they often suffer recurrent otitis media (inner ear infections), which should be treated as early as possible to prevent it from becoming a source of language difficulties. Common eye problems include myopia (nearsightedness) and a high incidence of "lazy eye." Orthopedic difficulties related to flat feet and joint laxity may occur. Twenty percent of males with Fragile X are prone to seizures, including petit mal, grand mal, and temporal lobe seizures. In addition, many children with Fragile X have digestive disorders, such as gastroesophageal reflux, that causes gagging, regurgitation, and discomfort.

Education of Children with Fragile X

Even at a young age, children with Fragile X tend to be good at imitation and to be very social. Consequently, they can benefit immensely from early intervention programs and prolonged contact with children who are developing normally. Congressional legislation (Public Law 99-457) mandates early intervention services for children with developmental delays, ages 3 to 5 years; in some states this includes younger children (for help finding local programs see Chapter 84— Resources for Information about Childhood Diseases).

Parents and educators should be aware that many children with Fragile X achieve above the level that would have been predicted from measured IQ, and it is important for parents and educators to help these children reach their maximum potential. Children with Fragile X with an IQ above 70 generally do best when mainstreamed into a well-organized classroom environment with individualized help from special education experts and other professionals. Cooperative instruction, using peers to help teach, often relieves some of the stress of the classroom environment and the teacher-child relationship.

Additional Therapies

To counter the sensory integration difficulties of children with Fragile X, a wide range of strategies has been employed. Minimizing exposure to noise and odors may prevent overstimulation. Therapeutic calming techniques, such as music therapy, can also be used. It may be helpful to make special efforts to provide structure in the immediate environment and in day-to-day activities. Children with Fragile X often develop their own routines. Occupational therapists specializing in sensory integration therapy can work with children with Fragile X to help them organize environmental stimuli and to improve their response to formal education.

The strength of their visual memory means that children with Fragile X process information better when they are presented with whole pictures rather than when information is presented orally or sequentially, as in normal reading. As a result, use of pictures, message boards, calculators, and other visual devices may be helpful. Some children with Fragile X learn sign language, a visual system. Computer software is now available for learning basic concepts in language and math using high-interest visual themes.

Psychology professionals warn against the tendency to assume that all characteristics of a child with Fragile X stem directly from the Fragile X syndrome. The emotional difficulties of an individual with Fragile X may include insecurity and anxiety related to having a disability.

These strategies are only a few that specialists have developed to help children with Fragile X. Parents and other individuals working with these children should make use of their assets, such as their positive outlook on life and love of other people. Children with Fragile X should be encouraged to express their feelings openly even when they have difficulty using words.

Future Research

Since the discovery of the Fragile X gene in 1991, there has been tremendous progress in the understanding of this disorder. Preimplantation genetic screening, using molecular genetic screening of *in vitro* fertilized embryos followed by implantation of embryos that are free of the disorder, may be available to would-be parents in the near future.

Some affected families argue that not enough research is being conducted on the treatment of Fragile X. In response, experts explain that it is difficult to treat Fragile X without first understanding more about the biology of the condition and the meaning of the DNA expansions. It has been particularly difficult to investigate these questions in the absence of an animal model. The nature of the Fragile X mutation may itself be a source of the difficulty scientists are having in developing an animal model of the disease. The excess genetic material of the Fragile X defect is so voluminous and so fragile that inserting the Fragile X DNA into animal cells has been a problem for laboratory scientists. However, there has been some recent progress in this area, and continued research is likely to bring success.

Once an animal model is developed, researchers will be able to learn more about the basis of the Fragile X mutation and the mechanisms that contribute to its unstable character. Ongoing analysis of the FMR-1 gene and its protein product may help researchers understand the normal function of this protein and perhaps find a way to intervene when its functioning goes awry.

Chapter 69

Down Syndrome

Named after John Langdon Down, the first physician to identify the syndrome, Down syndrome is the most frequent genetic cause of mild to moderate mental retardation and associated medical problems and occurs in one out of 800 live births, in all races and economic groups. Down syndrome is a chromosomal disorder caused by an error in cell division that results in the presence of an additional third chromosome 21 or "trisomy 21."

The Chromosomal Basis of Down Syndrome

To understand why Down syndrome occurs, the structure and function of the human chromosome must be understood. The human body is made of cells; all cells contain chromosomes, structures that transmit genetic information. Most cells of the human body contain 23 pairs of chromosomes, half of which are inherited from each parent. Only the human reproductive cells, the sperm cells in males and the ovum in females, have 23 individual chromosomes, not pairs. Scientists identify these chromosome pairs as the XX pair, present in females, and the XY pair, present in males, and number them 1 through 22.

When the reproductive cells, the sperm and ovum, combine at fertilization, the fertilized egg that results contains 23 chromosome pairs. A fertilized egg that will develop into a female contains chromosome

Excerpted from "Facts About Down Syndrome," National Institute of Child Health and Human Development (NICHD), National Institutes of Health (NIH), http://www.nichd.nih.gov/publications/pubs/downsyndrome/down.htm, 2002.

pairs 1 through 22, and the XX pair. A fertilized egg that will develop into a male contains chromosome pairs 1 through 22, and the XY pair. When the fertilized egg contains extra material from chromosome number 21, this results in Down syndrome.

The Occurrence of Down Syndrome

Most of the time, the occurrence of Down syndrome is due to a random event that occurred during formation of the reproductive cells, the ovum or sperm. As far as we know, Down syndrome is not attributable to any behavioral activity of the parents or environmental factors. The probability that another child with Down syndrome will be born in a subsequent pregnancy is about 1 percent, regardless of maternal age.

Down Syndrome and Maternal Age

Researchers have established that the likelihood that a reproductive cell will contain an extra copy of chromosome 21 increases dramatically as a woman ages. Therefore, an older mother is more likely than a younger mother to have a baby with Down syndrome. However, of the total population, older mothers have fewer babies; about 75% of babies with Down syndrome are born to younger women because more younger women than older women have babies. Only about nine percent of total pregnancies occur in women 35 years or older each year, but about 25% of babies with Down syndrome are born to women in this age group.

The incidence of Down syndrome rises with increasing maternal age. Many specialists recommend that women who become pregnant at age 35 or older undergo prenatal testing for Down syndrome. The likelihood that a woman under 30 who becomes pregnant will have a baby with Down syndrome is less than 1 in 1,000, but the chance of having a baby with Down syndrome increases to 1 in 400 for women who become pregnant at age 35. The likelihood of Down syndrome continues to increase as a woman ages, so that by age 42, the chance is 1 in 60 that a pregnant woman will have a baby with Down syndrome, and by age 49, the chance is 1 in 12. But using maternal age alone will not detect over 75% of pregnancies that will result in Down syndrome.

Prenatal Screening for Down Syndrome

Prenatal screening for Down syndrome is available. There is a relatively simple, noninvasive screening test that examines a drop of the mother's blood to determine if there is an increased likelihood for Down syndrome. This blood test measures the levels of three markers for Down syndrome: serum alpha fetoprotein (MSAFP), chorionic gonadotropin (hCG), and unconjugated estriol (uE3). While these measurements are not a definitive test for Down syndrome, a lower MSAFP value, a lower uE3 level, and an elevated hCG level, on average, suggests an increased likelihood of a Down syndrome fetus, and additional diagnostic testing may be desired.

A Diagnosis of Down Syndrome

A newborn baby with Down syndrome often has physical features the attending physician will most likely recognize in the delivery room. These may include a flat facial profile, an upward slant to the eye, a short neck, abnormally shaped ears, white spots on the iris of the eye (called Brushfield spots), and a single, deep transverse crease on the palm of the hand. However, a child with Down syndrome may not possess all of these features; some of these features can even be found in the general population.

To confirm the diagnosis, the doctor will request a blood test called a chromosomal karyotype. This involves "growing" the cells from the baby's blood for about two weeks, followed by a microscopic visualization of the chromosomes to determine if extra material from chromosome 21 is present.

When parents are told that their newborn baby has Down syndrome, it is not unusual for them to have feelings of sadness and disappointment. Many parents report that at the time their child is first diagnosed with Down syndrome and during the weeks that follow, they feel overwhelmed by feelings of loss and anxiety. While caring for a child with Down syndrome frequently requires more time and energy, parents of newborn children with Down syndrome should seek the advice of a knowledgeable pediatrician and/or the many Down syndrome support groups and organizations available.

The doctor making the initial diagnosis of Down syndrome has no way of knowing the intellectual or physical capabilities this child, or any other child, may have. Children and adults with Down syndrome have a wide range of abilities. A person with Down syndrome may be very healthy or they may present unusual and demanding medical and social problems at virtually every stage of life. However, every person with Down syndrome is a unique individual, and not all people with Down syndrome will develop all the medical disorders discussed below.

Down Syndrome and Associated Medical Disorders

During the first days and months of life, some disorders may be immediately diagnosed. Congenital hypothyroidism, characterized by a reduced basal metabolism, an enlargement of the thyroid gland, and disturbances in the autonomic nervous system, occurs slightly more frequently in babies with Down syndrome. A routine blood test for hypothyroidism that is performed on newborns will detect this condition if present.

Several other well-known medical conditions, including hearing loss, congenital heart disease, and vision disorders, are more prevalent among those with Down syndrome.

Recent studies indicate that 66 to 89% of children with Down syndrome have a hearing loss of greater than 15 to 20 decibels in at least one ear, due to the fact that the external ear and the bones of the middle and inner ear may develop differently in children with Down syndrome. Many hearing problems can be corrected. But, because of the high prevalence of hearing loss in children with Down syndrome, an objective measure of hearing should be taken to establish hearing status. In addition to hearing disorders, visual problems also may be present early in life. Cataracts occur in approximately 3% of children with Down syndrome, but can be surgically removed.

Approximately half of the children with Down syndrome have congenital heart disease and associated early onset of pulmonary hypertension, or high blood pressure in the lungs. Echocardiography may be indicated to identify any congenital heart disease. If the defects have been identified before the onset of pulmonary hypertension, surgery has provided favorable results.

Seizure disorders, though less prevalent than some of the other associated medical conditions, still affect between 5 and 13% of individuals with Down syndrome, a 10-fold greater incidence than in the general population. There is an unusually high incidence of infantile spasms or seizures in children less than one year of age, some of which are precipitated by neonatal complications and infections and cardiovascular disease. However, these seizures can be treated with anti-epileptic drugs.

The incidence and severity of these associated medical ailments will vary in babies with Down syndrome and some may require surgery.

Infants and Preschool Children

Medical care for infants with Down syndrome should include the same well-baby care that other children receive during the first years of life, as well as attention to some problems that are more common in children with Down syndrome. If heart, digestive, orthopedic or other medical conditions were identified during the neonatal period, these problems should continue to be monitored.

During the early years of life, children with Down syndrome are 10–15 times more likely than other children to develop leukemia, a potentially fatal disease. These children should receive an appropriate cancer therapy, such as chemotherapy. Infants with Down syndrome are also more susceptible to transient myelodysplasia, or the defective development of the spinal cord.

Compared to the general population, individuals with Down syndrome have a 12-fold higher mortality rate from infectious diseases, if these infections are left untreated and unmonitored. These infections are due to abnormalities in their immune systems, usually the t-cell and antibody-mediated immunity functions that fight off infections. Children with Down syndrome are also more likely to develop chronic respiratory infections, middle ear infections, and recurrent tonsillitis. In addition, there is a 62-fold higher incidence of pneumonia in children with Down syndrome than in the general population.

Children with Down syndrome may be developmentally delayed. A child with Down syndrome is often slow to turn over, sit, stand, and respond. This may be related to the child's poor muscle tone. Development of speech and language abilities may take longer than expected and may not occur as fully as parents would like. However, children with Down syndrome do develop the communication skills they need.

Parents of other children with Down syndrome are often valuable sources of information and support. Parents should keep in mind that children with Down syndrome have a wide range of abilities and talents, and each child develops at his or her own particular pace. It may take children with Down syndrome longer than other children to reach developmental milestones, but many of these milestones will eventually be met. Parents should make a concerted effort not to compare the developmental progress of a child with Down syndrome to the progress of other siblings or even to other children with Down syndrome.

Early Intervention and Education

The term "early intervention" refers to an array of specialized programs and related resources that are made available by health care professionals to the child with Down syndrome. These health care professionals may include special educators, speech therapists, occupational therapists, and social workers. It is recommended that stimulation and encouragement be provided to children with Down syndrome.

The evaluation of early intervention programs for children with Down syndrome is difficult, due to the wide variety of experimental designs used in interventions, the limited existing measures available that chart the progress of disabled infants, and the tremendous variability in the developmental progress among children with Down syndrome, a consequence in part of the many complicating medical factors. While many studies have been conducted to assess the effects of early intervention, the information is limited and contradictory regarding the long-term success of early intervention for children with Down syndrome.

However, federal laws (Public Law 94-12) are in place to ensure each state has as a goal that "all handicapped children have available to them a free public education and related services designed to meet their unique needs." The decision of what type of school a child with Down syndrome should attend is an important one, made by the parents in consultation with health and education professionals. A parent must decide between enrolling the child in a school where most of the children do not have disabilities (inclusion) or sending the child to a school for children with special needs. Inclusion has become more common over the past decade.

Adolescence

Like all teenagers, individuals with Down syndrome undergo hormonal changes during adolescence. Therefore, teenagers with Down syndrome should be educated about their sexual drives. Scientists have medical evidence that males with Down syndrome generally have a reduced sperm count and rarely father children. Females with Down syndrome have regular menstrual periods and are capable of becoming pregnant and carrying a baby to term.

Adults with Down Syndrome

The life expectancy for people with Down syndrome has increased substantially. In 1929, the average life span of a person with Down syndrome was nine years. Today, it is common for a person with Down syndrome to live to age fifty and beyond. In addition to living longer, people with Down syndrome are now living fuller, richer lives than ever before as family members and contributors to their community.

Many people with Down syndrome form meaningful relationships and eventually marry. Now that people with Down syndrome are living longer, the needs of adults with Down syndrome are receiving greater attention. With assistance from family and caretakers, many adults with Down syndrome have developed the skills required to hold jobs and to live semi-independently.

Premature aging is a characteristic of adults with Down syndrome. In addition, dementia, or memory loss and impaired judgment similar to that occurring in Alzheimer disease patients, may appear in adults with Down syndrome. This condition often occurs when the person is younger than forty years old. Family members and caretakers of an adult with Down syndrome must be prepared to intervene if the individual begins to lose the skills required for independent living.

Future Directions in Down Syndrome Research

Recently, it has been suggested that children with Down syndrome might benefit from medical intervention that includes amino acid supplements and a drug known as Piracetam. Piracetam is a psychoactive drug that some believe may improve cognitive function. However, there have been no controlled clinical studies conducted to date using Piracetam to treat Down syndrome in the U.S. or elsewhere that show its safety and efficacy.

Down syndrome researchers have developed a mouse model to analyze the developmental consequences of Down syndrome. Mice are used because a large stretch of mouse chromosome 16 has many genes in common with those on human chromosome 21. Studying these models at varying stages of development will enhance our basic understanding of Down syndrome and facilitate the development of effective interventions and treatment strategies.

Questions and Answers about Down Syndrome

Is Down syndrome a rare genetic disorder?

Down syndrome occurs in 1 in 800 births.

Do only older women give birth to babies with Down syndrome?

Researchers have established that the likelihood that a reproductive cell will contain an extra copy of chromosome 21 increases dramatically as a woman ages. Therefore, an older mother is more likely than a younger mother to have a baby with Down syndrome, but older mothers account for only about 9% of all live births each year and 25% of Down syndrome births.

Are all people with Down syndrome severely retarded?

Most people with Down syndrome have IQ's that fall in the mild to moderate range of retardation. Some are so mildly affected that they live independently and are gainfully employed.

Can people with Down syndrome receive proper care at home?

Home-based care and community living give them the opportunity to socialize and benefit from such interactions.

Should all children with Down syndrome be placed in special education classrooms?

While federal laws have been established to insure that all handi-capped children have access to public education, children with Down syndrome can and have been included into a regular classroom.

Is there a cure for Down syndrome?

Researchers have identified the genes that cause the characteristics of Down syndrome and are working to further develop mouse models, at varying stages of development, in order to enhance their basic understanding of Down syndrome and facilitate the development of effective interventions and treatment strategies.

Chapter 70

Autism

Introduction

Isolated in worlds of their own, people with autism appear indifferent and remote and are unable to form emotional bonds with others. Although people with this baffling brain disorder can display a wide range of symptoms and disability, many are incapable of understanding other people's thoughts, feelings, and needs. Often, language and intelligence fail to develop fully, making communication and social relationships difficult. Many people with autism engage in repetitive activities, like rocking or banging their heads, or rigidly following familiar patterns in their everyday routines. Some are painfully sensitive to sound, touch, sight, or smell.

Children with autism do not follow the typical patterns of child development. In some children, hints of future problems may be apparent from birth. In most cases, the problems become more noticeable as the child slips farther behind other children the same age. Other children start off well enough. But between 18 and 36 months old, they suddenly reject people, act strangely, and lose language and social skills they had already acquired.

As a parent, teacher, or care giver you may know the frustration of trying to communicate and connect with children or adults who have autism. You may feel ignored as they engage in endlessly repetitive

Excerpted from "Autism," National Institute of Mental Health (NIMH), NIH Pub. No. 97-4023, September 1997, updated June 1999. Available online at http://www.nimh.nih.gov/publicat/autism.cfm.

behaviors. You may despair at the bizarre ways they express their inner needs. And you may feel sorrow that your hopes and dreams for them may never materialize.

But there is help—and hope. Gone are the days when people with autism were isolated, typically sent away to institutions. Today, many youngsters can be helped to attend school with other children. Methods are available to help improve their social, language, and academic skills. Even though more than 60 percent of adults with autism continue to need care throughout their lives, some programs are beginning to demonstrate that with appropriate support, many people with autism can be trained to do meaningful work and participate in the life of the community.

Autism is found in every country and region of the world, and in families of all racial, ethnic, religious, and economic backgrounds. Emerging in childhood, it affects about 1 or 2 people in every thousand and is three to four times more common in boys than girls. Girls with the disorder, however, tend to have more severe symptoms and lower intelligence. In addition to loss of personal potential, the cost of health and educational services to those affected exceeds $3 billion each year. So, at some level, autism affects us all.

What Is Autism?

Autism is a brain disorder that typically affects a person's ability to communicate, form relationships with others, and respond appropriately to the environment. Some people with autism are relatively high-functioning, with speech and intelligence intact. Others are mentally retarded, mute, or have serious language delays. For some, autism makes them seem closed off and shut down; others seem locked into repetitive behaviors and rigid patterns of thinking.

Although people with autism do not have exactly the same symptoms and deficits, they tend to share certain social, communication, motor, and sensory problems that affect their behavior in predictable ways.

Social Symptoms

From the start, most infants are social beings. Early in life, they gaze at people, turn toward voices, endearingly grasp a finger, and even smile.

In contrast, most children with autism seem to have tremendous difficulty learning to engage in the give-and-take of everyday human interaction. Even in the first few months of life, many do not interact and they avoid eye contact. They seem to prefer being alone. They may resist attention and affection or passively accept hugs and cuddling. Later, they seldom seek comfort or respond to anger or affection. Unlike other children, they rarely become upset when the parent leaves or show pleasure when the parent returns.

Parents who looked forward to the joys of cuddling, teaching, and playing with their child may feel crushed by this lack of response.

Children with autism also take longer to learn to interpret what others are thinking and feeling. Subtle social cues—whether a smile, a wink, or a grimace—may have little meaning. To a child who misses these cues, "Come here," always means the same thing, whether the speaker is smiling and extending her arms for a hug or squinting and planting her fists on her hips. Without the ability to interpret gestures and facial expressions, the social world may seem bewildering.

To compound the problem, people with autism have problems seeing things from another person's perspective. Most 5-year-olds understand that other people have different information, feelings, and goals than they have. A person with autism may lack such understanding. This inability leaves them unable to predict or understand other people's actions.

Some people with autism also tend to be physically aggressive at times, making social relationships still more difficult. Some lose control, particularly when they're in a strange or overwhelming environment, or when angry and frustrated. They are capable at times of breaking things, attacking others, or harming themselves. Others are self-destructive, banging their heads, pulling their hair, or biting their arms.

Language Difficulties

By age 3, most children have passed several predictable milestones on the path to learning language. One of the earliest is babbling. By the first birthday, a typical toddler says words, turns when he hears his name, points when he wants a toy, and when offered something distasteful, makes it very clear that his answer is no. By age 2, most children begin to put together sentences like "See doggie," or "More cookie," and can follow simple directions.

Research shows that about half of the children diagnosed with autism remain mute throughout their lives. Some infants who later show signs of autism do coo and babble during the first 6 months of life. But they soon stop. Although they may learn to communicate using sign language or special electronic equipment, they may never speak. Others may be delayed, developing language as late as age 5 to 8.

Those who do speak often use language in unusual ways. Some seem unable to combine words into meaningful sentences. Some speak only single words. Others repeat the same phrase no matter what the situation.

Some children with autism are only able to parrot what they hear, a condition called echolalia. Without persistent training, echoing other people's phrases may be the only language that people with autism ever acquire. What they repeat might be a question they were just asked, or an advertisement on television. Or out of the blue, a child may shout, "Stay on your own side of the road!"—something he heard his father say weeks before. Although children without autism go through a stage where they repeat what they hear, it normally passes by the time they are 3.

It can be equally difficult to understand the body language of a person with autism. Most of us smile when we talk about things we enjoy, or shrug when we can't answer a question. But for children with autism, facial expressions, movements, and gestures rarely match what they are saying. Their tone of voice also fails to reflect their feelings. A high-pitched, sing-song, or flat, robot-like voice is common.

Without meaningful gestures or the language to ask for things, people with autism are at a loss to let others know what they need. As a result, children with autism may simply scream or grab what they want. Temple Grandin, an exceptional woman with autism who has written two books about her disorder, admits, "Not being able to speak was utter frustration. Screaming was the only way I could communicate." Often she would logically think to herself, "I am going to scream now because I want to tell somebody I don't want to do something." Until they are taught better means of expressing their needs, people with autism do whatever they can to get through to others.

Repetitive Behaviors and Obsessions

Although children with autism usually appear physically normal and have good muscle control, odd repetitive motions may set them off from other children. A child might spend hours repeatedly flicking or flapping her fingers or rocking back and forth. Many flail their arms or walk on their toes. Some suddenly freeze in position. Experts call such behaviors stereotypies or self-stimulation. Some people with autism also tend to repeat certain actions over and over. A child might spend hours lining up pretzel sticks.

Some children with autism develop troublesome fixations with specific objects, which can lead to unhealthy or dangerous behaviors. For example, one child insists on carrying feces from the bathroom into her classroom.

Other behaviors are simply startling, humorous, or embarrassing to those around them. One girl, obsessed with digital watches, grabs the arms of strangers to look at their wrists.

For unexplained reasons, people with autism demand consistency in their environment. Many insist on eating the same foods, at the same time, sitting at precisely the same place at the table every day. They may get furious if a picture is tilted on the wall, or wildly upset if their toothbrush has been moved even slightly. A minor change in their routine, like taking a different route to school, may be tremendously upsetting.

Scientists are exploring several possible explanations for such repetitive, obsessive behavior. Perhaps the order and sameness lends some stability in a world of sensory confusion. Perhaps focused behaviors help them to block out painful stimuli. Yet another theory is that these behaviors are linked to the senses that work well or poorly. A child who sniffs everything in sight may be using a stable sense of smell to explore his environment. Or perhaps the reverse is true: he may be trying to stimulate a sense that is dim.

Imaginative play, too, is limited by these repetitive behaviors and obsessions. Most children, as early as age 2, use their imagination to pretend. They create new uses for an object, perhaps using a bowl for a hat. Or they pretend to be someone else, like a mother cooking dinner for her "family" of dolls. In contrast, children with autism rarely pretend. Rather than rocking a doll or rolling a toy car, they may simply hold it, smell it, or spin it for hours on end.

Sensory Symptoms

When children's perceptions are accurate, they can learn from what they see, feel, or hear. On the other hand, if sensory information is faulty or if the input from the various senses fails to merge into a coherent picture, the child's experiences of the world can be confusing. People with autism seem to have one or both of these problems. There may be problems in the sensory signals that reach the brain or in the integration of the sensory signals—and quite possibly, both.

Apparently, as a result of a brain malfunction, many children with autism are highly attuned or even painfully sensitive to certain sounds, textures, tastes, and smells. Some children find the feel of clothes touching their skin so disturbing that they can't focus on anything else. For others, a gentle hug may be overwhelming. Some children cover their ears and scream at the sound of a vacuum cleaner, a distant airplane, a telephone ring, or even the wind. Temple Grandin says, "It was like having a hearing aid that picks up everything, with the volume control stuck on super loud." Because any noise was so painful, she often chose to withdraw and tuned out sounds to the point of seeming deaf.

In autism, the brain also seems unable to balance the senses appropriately. Some children with autism seem oblivious to extreme cold or pain, but react hysterically to things that wouldn't bother other children. A child with autism may break her arm in a fall and never cry. Another child might bash his head on the wall without a wince. On the other hand, a light touch may make the child scream with alarm.

In some people, the senses are even scrambled. One child gags when she feels a certain texture. A man with autism hears a sound when someone touches a point on his chin. Another experiences certain sounds as colors.

Unusual Abilities

Some people with autism display remarkable abilities. A few demonstrate skills far out of the ordinary. At a young age, when other children are drawing straight lines and scribbling, some children with autism are able to draw detailed, realistic pictures in three-dimensional perspective. Some toddlers who are autistic are so visually skilled that they can put complex jigsaw puzzles together. Many begin to read exceptionally early—sometimes even before they begin to speak. Some who have a keenly developed sense of hearing can play musical instruments they have never been taught, play a song accurately after hearing it once, or name any note they hear. Like the person played by Dustin Hoffman in the movie Rain Man, some people with autism can memorize entire television shows, pages of the phone book, or the scores of every major league baseball game for the past 20 years. However, such skills, known as islets of intelligence or savant skills are rare.

How Is Autism Diagnosed?

Parents are usually the first to notice unusual behaviors in their child. In many cases, their baby seemed different from birth—being unresponsive to people and toys, or focusing intently on one item for long periods of time. The first signs of autism may also appear in children who had been developing normally. When an affectionate, babbling toddler suddenly becomes silent, withdrawn, violent, or self-abusive, something is wrong.

Even so, years may go by before the family seeks a diagnosis. Well-meaning friends and relatives sometimes help parents ignore the problems with reassurances that "Every child is different," or "Janie can talk—she just doesn't want to!" Unfortunately, this only delays getting appropriate assessment and treatment.

Diagnostic Procedures

To date, there are no medical tests like x-rays or blood tests that detect autism. And no two children with the disorder behave the same way. In addition, several conditions can cause symptoms that resemble those of autism. So parents and the child's pediatrician need to rule out other disorders, including hearing loss, speech problems, mental retardation, and neurological problems. But once these possibilities have been eliminated, a visit to a professional who specializes in autism is necessary. Such specialists include people with the professional titles of child psychiatrist, child psychologist, developmental pediatrician, or pediatric neurologist.

What Causes Autism?

It is generally accepted that autism is caused by abnormalities in brain structures or functions. Using a variety of new research tools to study human and animal brain growth, scientists are discovering more about normal development and how abnormalities occur.

The brain of a fetus develops throughout pregnancy. Starting out with a few cells, the cells grow and divide until the brain contains billions of specialized cells, called neurons. Research sponsored by the National Institute of Mental Health (NIMH) and other components at the National Institutes of Health is playing a key role in showing how cells find their way to a specific area of the brain and take on special functions. Once in place, each neuron sends out long fibers that connect with other neurons. In this way, lines of communication are established between various areas of the brain and between the brain and the rest of the body. As each neuron receives a signal it releases chemicals called neurotransmitters, which pass the signal to the next neuron. By birth, the brain has evolved into a complex organ with several distinct regions and subregions, each with a precise set of functions and responsibilities.

But brain development does not stop at birth. The brain continues to change during the first few years of life, as new neurotransmitters become activated and additional lines of communication are established. Neural networks are forming and creating a foundation for processing language, emotions, and thought.

However, scientists now know that a number of problems may interfere with normal brain development. Cells may migrate to the wrong place in the brain. Or, due to problems with the neural pathways or the neurotransmitters, some parts of the communication network may fail to perform. A problem with the communication network may interfere with the overall task of coordinating sensory information, thoughts, feelings, and actions.

Is There Reason for Hope?

When parents learn that their child is autistic, most wish they could magically make the problem go away. They looked forward to having a baby and watching their child learn and grow. Instead, they must face the fact that they have a child who may not live up to their dreams and will daily challenge their patience. Some families deny the problem or fantasize about an instant cure. They may take the child from one specialist to another, hoping for a different diagnosis. It is important for the family to eventually overcome their pain and deal with the problem, while still cherishing hopes for their child's future. Most families realize that their lives can move on.

Today, more than ever before, people with autism can be helped. A combination of early intervention, special education, family support, and in some cases, medication, is helping increasing numbers of children with autism to live more normal lives. Special interventions and education programs can expand their capacity to learn, communicate, and relate to others, while reducing the severity and frequency of disruptive behaviors. Medications can be used to help alleviate certain symptoms. Older children and adults may also benefit from the treatments that are available today. So, while no cure is in sight, it is possible to greatly improve the day-to-day life of children and adults with autism.

Today, a child who receives effective therapy and education has every hope of using his or her unique capacity to learn. Even some who are seriously mentally retarded can often master many self-help skills like cooking, dressing, doing laundry, and handling money. For such children, greater independence and self-care may be the primary training goals. Other youngsters may go on to learn basic academic skills, like reading, writing, and simple math. Many complete high school. Some, like Temple Grandin, may even earn college degrees. Like anyone else, their personal interests provide strong incentives to learn. Clearly, an important factor in developing a child's long-term potential for independence and success is early intervention. The sooner a child begins to receive help, the more opportunity for learning. Furthermore, because a young child's brain is still forming, scientists believe that early intervention gives children the best chance of developing their full potential. Even so, no matter when the child is diagnosed, it's never too late to begin treatment.

Selecting a Treatment Program

Parents are often disappointed to learn that there is no single best treatment for all children with autism; possibly not even for a specific child.

Even after a child has been thoroughly tested and formally diagnosed, there is no clear "right" course of action. The diagnostic team may suggest treatment methods and service providers, but ultimately it is up to the parents to consider their child's unique needs, research the various options, and decide.

Above all, parents should consider their own sense of what will work for their child. Keeping in mind that autism takes many forms, parents need to consider whether a specific program has helped children like their own.

Chapter 71

Tic Disorders and Tourette Syndrome

Tic Disorders

A tic is a problem in which a part of the body moves repeatedly, quickly, suddenly, and uncontrollably. Tics can occur in any body part, such as the face, shoulders, hands, or legs. They can be stopped voluntarily for brief periods. Sounds that are made involuntarily (such as throat clearing) are called vocal tics. Most tics are mild and hardly noticeable. However, in some cases they are frequent and severe, and can affect many areas of a child's life.

The most common tic disorder is called transient tic disorder, which may affect up to 10 percent of children during the early school years. Teachers or others may notice the tics and wonder if the youth is under stress or nervous. Transient tics go away by themselves. Some may get worse with anxiety, tiredness, and some medications.

Some tics do not go away. Tics which last one year or more are called chronic tics. Chronic tics affect less than one percent of youth and may be related to a special, more unusual tic disorder called Tourette syndrome.

This chapter contains text reprinted with permission from "Tic Disorders," part of the American Academy of Child and Adolescent Psychiatry's *Facts for Families Series*. © 2000. For more information about issues related to child and adolescent psychiatry, or for information about how to get help in your area, visit the Referral Directory on the AACAP website at http://www.aacap. org/ReferralDirectory/index.htm. This chapter also includes "Tourette Syndrome Fact Sheet," National Institute of Neurological Disorders and Stroke (NINDS), National Institutes of Health (NIH), reviewed July 2001.

Children with Tourette syndrome have both body and vocal tics (throat clearing). Some tics disappear by early adulthood, and some continue. Children with Tourette syndrome may have problems with attention, concentration, and may have learning disabilities as well. They may act impulsively, or develop obsessions and compulsions.

Sometimes people with Tourette syndrome may blurt out obscene words, insult others, or make obscene gestures or movements. They cannot control these sounds and movements and should not be blamed for them. Punishment by parents, teasing by classmates, and scolding by teachers will not help the youth to control the tics but will hurt the youth's self-esteem.

Through a comprehensive medical evaluation, often involving pediatric and/or neurologic consultation, a child and adolescent psychiatrist can determine whether the youth has Tourette syndrome or another tic disorder. Treatment for the youth with a tic disorder may include medication to help control the symptoms. The child and adolescent psychiatrist can also advise the family about how to provide emotional support and the appropriate educational environment for the youngster.

Tourette's Syndrome

What is Tourette's syndrome?

Tourette syndrome (TS) is an inherited, neurological disorder characterized by multiple involuntary movements and uncontrollable vocalizations called tics that come and go over years.

The disorder is named for Dr. Georges Gilles de la Tourette, the pioneering French neurologist who first described an 86-year-old French noblewoman with the condition in 1885.

The symptoms of TS generally appear before the individual is 18 years old. TS can affect people of all ethnic groups; males are affected 3 to 4 times more often than females. It is estimated that 100,000 Americans have full-blown TS, and that perhaps as many as 1 in 200 show a partial expression of the disorder, such as chronic multiple tics or transient childhood tics.

The natural course of TS varies from patient to patient. Although TS symptoms range from very mild to quite severe, the majority of cases fall in the mild category.

What are the symptoms?

The first symptoms of TS are usually facial tics—commonly eye blinking. However, facial tics can also include nose twitching or grimaces.

With time, other motor tics may appear such as head jerking, neck stretching, foot stamping, or body twisting and bending.

TS patients may utter strange and unacceptable sounds, words, or phrases. It is not uncommon for a person with TS to continuously clear his or her throat, cough, sniff, grunt, yelp, bark, or shout.

People with TS may involuntarily shout obscenities (coprolalia) or constantly repeat the words of other people (echolalia). They may touch other people excessively or repeat actions obsessively and unnecessarily. A few patients with severe TS demonstrate self-harming behaviors such as lip and cheek biting and head banging against hard objects. However, these behaviors are extremely rare.

Tics alternately increase and decrease in severity, and periodically change in number, frequency, type, and location. Symptoms may subside for weeks or months at a time and later recur.

How are tics classified?

There are two categories of tics: simple and complex. Simple tics are sudden, brief movements that involve a limited number of muscle groups. They occur in a single or isolated fashion and are often repetitive. Some of the more common examples of simple tics include eye blinking, shoulder shrugging, facial grimacing, head jerking, yelping, and sniffing. Complex tics are distinct, coordinated patterns of successive movements involving several muscle groups. Complex tics might include jumping, smelling objects, touching the nose, touching other people, coprolalia, echolalia, or self-harming behaviors.

Can people with TS control their tics?

People with TS can sometimes suppress their tics for a short time, but the effort is similar to that of holding back a sneeze. Eventually tension mounts to the point where the tic escapes. Tics worsen in stressful situations; however they improve when the person is relaxed or absorbed in an activity. In most cases tics decrease markedly during sleep.

What causes TS?

Although the basic cause of TS is unknown, current research suggests that there is an abnormality in the gene(s) affecting the brain's metabolism of neurotransmitters such as dopamine, serotonin, and norepinephrine. Neurotransmitters are chemicals in the brain that carry signals from one nerve cell to another.

How is TS diagnosed?

Generally, TS is diagnosed by obtaining a description of the tics and evaluating family history. For a diagnosis of TS to be made, both motor and phonic tics must be present for at least one year. Neuro-imaging studies, such as magnetic resonance imaging (MRI), comput-erized tomography (CT), and electroencephalogram (EEG) scans, or certain blood tests may be used to rule out other conditions that might be confused with TS. However, TS is a clinical diagnosis. There are no blood tests or other laboratory tests that definitively diagnose the disorder.

Studies show that correct diagnosis of TS is frequently delayed after the start of symptoms because many physicians may not be fa-miliar with the disorder. The behavioral symptoms and tics are eas-ily misinterpreted, often causing children with TS to be misunderstood at school, at home, and even in the doctor's office. Parents, relatives, and peers who are unfamiliar with the disorder may incorrectly at-tribute the tics and other symptoms to psychological problems, thereby increasing the social isolation of those with the disorder. And because tics can wax and wane in severity and can also be suppressed, they are often absent during doctor visits, which further complicates mak-ing a diagnosis.

In many cases, parents, relatives, friends, or even the patients themselves become aware of the disorder based on information they have heard or read in the popular media.

How is TS treated?

Because symptoms do not impair most patients and development usually proceeds normally, the majority of people with TS require no medication. However, medications are available to help when symp-toms interfere with functioning. Unfortunately, there is no one medi-cation that is helpful to all persons with TS, nor does any medication completely eliminate symptoms; in addition, all medications have side effects. Instead, the available TS medications are only able to help reduce specific symptoms.

Some patients who require medication to reduce the frequency and intensity of the tic symptoms may be treated with neuroleptic drugs such as haloperidol and pimozide. These medications are usually given in very small doses that are increased slowly until the best possible balance between symptoms and side effects is achieved.

Recently scientists have discovered that long-term use of neuro-leptic drugs may cause an involuntary movement disorder called tardive dyskinesia. However, this condition usually disappears when medication is discontinued. Short-term side effects of haloperidol and pimozide include muscular rigidity, drooling, tremor, lack of facial expression, slow movement, and restlessness. These side effects can be reduced by drugs commonly used to treat Parkinson's disease. Other side effects such as fatigue, depression, anxiety, weight gain, and difficulties in thinking clearly may be more troublesome.

Clonidine, an antihypertensive drug, is also used in the treatment of tics. Studies show that it is more effective in reducing motor tics than reducing vocal tics. Fatigue, dry mouth, irritability, dizziness, headache, and insomnia are common side effects associated with clonidine use. Fluphenazine and clonazepam may also be prescribed to help control tic symptoms.

Other types of therapy may also be helpful. Although psychological problems do not cause TS, psychotherapy may help the person better cope with the disorder and deal with the secondary social and emotional problems that sometimes occur. Psychotherapy does not help suppress the patient's tics.

Relaxation techniques and biofeedback may be useful in alleviating stress which can lead to an increase in tic symptoms.

Is TS inherited?

Evidence from genetic studies suggests that TS is inherited in a dominant mode and the gene(s) involved can cause a variable range of symptoms in different family members. A person with TS has about a 50-50 chance of passing on the gene(s) to one of his or her offspring. However, that genetic predisposition may not necessarily result in full-blown TS; instead, it may express itself as a milder tic disorder or as obsessive compulsive behaviors or possibly attention deficit-hyperactivity disorder with few or no tics at all. It is also possible that the gene-carrying offspring will not develop any TS symptoms. A higher than normal incidence of milder tic disorders and obsessive compulsive behaviors has been found in families of individuals with TS.

Gender also plays an important role in TS gene expression. If the gene-carrying offspring of a TS patient is male, then the risk of developing symptoms is 3 to 4 times higher. However, most people who inherit the gene(s) will not develop symptoms severe enough to warrant medical attention. In some cases of TS, inheritance cannot be determined. These cases are called sporadic and their cause is unknown.

What is the prognosis?

There is no cure for TS; however, the condition in many individuals improves as they mature. Individuals with TS can expect to live a normal life span. Although the disorder is generally lifelong and chronic, it is not a degenerative condition. TS does not impair intelligence. Tics tend to decrease with age, enabling some patients to discontinue using medication. In a few cases, complete remission occurs after adolescence. Although tic symptoms tend to decrease with age, it is possible that neuropsychiatric disorders such as depression, panic attacks, mood swings, and antisocial behaviors may increase.

What is the best educational setting for children with TS?

Although students with TS often function well in the regular classroom, it is estimated that many may have some kind of learning disability. When attention deficit-hyperactivity disorder, obsessive compulsive disorder, and frequent tics greatly interfere with academic performance or social adjustment, students should be placed in an educational setting that meets their individual needs. These students may require tutoring, smaller or special classes, and in some cases special schools.

All students with TS need a tolerant and compassionate setting that both encourages them to work to their full potential and is flexible enough to accommodate their special needs. This setting may include a private study area, exams outside the regular classroom, or even oral exams when the child's symptoms interfere with his or her ability to write. Untimed testing reduces stress for students with TS.

What research is being done?

Recent research has led to several notable advances in the understanding of TS. Already scientists have learned that TS is inherited from a dominant gene(s) that causes different symptoms from patient to patient, and that the disorder is more common than was previously thought.

Genetic studies. Currently, investigators are conducting genetic linkage studies in large multigenerational families affected with TS in an effort to find the chromosomal location of the TS gene(s). Finding a genetic marker (a biochemical abnormality that all TS patients might share) for TS would be a major step toward understanding the genetic risk factors for TS. Once the marker is found, research efforts would then focus on locating the TS gene(s). Understanding the genetics of TS will directly benefit patients who are concerned about recurrence in their families and will ultimately help to clarify the development of the disorder. Localization of the TS gene will strengthen clinical diagnosis, improve genetic counseling, lead to the clarification of pathophysiology, and provide clues for more effective therapies.

Neurotransmitter studies. Investigators continue to study certain neurotransmitters to increase our understanding of the syndrome, explore the role they play in the disease process, and provide more effective therapies.

Environmental studies. Other research projects currently under way include analyzing young unaffected children at high risk for TS in order to identify environmental factors such as life stresses or exposure to certain medications that may influence the expression of the disorder.

Scientists are also conducting neuropsychological tests and neuroimaging studies of brain activity and structure to determine the extent to which specific environmental exposures may affect the emergence of tics and/or obsessive compulsive symptoms.

Chapter 72

Does Your Child Have Obsessive-Compulsive Disorder?

Facts about Obsessive-Compulsive Disorder

People with obsessive-compulsive disorder (OCD) suffer intensely from recurrent, unwanted thoughts (obsessions) or rituals (compulsions), which they feel they cannot control. Rituals such as hand-washing, counting, checking, or cleaning are often performed with the hope of preventing obsessive thoughts or making them go away. Performing these rituals, however, provides only temporary relief, and not performing them markedly increases anxiety. Left untreated, obsessions and the need to perform rituals can take over a person's life. OCD is often a chronic, relapsing illness. Fortunately, through research supported by the National Institute of Mental Health (NIMH) and by industry, effective treatments have been developed to help people with OCD.

OCD typically begins during adolescence or early childhood; at least one-third of the cases of adult OCD began in childhood. OCD is not caused by family problems or attitudes learned in childhood, such

This chapter includes excerpts from "Facts about Obsessive-Compulsive Disorder," National Institute of Mental Health (NIMH), Pub. No. OM-99 4154, updated June 28, 2002 and "Treatments Reduce Strep-Triggered Symptoms of OCD and Tics in Some Children," NIMH Press Release, September 20, 1999. The section titled "The Silent Tragedy of OCD in Children," is reprinted with permission from "Obsessive Compulsive Disorder in Children: The Silent Tragedy," by Connie Foster. This article originally appeared in the Winter 1998 issue of *Because Kids Grow Up*, a publication of the National Alliance for the Mentally Ill. © 1998.

as an inordinate emphasis on cleanliness, or a belief that certain thoughts are dangerous or unacceptable.

There is growing evidence that OCD represents abnormal functioning of brain circuitry, probably involving a part of the brain called the striatum. Brain imaging studies using a technique called positron emission tomography (PET) have compared people with and without OCD. Those with OCD have patterns of brain activity that differ from people with other mental illnesses or people with no mental illness at all. In addition, PET scans show that in patients with OCD, both behavioral therapy and medication produce changes in the striatum. This is graphic evidence that both psychotherapy and medication affect the brain.

OCD is sometimes accompanied by depression, eating disorders, substance abuse, attention deficit hyperactivity disorder, or other anxiety disorders. When a person also has other disorders, OCD is often more difficult to diagnose and treat. Symptoms of OCD can also coexist and may even be part of a spectrum of other brain disorders, such as Tourette syndrome. Appropriate diagnosis and treatment of other disorders are important to successful treatment of OCD.

The Silent Tragedy of OCD in Children

A neurobiological illness like obsessive-compulsive disorder can often times have you residing in a land of limbo. At the very best, it's like having a bad itch that must be occasionally yet vigorously scratched in order to go away. Conversely, at its worst, OCD can hold you trapped. Locked in a perpetual cycle, doomed to repeat and repeat and repeat, in an endless process of demanding and all-consuming rituals that can leave its participants believing they are destined to carry on into infinity, and possibly beyond.

OCD, like all neurobiological diseases, tends to lie somewhere beyond the limits of tolerance for acceptable behaviors. Consequently, our children learn at an early age to keep it (and sometimes themselves) well hidden from judgmental eyes. As parents and educators of OCD children, we desperately need to recognize this chemical imbalance of the brain that is far more prevalent than many other better-known childhood ailments, such as juvenile diabetes.

Many American children suffer in lonely and excruciating silence due to the embarrassing stigmas, myths, and misconceptions of having a neurobiological disease. A neurobiological disease can make your behavior unacceptable, but chemical and behavioral treatments are available. Medication, one feels more at ease. There is a new-found measure of self-respect. It is not necessary to check the locks anymore or wash your hands over and over. There is less worrying and more acceptance of the disorder. There are fewer fear-filled dreams and more rest.

These children's successes are their own, and they are both powerful and wonderful. In time, they will gain their strength and individual sense of self from these successes and slowly use them to compile those behaviors that others take so easily for granted. It is up to the adults, parents and teachers alike, to seek and acquire the knowledge that is needed in order to gently and successfully guide our OCD children into becoming fully contributing members of society.

What Treatments Are Available for OCD?

Treatments, which combine medications and behavioral therapy (a specific type of psychotherapy), are often effective. Several medications have been proven effective in helping people with OCD: clomipramine, fluoxetine, fluvoxamine, sertraline, and paroxetine. If one drug is not effective, others should be tried. A number of other medications are currently being studied. A type of behavioral therapy known as "exposure and response prevention" is very useful for treating OCD. In this approach, a person is deliberately and voluntarily exposed to whatever triggers the obsessive thoughts, and then is taught techniques to avoid performing the compulsive rituals and to deal with the anxiety.

Treatments Reduce Strep-Triggered Symptoms of OCD and Tics in Some Children

National Institute of Mental Health (NIMH) researchers report that some children whose symptoms of obsessive-compulsive disorder (OCD) and tic disorders were worsened by a common strep infection have been successfully treated with plasma exchange (PEX) and intravenous immunoglobulin (IVIG). Dr. Susan Swedo and colleagues at the National Institutes of Health reported their findings in the October 2, 1999 issue of *Lancet*.

In previous studies, Dr. Swedo and others observed that in a small number of children suffering from the obsessional thoughts and compulsive behaviors typical of OCD and tic disorders, symptoms suddenly became worse following infection with Group A beta hemolytic streptococci. Evidence pointed to an autoimmune response to the infection, in which antibodies attack healthy as well as infected cells, leading to inflammation in the brain's basal ganglia, an area involving movement and motor control. The syndrome, known as PANDAS, or Pediatric Autoimmune Neuropsychiatric Disorders Associated with Streptococcal Infections, typically occurs in young children and is noted for its dramatic, sudden onset or exacerbation of symptoms and episodic course, in which periods of symptom worsening follow strep infections.

The investigation shows that plasma exchange and IVIG relieve neuropsychiatric symptoms in this subgroup of children with tics and obsessive-compulsive disorder. "A few children were even able to discontinue all psychotropic medications after treatment," Dr. Swedo said. "The study does not, however, support using PEX and IVIG for all cases of tics or OCD. Nor does it suggest that all children with untreated strep infections will get OCD, tics, or Tourette syndrome. In fact, strep infections are very common and strep-triggered neuropsychiatric disorders are quite rare, so the vast majority of children with strep infections are not at risk for developing these disorders, particularly with prompt attention and treatment," according to Dr. Swedo.

For More Information

The Anxiety Disorders Education Program
National Institute of Mental Health
6001 Executive Blvd.
Room 8184, MSC 9663
Bethesda, MD 20892-9663
Phone: 301-443-4513

Publications and other information are also available online from the NIMH website at http://www.nimh.nih.gov or by calling toll-free 88-88-ANXIETY (888-826-9438).

National Alliance for the Mentally Ill (NAMI)
Colonial Place Three
2107 Wilson Blvd., Suite 300
Arlington, VA 22201
Toll-Free: 800-950-NAMI (HelpLine)
Phone: 703-524-7600
Website: http://www.nami.org

Chapter 73

Epilepsy in Children

Facts about Epilepsy

About two million Americans have epilepsy; of the 125,000 new cases that develop each year, up to 50% are in children and adolescents.

According to the Epilepsy Foundation of America, epilepsy is a physical condition that occurs when there is a sudden, brief change in how the brain works. When brain cells are not working properly, a person's consciousness, movement, or actions may be altered for a short time. These physical changes are called epileptic seizures. Epilepsy is therefore sometimes called a seizure disorder. Epilepsy affects people in all nations and of all races.

Some people can experience a seizure and not have epilepsy. For example, many young children have convulsions from fevers. These febrile convulsions are one type of seizure. Other types of seizures not classified as epilepsy include those caused by an imbalance of body fluids or chemicals or by alcohol or drug withdrawal. A single seizure does not mean that the person has epilepsy.

This chapter includes text from "Epilepsy," National Information Center for Children and Youth with Disabilities (NICHCY), August 2002. Additional information from NICHCY can be found online at www.nichcy.org or by calling 800-695-0285. The section titled "Questions and Answers about Epilepsy and Its Treatment," is excerpted from "Pediatric Epilepsy Surgery," by Harley I. Kornblum, M.D., Ph.D., reviewed April 2002, copyright MedicineNet, Inc. (http://www.medicinenet.com); reprinted with permission.

Although the symptoms listed below are not necessarily indicators of epilepsy, it is wise to consult a doctor if you or a member of your family experiences one or more of them:

- "Blackouts" or periods of confused memory;

- Episodes of staring or unexplained periods of unresponsiveness;

- Involuntary movement of arms and legs;

- "Fainting spells" with incontinence or followed by excessive fatigue; or

- Odd sounds, distorted perceptions, episodic feelings of fear that cannot be explained.

Seizures can be generalized, meaning that all brain cells are involved. One type of generalized seizure consists of a convulsion with a complete loss of consciousness. Another type looks like a brief period of fixed staring.

Seizures are partial when those brain cells not working properly are limited to one part of the brain. Such partial seizures may cause periods of "automatic behavior" and altered consciousness. This is typified by purposeful-looking behavior, such as buttoning or unbuttoning a shirt. Such behavior, however, is unconscious, may be repetitive, and is usually not recalled.

Questions and Answers about Epilepsy and Its Treatment

What is epilepsy?

Epilepsy is the tendency to have seizures. Pediatric epilepsy is the occurrence of these convulsions in children. Seizures can be of several types. The most familiar type is the generalized tonic clonic (grand mal) convulsion, in which there is a loss of consciousness and the whole body shakes rhythmically. An absence (petit mal) seizure involves a brief loss of awareness, which can be accompanied by blinking or mouth twitching. Petit mal seizures have a very characteristic appearance on an electroencephalogram (EEG). Partial seizures occur when the convulsion starts in one area of the brain. Simple partial seizures do not cause an alteration of consciousness, whereas complex partial seizures involve some alteration of consciousness. The manifestations, or symptoms, of the seizure depend on where in the brain it starts. For example, a partial seizure originating in the area of the brain that controls hand movements will result in hand twitching. A partial seizure that starts in the area of the brain controlling emotion may result in a fearful feeling. Sometimes, it is difficult to distinguish a partial seizure from a petit mal seizure, but they can be differentiated on an EEG.

What causes epilepsy in children?

Epilepsy can be caused by numerous factors. Many people who have epilepsy begin having seizures in childhood. Epilepsy in children can result from anything that interferes with brain development or function. Some babies suffer a lack of oxygen to the brain before or during birth. This oxygen deprivation can cause cerebral palsy and epilepsy. Some children have bleeding in the brain as a result of prematurity or abnormal blood vessels in the brain (arteriovenous malformations). The bleeding can then result in seizures.

Epilepsy can also be caused by genetic changes. Some children are born with epilepsy genes that cause them to have seizures. These seizures may occur early in life or start later—even as late as the third decade of life. Usually, genetically caused seizures are generalized. This means that they do not start in a specific part of the brain, but affect the entire brain all at once. Other causes of childhood epilepsy include brain tumors, infection in the brain (encephalitis), head trauma (injury), and errors in the chemical processes of the body and the brain. In all cases, it must be remembered that the brain of a child is more prone to seizures than is the brain of an adult.

Are seizures bad for children?

Seizures, in and of themselves, can be life-threatening, but this is relatively rare. Children who have prolonged seizures (more than 30 minutes of convulsion) can also have brain damage that is caused by the seizure, but this is also probably rare. However, uncontrolled seizures in children result in severe learning and developmental problems. The goal of treatment in pediatric epilepsy is not only to control seizures, but to improve the developmental potential of the child.

How is epilepsy treated?

The majority of patients who have seizures are relatively easily treated with medication (70 to 80%). Numerous anti-epileptic drugs (AEDs) are now available. The choice of the medication depends on several factors, including the kind of seizures, the age of the child, other medical problems, and the potential side effects of the medicine. Some patients, however, do not respond to the usual medical treatments and are then considered for epilepsy surgery or other treatments.

What is epilepsy surgery?

Epilepsy surgery is a surgical operation to control seizures. There are currently three major categories of epilepsy surgery:

- Resective surgery; in which the part of the brain that causes partial-onset seizures is removed.

- Corpus callosotomy; in which the major connection between the two sides of the brain is severed (cut) in order to lessen the severity of some types of seizures.

- Vagus nerve stimulator; in which a small wire electrically shocks the vagus nerve in the neck. This surgery is also performed to limit the severity of seizures.

Who performs pediatric epilepsy surgery?

Pediatric epilepsy surgery must be performed by a neurosurgeon with specialized training and experience in pediatric epilepsy surgery. Most cases are performed in large academic medical centers with affiliations to medical schools. Prior to the surgery, however, the patient must be evaluated by a competent pediatric epileptologist—usually a neurologist with specialized training in pediatric EEG and epilepsy. The team of epileptologists and neurosurgeons tailor the surgery for each child on an individual basis.

Educational Implications for Children with Epilepsy

Students with epilepsy or seizure disorders are eligible for special education and related services under the Individuals with Disabilities Education Act (IDEA). Epilepsy is classified as "other health impaired" and an Individualized Education Program (IEP) would be developed to specify appropriate services. Some students may have additional conditions such as learning disabilities along with the seizure disorders.

Seizures may interfere with the child's ability to learn. If the student has the type of seizure characterized by a brief period of fixed staring, he or she may be missing parts of what the teacher is saying.

It is important that the teacher observe and document these episodes and report them promptly to parents and to school nurses.

Depending on the type of seizure or how often they occur, some children may need additional assistance to help them keep up with classmates. Assistance can include adaptations in classroom instruction, first aid instruction on seizure management to the student's teachers, and counseling, all of which should be written in the IEP.

It is important that the teachers and school staff are informed about the child's condition, possible effects of medication, and what to do in case a seizure occurs at school. Most parents find that a friendly conversation with the teacher(s) at the beginning of the school year is the best way to handle the situation. Even if a child has seizures that are largely controlled by medication, it is still best to notify the school staff about the condition.

School personnel and the family should work together to monitor the effectiveness of medication as well as any side effects. If a child's physical or intellectual skills seem to change, it is important to tell the doctor. There may also be associated hearing or perception problems caused by the brain changes. Written observations of both the family and school staff will be helpful in discussions with the child's doctor.

Children and youth with epilepsy must also deal with the psychological and social aspects of the condition. These include public misperceptions and fear of seizures, uncertain occurrence, loss of self control during the seizure episode, and compliance with medications. To help children feel more confident about themselves and accept their epilepsy, the school can assist by providing epilepsy education programs for staff and students, including information on seizure recognition and first aid.

Students can benefit the most when both the family and school are working together. There are many materials available for families and teachers so that they can understand how to work most effectively as a team.

Chapter 74

Cerebral Palsy

What Is Cerebral Palsy?

Cerebral palsy is an umbrella-like term used to describe a group of chronic disorders impairing control of movement that appear in the first few years of life and generally do not worsen over time. The term cerebral refers to the brain's two halves, or hemispheres, and palsy describes any disorder that impairs control of body movement. Thus, these disorders are not caused by problems in the muscles or nerves. Instead, faulty development or damage to motor areas in the brain disrupts the brain's ability to adequately control movement and posture.

Symptoms of cerebral palsy lie along a spectrum of varying severity. An individual with cerebral palsy may have difficulty with fine motor tasks, such as writing or cutting with scissors; experience trouble with maintaining balance and walking; or be affected by involuntary movements, such as uncontrollable writhing motion of the hands or drooling. The symptoms differ from one person to the next, and may even change over time in the individual. Some people with cerebral palsy are also affected by other medical disorders, including seizures or mental impairment. Contrary to common belief, however, cerebral palsy does not always cause profound handicap. While a child with severe cerebral palsy might be unable to walk and need extensive, lifelong care, a child with mild cerebral palsy might only be

Excerpted from "Cerebral Palsy: Hope Through Research," National Institute of Neurological Disorders and Stroke (NINDS), NIH Pub. No. 93-159, reviewed July 2001.

slightly awkward and require no special assistance. Cerebral palsy is not contagious nor is it usually inherited from one generation to the next. At this time, it cannot be cured, although scientific research continues to yield improved treatments and methods of prevention.

What Are the Different Forms?

Spastic diplegia, the disorder first described by Dr. Little in the 1860s, is only one of several disorders called cerebral palsy. Today, doctors classify cerebral palsy into four broad categories—spastic, athetoid, ataxic, and mixed forms—according to the type of movement disturbance.

Spastic cerebral palsy. In this form of cerebral palsy, which affects 70 to 80 percent of patients, the muscles are stiffly and permanently contracted. Doctors will often describe which type of spastic cerebral palsy a patient has based on which limbs are affected. The names given to these types combine a Latin description of affected limbs with the term plegia or paresis, meaning paralyzed or weak.

Athetoid, or dyskinetic, cerebral palsy. This form of cerebral palsy is characterized by uncontrolled, slow, writhing movements. These abnormal movements usually affect the hands, feet, arms, or legs and, in some cases, the muscles of the face and tongue, causing grimacing or drooling. The movements often increase during periods of emotional stress and disappear during sleep. Patients may also have problems coordinating the muscle movements needed for speech, a condition known as dysarthria. Athetoid cerebral palsy affects about 10 to 20 percent of patients.

Ataxic cerebral palsy. This rare form affects the sense of balance and depth perception. Affected persons often have poor coordination; walk unsteadily with a wide-based gait, placing their feet unusually far apart; and experience difficulty when attempting quick or precise movements, such as writing or buttoning a shirt. They may also have intention tremor. In this form of tremor, beginning a voluntary movement, such as reaching for a book, causes a trembling that affects the body part being used and that worsens as the individual gets nearer to the desired object. The ataxic form affects an estimated 5 to 10 percent of cerebral palsy patients.

Mixed forms. It is common for patients to have symptoms of more than one of the previous three forms. The most common mixed form includes spasticity and athetoid movements but other combinations are also possible.

What Other Medical Disorders Are Associated with Cerebral Palsy?

Many individuals who have cerebral palsy have no associated medical disorders. However, disorders that involve the brain and impair its motor function can also cause seizures and impair an individual's intellectual development, attentiveness to the outside world, activity and behavior, and vision and hearing. Medical disorders associated with cerebral palsy include mental impairment, seizures or epilepsy, growth problems, impaired vision or hearing, and abnormal sensation and perception.

What Causes Cerebral Palsy?

Cerebral palsy is not one disease with a single cause, like chicken pox or measles. It is a group of disorders with similar problems in control of movement, but probably with different causes. When physicians try to uncover the cause of cerebral palsy in an individual child, they look at the form of cerebral palsy, the mother's and child's medical history, and the onset of the disorder.

In the United States, about 10 to 20 percent of children who have cerebral palsy acquire the disorder after birth (the figures are higher in underdeveloped countries). Acquired cerebral palsy results from brain damage in the first few months or years of life and can follow brain infections, such as bacterial meningitis or viral encephalitis, or results from head injury—most often from a motor vehicle accident, a fall, or child abuse.

Congenital cerebral palsy, on the other hand, is present at birth, although it may not be detected for months. In most cases, the cause of congenital cerebral palsy is unknown. Thanks to research, however, scientists have pinpointed some specific events during pregnancy or around the time of birth that can damage motor centers in the developing brain. Some of these causes of congenital cerebral palsy include:

- Infections during pregnancy.

- Jaundice in the infant.

- Rh incompatibility.

- Severe oxygen shortage in the brain or trauma to the head during labor and delivery.

- Stroke.

What Are the Risk Factors?

Research scientists have examined thousands of expectant mothers, followed them through childbirth, and monitored their children's early neurological development. As a result, they have uncovered certain characteristics, called risk factors, that increase the possibility that a child will later be diagnosed with cerebral palsy:

- Breech presentation.
- Complicated labor and delivery.
- Low Apgar score.
- Low birth weight and premature birth.
- Multiple births.
- Nervous system malformations.
- Maternal bleeding or severe proteinuria late in pregnancy.
- Maternal hyperthyroidism, mental retardation, or seizures.
- Seizures in the newborn.

Knowing these warning signs helps doctors keep a close eye on children who face a higher risk for long-term problems in the nervous system. However, parents should not become too alarmed if their child has one or more of these factors. Most such children do not have and do not develop cerebral palsy.

Can Cerebral Palsy Be Prevented?

Several of the causes of cerebral palsy that have been identified through research are preventable or treatable:

- Head injury can be prevented by regular use of child safety seats when driving in a car and helmets during bicycle rides, and elimination of child abuse. In addition, common sense measures around the household—like close supervision during bathing and keeping poisons out of reach—can reduce the risk of accidental injury.

- Jaundice of newborn infants can be treated with phototherapy. In phototherapy, babies are exposed to special blue lights that break down bile pigments, preventing them from building up and threatening the brain. In the few cases in which this treatment is not enough, physicians can correct the condition with a special form of blood transfusion.

- Rh incompatibility is easily identified by a simple blood test routinely performed on expectant mothers and, if indicated, expectant fathers. This incompatibility in blood types does not usually cause problems during a woman's first pregnancy, since the mother's body generally does not produce the unwanted antibodies until after delivery. In most cases, a special serum given after each childbirth can prevent the unwanted production of antibodies. In unusual cases, such as when a pregnant woman develops the antibodies during her first pregnancy or antibody production is not prevented, doctors can help minimize problems by closely watching the developing baby and, when needed, performing a transfusion to the baby while in the womb or an exchange transfusion (in which a large volume of the baby's blood is removed and replaced) after birth.

- Rubella, or German measles, can be prevented if women are vaccinated against this disease before becoming pregnant.

In addition, it is always good to work toward a healthy pregnancy through regular prenatal care and good nutrition and by eliminating smoking, alcohol consumption, and drug abuse. Despite the best efforts of parents and physicians, however, children will still be born with cerebral palsy. Since in most cases the cause of cerebral palsy is unknown, little can currently be done to prevent it. As investigators learn more about the causes of cerebral palsy through basic and clinical research, doctors and parents will be better equipped to help prevent this disorder.

What Are the Early Signs?

Early signs of cerebral palsy usually appear before 3 years of age, and parents are often the first to suspect that their infant is not developing motor skills normally. Infants with cerebral palsy are frequently slow to reach developmental milestones, such as learning to roll over, sit, crawl, smile, or walk. This is sometimes called developmental delay.

Some affected children have abnormal muscle tone. Decreased muscle tone is called hypotonia; the baby may seem flaccid and relaxed, even floppy. Increased muscle tone is called hypertonia, and the baby may seem stiff or rigid. In some cases, the baby has an early period of hypotonia that progresses to hypertonia after the first 2 to 3 months of life. Affected children may also have unusual posture or favor one side of their body.

Parents who are concerned about their baby's development for any reason should contact their physician, who can help distinguish normal variation in development from a developmental disorder.

How Is Cerebral Palsy Diagnosed?

Doctors diagnose cerebral palsy by testing an infant's motor skills and looking carefully at the infant's medical history. In addition to checking for those symptoms described above—slow development, abnormal muscle tone, and unusual posture—a physician also tests the infant's reflexes and looks for early development of hand preference.

Reflexes are movements that the body makes automatically in response to a specific cue. For example, if a newborn baby is held on its back and tilted so the legs are above its head, the baby will automatically extend its arms in a gesture, called the Moro reflex, that looks like an embrace. Babies normally lose this reflex after they reach 6 months, but those with cerebral palsy may retain it for abnormally long periods. This is just one of several reflexes that a physician can check.

Doctors can also look for hand preference—a tendency to use either the right or left hand more often. When the doctor holds an object in front and to the side of the infant, an infant with hand preference will use the favored hand to reach for the object, even when it is held closer to the opposite hand. During the first 12 months of life, babies do not usually show hand preference. But infants with spastic hemiplegia, in particular, may develop a preference much earlier, since the hand on the unaffected side of their body is stronger and more useful.

The next step in diagnosing cerebral palsy is to rule out other disorders that can cause movement problems. Most important, doctors must determine that the child's condition is not getting worse. Although its symptoms may change over time, cerebral palsy by definition is not progressive. If a child is continuously losing motor skills, the problem more likely springs from elsewhere—including genetic diseases, muscle diseases, disorders of metabolism, or tumors in the nervous system. The child's medical history, special diagnostic tests, and, in some cases, repeated check-ups can help confirm that other disorders are not at fault.

The doctor may also order specialized tests to learn more about the possible cause of cerebral palsy. One such test is computed tomography, or CT, a sophisticated imaging technique that uses X rays and a computer to create an anatomical picture of the brain's tissues and structures. A CT scan may reveal brain areas that are underdeveloped, abnormal cysts (sacs that are often filled with liquid) in the brain, or other physical problems. With the information from CT scans, doctors may be better equipped to judge the long-term outlook for an affected child.

Magnetic resonance imaging, or MRI, is a relatively new brain imaging technique that is rapidly gaining widespread use for identifying brain disorders. This technique uses a magnetic field and radio waves, rather than X-rays. MRI gives better pictures of structures or abnormal areas located near bone than CT.

A third test that can expose problems in brain tissues is ultrasonography. This technique bounces sound waves off the brain and uses the pattern of echoes to form a picture, or sonogram, of its structures. Ultrasonography can be used in infants before the bones of the skull harden and close. Although it is less precise than CT and MRI scanning, this technique can detect cysts and structures in the brain, is less expensive, and does not require long periods of immobility.

Finally, physicians may want to look for other conditions that are linked to cerebral palsy, including seizure disorders, mental impairment, and vision or hearing problems.

When the doctor suspects a seizure disorder, an electroencephalogram, or EEG, may be ordered. An EEG uses special patches called electrodes placed on the scalp to record the natural electrical currents inside the brain. This recording can help the doctor see telltale patterns in the brain's electrical activity that suggest a seizure disorder.

Intelligence tests are often used to determine if a child with cerebral palsy is mentally impaired. Sometimes, however, a child's intelligence may be underestimated because problems with movement, sensation, or speech due to cerebral palsy make it difficult for him or her to perform well on these tests.

If problems with vision are suspected, the doctor may refer the patient to an ophthalmologist for examination; if hearing impairment seems likely, an otologist may be called in.

Identifying these accompanying conditions is important and is becoming more accurate as ongoing research yields advances that make diagnosis easier. Many of these conditions can then be addressed through specific treatments, improving the long-term outlook for those with cerebral palsy.

How Is Cerebral Palsy Managed?

Cerebral palsy can not be cured, but treatment can often improve a child's capabilities. In fact, progress due to medical research now means that many patients can enjoy near-normal lives if their neurological problems are properly managed. There is no standard therapy that works for all patients. Instead, the physician must work with a team of health care professionals first to identify a child's unique needs and impairments and then to create an individual treatment plan that addresses them.

Individuals who have cerebral palsy and their family or caregivers are also key members of the treatment team, and they should be intimately involved in all steps of planning, making decisions, and applying treatments. Studies have shown that family support and personal determination are two of the most important predictors of individuals who have cerebral palsy who achieve long-term goals.

Too often, however, physicians and parents may focus primarily on an individual symptom—especially the inability to walk. While mastering specific skills is an important focus of treatment on a day-to-day basis, the ultimate goal is to help individuals grow to adulthood and have maximum independence in society. In the words of one physician, "After all, the real point of walking is to get from point A to point B. Even if a child needs a wheelchair, what's important is that they're able to achieve this goal."

What Specific Treatments Are Available?

Physical, Behavioral, and Other Therapies

Therapy—whether for movement, speech, or practical tasks—is a cornerstone of cerebral palsy treatment. The skills a 2-year-old needs to explore the world are very different from those that a child needs in the classroom or a young adult needs to become independent. Cerebral palsy therapy should be tailored to reflect these changing demands.

Physical therapy usually begins in the first few years of life, soon after the diagnosis is made. Physical therapy programs use specific sets of exercises to work toward two important goals: preventing the weakening or deterioration of muscles that can follow lack of use (called disuse atrophy) and avoiding contracture, in which muscles become fixed in a rigid, abnormal position. A third goal of some physical therapy programs is to improve the child's motor development.

Behavioral therapy provides yet another avenue to increase a child's abilities. This therapy, which uses psychological theory and techniques, can complement physical, speech, or occupational therapy.

Regardless of the patient's age and which forms of therapy are used, treatment does not end when the patient leaves the office or treatment center. In fact, most of the work is often done at home. The therapist functions as a coach, providing parents and patients with the strategy and drills that can help improve performance at home, at school, and in the world. As research continues, doctors and parents can expect new forms of therapy and better information about which forms of therapy are most effective for individuals with cerebral palsy.

Drug Therapy

Physicians usually prescribe drugs for those who have seizures associated with cerebral palsy, and these medications are very effective in preventing seizures in many patients. In general, the drugs given to individual patients are chosen based on the type of seizures, since no one drug controls all types. However, different people with the same type of seizure may do better on different drugs, and some individuals may need a combination of two or more drugs to achieve good seizure control. Drugs are also sometimes used to control spasticity, particularly following surgery. Additionally, patients with athetoid cerebral palsy may sometimes be given drugs that help reduce abnormal movements.

Surgery

Surgery is often recommended when contractures are severe enough to cause movement problems. In the operating room, surgeons can lengthen muscles and tendons that are proportionately too short.

Mechanical Aids

Whether they are as humble as Velcro shoes or as advanced as computerized communication devices, special machines and gadgets in the home, school, and workplace can help the child with cerebral palsy overcome limitations.

Chapter 75

Muscular Dystrophy

The muscular dystrophies refer to a group of genetic diseases characterized by progressive weakness and degeneration of the skeletal or voluntary muscles. This is due to the muscles lacking a key protein that is needed to function properly. As the muscle tissue weakens and degenerates, it is replaced with fat tissue, making the muscles appear larger than normal. Approximately 33 percent of muscle mass has to be lost for function to be impaired. The muscles of the heart and some other involuntary muscles are also affected in some forms of muscular dystrophy (MD), and a few forms involve other organs as well. The major forms of MD include:

- Myotonic
- Duchenne
- Becker
- Limb-girdle
- Facioscapulohumeral
- Congenital
- Distal
- Emery-Dreifuss

MD can affect people of all ages. Although some forms first become apparent in infancy or childhood, others may not appear until middle age or later. Duchenne muscular dystrophy is the most common form affecting children, while myotonic MD is the most common form affecting adults.

There are three primary types of inheritance in which the faulty gene that causes MD can be passed along to offspring:

- **X-linked recessive:** Genes that are X-linked recessive are carried by the female on one of the X chromosomes that determine the sex of the child. As such, only boys will inherit conditions determined by these genes. Their mothers, known as carriers, will usually not show signs of the disease. A son of a carrier of MD has about a 50 percent chance of developing the disease, while a daughter of a carrier has a 50 percent chance of being a carrier. If a boy is unaffected, he cannot pass on MD, however daughters from a man with an X-linked dystrophy will all be carriers.

- **Autosomal recessive:** For this type of inheritance, both parents must carry and pass on the faulty gene. Neither parent shows any symptoms, but each of their offspring, regardless of gender, will have a 25 percent chance of developing the disease.

- **Autosomal dominant:** In the case of autosomal dominant inheritance, an affected person will have MD even though only one faulty gene has been passed along. This faulty gene can come from either parent, and it can affect either sex. Each child of an affected parent will have a 50 percent chance of developing MD. For this type of inheritance, the severity of MD can vary greatly. It can be so mild that it is not recognized but it can also be severe.

Diagnosis

After carefully evaluating a patient's medical history, the doctor will perform a thorough physical exam to rule out other causes. If MD is suspected, there are a variety of laboratory tests that can be used to solidify a diagnosis. These tests may include:

- **Blood tests:** When blood tests are performed to test for MD, the doctors are looking for an enzyme called creatine kinase (CK). This enzyme rises in the blood due to muscle damage or deterioration and may reveal some forms of MD before any physical symptoms appear.

- **Muscle biopsy:** During a muscle biopsy, a small piece of muscle tissue is removed and then examined under a microscope. If MD is present, changes in the structure of muscle cells and other characteristics of the different forms of MD can be detected. The sample can also be stained to detect the presence or absence of particular proteins.

- **Electromyogram (EMG):** An EMG is a test that measures the muscle's response to stimulation of its nerve supply (nerve conduction study) and the electrical activity in the muscle (needle electrode examination). Both components of the EMG are very useful in diagnosing MD.

- **Genetic tests:** Several of the muscular dystrophies can be positively diagnosed by testing for the mutated gene involved. These include Duchenne, Becker, Distal and some forms of Limb-girdle and Emery-Dreifuss dystrophies.

Treatment

There is no cure for muscular dystrophy, although some drugs still in the trial stage have shown promise in slowing or delaying the progression of the disease. For the time being, treatment is aimed at preventing complications due to the effects of weakness, decreased mobility, contractures, scoliosis, heart defects and respiratory weakness.

- **Physical therapy:** Physical therapy, especially regular stretching, is important in helping to maintain the range of motion for affected muscles and to prevent or delay contractures. Strengthening other muscles to compensate for weakness in affected muscles may be of benefit also, especially in earlier stages of milder MD. Regular exercise is important in maintaining good, overall health, but strenuous exercise may damage muscles further. For patients whose leg muscles are affected, braces may help lengthen the period of time that they can walk independently.

- **Surgery:** If a patient's contractures have become more pronounced, surgery may be used to relieve the tension by cutting the tendon of the affected muscle then bracing it in a normal resting position while it regrows. Other surgeries are used compensate for shoulder weakness in facioscapulohumeral MD, and to keep the breathing airway open for people with distal MD who sometimes experience sleep apnea. Surgery for scoliosis is often needed for patients with Duchenne MD.

Table 75.1. Muscular Dystrophies that May Have an Onset in Childhood (contiuned on next page)

Alternate names and commonly used abbreviations are given in parentheses.

Becker Muscular Dystrophy (BMD)

Onset: Adolescence or adulthood.

Symptoms: Almost identical to Duchenne (see below) but often much less severe. Can be significant heart involvements.

Progression: Slower and more variable than Duchenne with survival well into mid to late adulthood.

Inheritance: X-linked recessive (females are carriers).

Congenital Muscular Dystrophy (CMD)

Onset: At birth.

Symptoms: Generalized muscle weakness with possible joint deformities.

Progression: Disease progresses very slowly. Fukuyama form is more severe and involves mental functions.

Inheritance: Autosomal recessive, autosomal dominant.

Duchenne Muscular Dystrophy (DMD) (also known as Pseudohypertrophic)

Onset: Early childhood until about 2 to 6 years.

Symptoms: Generalized weakness and muscle wasting affecting limb and trunk muscles first. Calves often enlarged.

Progression: Disease progresses slowly but will affect all voluntary muscles. Survival rare beyond late twenties.

Inheritance: X-linked recessive (females are carriers).

Emery-Dreifuss Muscular Dystrophy (EDMD)

Onset: Childhood to early teens.

Symptoms: Weakness and wasting of shoulder, upper arm, and shin muscles. Joint deformities are common.

Progression: Disease usually progresses slowly. Frequent cardiac complications are common.

Inheritance: X-linked recessive (females are carriers).

Facioscapulohumeral Muscular Dystrophy (FSH or FSHD) (also known as Landouzy-Dejerine)

Onset: Childhood to early adulthood.

Table 75.1. Muscular Dystrophies that May Have an Onset in Childhood (continued from previous page)

Alternate names and commonly used abbreviations are given in parentheses.

Facioscapulohumeral Muscular Dystrophy (FSH or FSHD) , continued

Symptoms: Facial muscle weakness, with weakness and wasting of the shoulders and upper arms.

Progression: Progresses slowly with some periods of rapid deterioration. Disease may span many decades.

Inheritance: Autosomal dominant.

Limb-Girdle Muscular Dystrophy (LGMD)

Onset: Childhood to middle age.

Symptoms: Weakness and wasting affecting shoulder and pelvic girdles first.

Progression: Usually progresses slowly with cardiopulmonary complications often occurring in later stages of the disease.

Inheritance: Autosomal recessive, X-linked recessive.

Myotonic Dystrophy (MMD) (also known as Steinert's Disease)

Onset: Childhood to middle age.

Symptoms: Generalized weakness and muscle wasting affecting face, feet, hands and neck first. Delayed relaxation of muscles after contraction. Congenital myotonic form is more severe.

Progression: Progression is slow, sometimes spanning 50 to 60 years.

Inheritance: Autosomal dominant.

For more information about muscular dystrophies or other neuromuscular diseases in the MDA program, contact:

Muscular Dystrophy Association
3300 East Sunrise Drive
Tucson, AZ 85718-3208
Toll Free: 800-572-1717
Website: http://www.mdausa.org

You can also look for the nearest local MDA office in your local phone book or by visiting "Clinics and Services" on the MDA website.

Source: Excerpted from "Neuromuscular Diseases in the MDA Program," updated January 29, 1999, © 1999 Muscular Dystrophy Association (MDA); reprinted with permission.

- **Occupational therapy:** Occupational therapy involves employing methods and tools to compensate for a patient's loss of strength and mobility. This may include modifications at home, dressing aids, wheelchair accessories, and communication aids.

- **Nutrition:** Nutrition has not been shown to treat any conditions of MD, but it is essential to maintaining good health.

- **Cardiac care:** Arrhythmias are often a symptom with Emery-Dreifuss and Becker MD and may need to be treated with special drugs. Pacemakers may also be needed in some cases and heart transplants are becoming more common for men with Becker MD.

- **Respiratory care:** When the muscles of the diaphragm and other respiratory muscles become too weak to function on their own, a patient may require a ventilator to continue breathing deeply enough. Air may also be administered through a tube or mouthpiece. It is, therefore, very important to maintain healthy lungs to reduce the risk of respiratory complications.

Like many other disorders, understanding and education about muscular dystrophy is the most important tool with which to manage and prevent complications.

Chapter 76

Scoliosis in Children and Adolescents

Scoliosis is a musculoskeletal disorder in which there is a sideways curvature of the spine, or backbone. The bones that make up the spine are called vertebrae. Some people who have scoliosis require treatment. Other people, who have milder curves, may only need to visit their doctor for periodic observation.

Who gets scoliosis?

People of all ages can have scoliosis, but this chapter focuses on children and adolescents. Of every 1,000 children, 3 to 5 develop spinal curves that are considered large enough to need treatment. Adolescent idiopathic scoliosis (scoliosis of unknown cause) is the most common type and occurs after the age of 10. Girls are more likely than boys to have this type of scoliosis. Since scoliosis can run in families, a child who has a parent, brother, or sister with idiopathic scoliosis should be checked regularly for scoliosis by the family physician.

Idiopathic scoliosis can also occur in children younger than 10 years of age, but is very rare. Early onset or infantile idiopathic scoliosis occurs in children less than 3 years old. It is more common in Europe than in the United States. Juvenile idiopathic scoliosis occurs in children between the ages of 3 and 10.

Excerpted from "Questions and Answers about Scoliosis in Children and Adolescents," National Institute of Arthritis and Musculoskeletal and Skin Diseases (NIAMS), NIH Pub. No. 01-4862, July 2001.

What causes scoliosis?

In 80 to 85 percent of people, the cause of scoliosis is unknown; this is called idiopathic scoliosis. Before concluding that a person has idiopathic scoliosis, the doctor looks for other possible causes, such as injury or infection. Causes of curves are classified as either nonstructural or structural.

- Nonstructural (functional) scoliosis—A structurally normal spine that appears curved. This is a temporary, changing curve. It is caused by an underlying condition such as a difference in leg length, muscle spasms, or inflammatory conditions such as appendicitis. Doctors treat this type of scoliosis by correcting the underlying problem.

- Structural scoliosis—A fixed curve that doctors treat case by case. Sometimes structural scoliosis is one part of a syndrome or disease, such as Marfan's syndrome, an inherited connective tissue disorder. In other cases, it occurs by itself. Structural scoliosis can be caused by neuromuscular diseases (such as cerebral palsy, poliomyelitis, or muscular dystrophy), birth defects (such as hemivertebra, in which one side of a vertebra fails to form normally before birth), injury, certain infections, tumors (such as those caused by neurofibromatosis, a birth defect sometimes associated with benign tumors on the spinal column), metabolic diseases, connective tissue disorders, rheumatic diseases, or unknown factors (idiopathic scoliosis).

How does the doctor diagnose scoliosis?

The doctor takes the following steps to evaluate a patient for scoliosis:

- Medical history—The doctor talks to the patient and the patient's parent or parents and reviews the patient's records to look for medical problems that might be causing the spine to curve, for example, birth defects, trauma, or other disorders that can be associated with scoliosis.

- Physical examination—The doctor looks at the patient's back, chest, pelvis, legs, feet, and skin. The doctor checks if the patient's shoulders are level, whether the head is centered, and whether opposite sides of the body look level. The doctor also examines the back muscles while the patient is bending forward to see if one side of the rib cage is higher than the other. If there is a significant asymmetry (difference between opposite sides of the body), the doctor will refer the patient to an orthopaedic spine specialist (a doctor who has experience treating people with scoliosis). Certain changes in the skin, such as so-called café au lait (coffee-with-milk-colored) spots, can suggest that the scoliosis is caused by a birth defect.

- X-ray evaluation—Patients with significant spinal curves, unusual back pain, or signs of involvement of the central nervous system (brain and spinal cord) such as bowel and bladder control problems need to have an x-ray. The x-ray should be done with the patient standing with his or her back to the x-ray machine. The view is of the entire spine on one long (36-inch) film. Occasionally, doctors ask for more tests to see if there are other problems.

- Curve measurement—The doctor measures the curve on the x-ray image. He or she finds the vertebrae at the beginning and end of the curve and measures the angle of the curve. Curves that are greater than 20 degrees require treatment. Doctors group curves of the spine by their location, shape, pattern, and cause. They use this information to decide how best to treat the scoliosis.

- Location—To identify a curve's location, doctors find the apex of the curve (the vertebra within the curve that is the most off-center); the location of the apex is the location of the curve. A thoracic curve has its apex in the thoracic area (the part of the spine to which the ribs attach). A lumbar curve has its apex in the lower back. A thoracolumbar curve has its apex where the thoracic and lumbar vertebrae join.

- Shape—The curve usually is S- or C-shaped.

- Pattern—Curves frequently follow patterns that have been studied in previous patients. The larger the curve is, the more likely it will progress (depending on the amount of growth remaining).

Does scoliosis have to be treated? What are the treatments?

Many children who are sent to the doctor by a school scoliosis screening program have very mild spinal curves that do not need treatment. When a child does need treatment, the doctor may send him or her to an orthopaedic spine specialist.

The doctor will suggest the best treatment for each patient based on the patient's age, how much more he or she is likely to grow, the degree and pattern of the curve, and the type of scoliosis. The doctor may recommend observation, bracing, or surgery.

- Observation—Doctors follow patients without treatment and re-examine them every 4 to 6 months when the patient is still growing (is skeletally immature) and has an idiopathic curve of less than 25 degrees.

- Bracing—Doctors advise patients to wear a brace to stop a curve from getting any worse. As a child nears the end of growth, the indications for bracing will depend on how the curve affects the child's appearance, whether the curve is getting worse, and the size of the curve. Doctors recommend bracing when the patient:

  - is still growing and has an idiopathic curve that is more than 25 to 30 degrees;

  - has at least 2 years of growth remaining, has an idiopathic curve that is between 20 and 29 degrees, and, if a girl, has not had her first menstrual period; or

  - is still growing and has an idiopathic curve between 20 and 29 degrees that is getting worse.

- Surgery—Doctors advise patients to have surgery to correct a curve or stop it from worsening when the patient is still growing, has a curve that is more than 45 degrees, and has a curve that is getting worse.

Are there other ways to treat scoliosis?

Some people have tried other ways to treat scoliosis, including manipulation by a chiropractor, electrical stimulation, dietary supplements, and corrective exercises. So far, studies of the following treatments have not been shown to prevent curve progression, or worsening:

- Chiropractic manipulation

- Electrical stimulation

- Nutritional supplementation

- Exercise—Studies have shown that exercise alone will not stop progressive curves. However, patients may wish to exercise for the effects on their general health and well-being.

Which brace is best?

The decision about which brace to wear depends on the type of curve and whether the patient will follow the doctor's directions about how many hours a day to wear the brace.

There are two main types of braces. Braces can be custom-made or can be made from a prefabricated mold. All must be selected for the specific curve problem and fitted to each patient. To have their intended effect (to keep a curve from getting worse), braces must be worn every day for the full number of hours prescribed by the doctor until the child stops growing.

- Milwaukee brace—Patients can wear this brace to correct any curve in the spine. This brace has a neck ring.

- Thoracolumbosacral orthosis (TLSO)—Patients can wear this brace to correct curves whose apex is at or below the eighth thoracic vertebra. The TLSO is an underarm brace, which means that it fits under the arm and around the rib cage, lower back, and hips.

If the doctor recommends surgery, which procedure is best?

Many surgical techniques can be used to correct the curves of scoliosis. The main surgical procedure is correction, stabilization, and fusion of the curve. Fusion is the joining of two or more vertebrae. Surgeons can choose different ways to straighten the spine and also different implants to keep the spine stable after surgery. (Implants are devices that remain in the patient after surgery to keep the spine aligned.) The decision about the type of implant will depend on the cost; the size of the implant, which depends on the size of the patient; the shape of the implant; its safety; and the experience of the surgeon. Each patient should discuss his or her options with at least two experienced surgeons.

Patients and parents who are thinking about surgery may want to ask the following questions:

- What are the benefits from surgery for scoliosis?
- What are the risks from surgery for scoliosis?
- What techniques will be used for the surgery?
- What devices will be used to keep the spine stable after surgery?
- Where will the incisions be made?

513

- How straight will the patient's spine be after surgery?
- How long will the hospital stay be?
- How long will it take to recover from surgery?
- Is there chronic back pain after surgery for scoliosis?
- Will the patient's growth be limited?
- How flexible will the spine remain?
- Can the curve worsen or progress after surgery?
- Will additional surgery be likely?
- Will the patient be able to do all the things he or she wants to do following surgery?

Can people with scoliosis exercise?

Although exercise programs have not been shown to affect the natural history of scoliosis, exercise is encouraged in patients with scoliosis to minimize any potential decrease in functional ability over time. It is very important for all people, including those with scoliosis, to exercise and remain physically fit. Girls have a higher risk than boys of developing osteoporosis (a disorder that results in weak bones that can break easily) later in life. The risk of osteoporosis is reduced in women who exercise regularly all their lives; and weight-bearing exercise, such as walking, running, soccer, and gymnastics, increases bone density and helps prevent osteoporosis. For both boys and girls, exercising and participating in sports also improves their general sense of well-being.

Part Eight

Allergies

Chapter 77

Allergy Tests

Chapter Contents

Section 77.1

What Is Allergy Testing?

You are sneezing, wheezing, and coughing. Your eyes are itchy and your nose is running. When you visit your doctor, she says you may have allergies. But to find out exactly what is making you sneeze, you'll need to have allergy testing done.

What Is Allergy Testing?

If you are allergic, you are reacting to a particular substance. Any substance that can trigger an allergic reaction is called an allergen. To determine which specific substances are triggering your allergies, your allergist will safely and effectively test your skin, or sometimes your blood, using tiny amounts of commonly troublesome allergens. Allergy tests are designed to gather the most specific information possible so your doctor can determine what you are allergic to and provide the best treatment.

Which Allergens Will I Be Tested for?

Because your physician has made a diagnosis of allergies, you know that one or more allergens is causing your allergic reaction—itching, swelling, sneezing, wheezing, and other symptoms. Your symptoms are probably caused by one of these common allergens:

- products from dust mites (tiny bugs you can't see) that live in your home

- proteins from furry pets, which are found in their skin secretions (dander), saliva, and urine (it's actually not their hair)

- molds in your home or in the air outside

- tree, grass, and weed pollen

- cockroach droppings

More serious allergic reactions can be caused by:

- venoms from the stings of bees, wasps, yellow jackets, fire ants, and other stinging insects

- foods

- natural rubber latex, such as gloves or balloons

- drugs, such as penicillin

All of these allergens are typically made up of proteins. Allergy tests find which of these proteins you may be reacting to.

The allergen extracts or vaccines used in allergy tests are made commercially and are standardized according to U.S. Food and Drug Administration (FDA) requirements. Your allergist is able to safely test you for allergies to substances listed above using these allergen extracts.

What Are Specific Types of Allergy Tests?

Scratch or puncture test. These tests are done on the surface of the skin. A tiny amount of allergen is scratched across or lightly pricked into the skin. If you have an allergy, the specific allergens that you are allergic to will cause a chain reaction to begin in your body.

People with allergies have an allergic antibody called IgE (immunoglobulin E) in their body. This chemical, which is only found in people with allergies, activates special cells called mast cells. These mast cells release chemicals called mediators, such as histamine, the chemical that causes redness and swelling. With testing, this swelling occurs only in the spots where the tiny amount of allergen to which you are allergic has been scratched onto your skin. So, if you are allergic to ragweed pollen but not to cats, the spot where the ragweed allergen scratched your skin will swell and itch a bit, forming a small dime-sized hive. The spot where the cat allergen scratched your skin will remain normal. This reaction happens quickly within your body.

Test results are available within 15 minutes of testing, so you don't have to wait long to find out what is triggering your allergies. And you won't have any other symptoms besides the slightly swollen, small hives where the test was done; this goes away within 30 minutes.

Intradermal test. This test is related to the scratch or puncture test, but is slightly more sensitive. It involves injecting a tiny amount of allergen under the skin, usually on the upper arms. Your allergist may do this test when your reaction to the scratch test cannot be clearly determined.

Blood (RAST) test. Sometimes your allergist will do a blood test, called a RAST (radioallergosorbent) test. Since this test involves drawing blood, it costs more, and the results are not available as rapidly as skin tests. RAST tests are generally used only in cases in which skin tests cannot be performed, such as on patients taking certain medications, or those with skin conditions that may interfere with skin testing.

Challenge tests. These tests are done only if specific allergy testing is not available, and the patient needs the food or medication to which they may be allergic. The test involves having the patient inhale or swallow a very small amount of the suspected allergen, such as milk or an antibiotic. If there is no reaction, the dose may be slowly increased. Since challenge tests may induce severe allergic reactions, they are only done when absolutely necessary, and must be closely supervised by an allergist.

The American Academy of Allergy, Asthma and Immunology (AAAAI), along with many other medical associations, considers some allergy testing methods to be unacceptable in medical practice. According to an AAAAI position statement, these unacceptable tests include cytotoxicity testing, urine autoinjection, skin titration (Rinkel method), provocative and neutralization (subcutaneous) testing or sublingual provocation. If your physician plans to conduct any of these tests on you, please see an AAAAI member allergist for proper allergy testing.

Who Can Be Tested for Allergies?

Adults and children of any age can be tested for allergies. Because different allergens bother different people, your allergist will take your medical history to determine which test is the best for you. Some medications can interfere with skin testing. Antihistamines, in particular, can inhibit some of the skin test reactions. Use of antihistamines should be stopped one to several days prior to skin testing.

Reasons for Allergy Testing

To help you manage your allergy symptoms most effectively, your allergist must first determine what is causing your allergy. For instance, you don't have to get rid of your cat if you are allergic to dust mites but not cats, and you don't need to take medication all year if you have a seasonal allergy to ragweed.

Allergy tests provide concrete information. And once you know the specific allergens causing your symptoms, you can try to:

- avoid exposure to the allergens

- get specific medical treatment

- if necessary, consider specific vaccination with the allergen, or allergy shots

Your allergist/immunologist can provide you with more information on allergy testing.

Section 77.2

Properly Diagnosing Allergies

Leonard Fromer, MD Addresses This Issue

A relatively new testing method can successfully detect specific allergies in children at any age, but many doctors do not know about the test because when they were in medical school it simply did not exist.

Leonard Fromer, MD, is an accredited allergist and family physician with specific expertise in the areas of allergy and asthma. He serves as advisor/consultant for such accredited professional organizations as American Academy of Family Physicians and the American

Medical Association, as well as Pharmacia Diagnostics, developer of the ImmunoCap allergy blood test, which is much more accurate than previous tests.

In a scheduled chat at the About Allergies site [http://allergies.about.com] on June 11, 2001, the advantages of the ImmunoCap test over previous testing techniques became apparent as Dr. Fromer answered questions from guest chatters. Here is an edited version of some of those questions and answers:

Vtmom: My son is 14 months and has asthma. He was recently diagnosed with eczema, too. I really would like him tested for allergies since we have a strong family history of allergies, including food allergies. My pediatrician says he is too young, that his immune system is not developed enough and tests will not be accurate (false negatives). The allergist will test for food allergies now, if I can get a referral, but will not test for inhaled allergens until he is two. Should I push for a referral now for food testing?

Accurate at Any Age

Dr. Fromer: Young children often exhibit allergies as eczema. They can be tested with a simple blood test that can be ordered by their pediatrician or family physician. This test can be done to check for allergies to inhaled pollens, dust, molds, and a variety of foods. This simple blood test can be ordered by your primary care physician.

This is known generically as the RAST test. The best available type of RAST test is the ImmunoCap RAST test. The test is accurate at any age. It tests for the presence of IgE antibodies in the serum directed at specific allergens.

The test can be ordered for specific foods, such as peanuts, and your pediatrician should speak to his reference lab for data on how accurate the test is.

There is research that shows the ImmunoCap RAST test is now as effective in diagnosing allergies as the best available skin testing technique.

Vtmom: Thanks Dr. Now I just need info to prove this to my pediatrician. Do you think getting my son tested would be worthwhile? Is there stuff about this test on the Internet I can print out and show him?

Dr. Fromer: Absolutely! You can find information at www.isit allergy.com.

At Almost Every Lab

Abby: My daughter just turned one. Is it too early to test for allergies? My pediatrician said we needed to wait until she was 3.

Dr. Fromer: No—she can be tested at that age. Your pediatrician is referring to the skin test which they usually wait until age 3 or 4. The pediatrician can run the ImmunoCap test at any age.

Abby: Do they all have access to that test now? Does this test tell all kinds of allergies or just a select few?

Dr. Fromer: The test is available at almost every lab that doctors send their specimens to. It can test for hundreds of different things, such as pollens, dust, dust mites, animal hairs, fabrics, molds, and foods.

Abby: My pediatrician says she probably has asthmatic/allergic tendencies but we need to wait. If there is something I can do now I want to do it. This test sounds wonderful. Allergies run high in both sides of our families. She gets sick and has to be put on Albuterol and steroids every time she gets a cold.

Dr. Fromer: Most doctors do not know about the test because they learned about blood testing for allergies in med school at a time when blood tests were not accurate. The newest version (ImmunoCap) has only been available for several years.

Testing Is Critical

Abby: My daughter is also on Claritin each day now that pollen season has hit North Carolina.

Dr. Fromer: Claritin and Astelin will help patients only if their symptoms are due to histamine related allergies. Approximately 60 percent of Americans who get allergy medications do not have true allergies.

Testing for allergies is critical to identify the truly allergic patient and what they are allergic to. Then appropriate medication can be prescribed. The ImmunoCap test can be done on patients of any age; it can be done at any time of the year because symptoms do not need to be present.

AllergiesADM: What makes the ImmunoCap different from the RAST?

Dr. Fromer: Great question. The ImmunoCap process affects the way the patient's serum and test medium react. This leads to a far more selective and sensitive result.

AllergiesADM: So you are saying it is the way the blood is processed?

Dr. Fromer: Yes, because the reagents and test media that are used lead to a result that is as accurate as the best available skin test.

Chapter 78

General Information about Airborne Allergies

Introduction

Sneezing is not always the symptom of a cold. Sometimes, it is an allergic reaction to something in the air. Experts estimate that 35 million Americans suffer from upper respiratory symptoms that are allergic reactions to airborne pollen. Pollen allergy, commonly called hay fever, is one of the most common chronic diseases in the United States. Worldwide, airborne dust causes the most problems for people with allergies. The respiratory symptoms of asthma, which affect approximately 15 million Americans, are often provoked by airborne allergens (substances that cause an allergic reaction).

Overall, allergic diseases are among the major causes of illness and disability in the United States, affecting as many as 40 to 50 million Americans. The National Institute of Allergy and Infectious Diseases, a component of the National Institutes of Health (NIH), conducts and supports research on allergic diseases. The goals of this research are to provide a better understanding of the causes of allergy, to improve the methods for diagnosing and treating allergic reactions, and eventually to prevent allergies. This text summarizes what is known about the causes and symptoms of allergic reactions to airborne allergens and how these reactions are diagnosed and treated.

Excerpted from "Something in the Air: Airborne Allergens," National Institute of Allergy and Infectious Diseases, February 1998, updated May 21, 2001. The full text of this document is available online at http://www.niaid.nih.gov/publications/allergens/full.htm.

What Is an Allergy?

An allergy is a specific immunologic reaction to a normally harmless substance, one that does not bother most people. People who have allergies often are sensitive to more than one substance. Types of allergens that cause allergic reactions include pollens, dust particles, mold spores, food, latex rubber, insect venom, or medicines.

Why Are Some People Allergic to These Substances While Others Are Not?

Scientists think that people inherit a tendency to be allergic, meaning an increased likelihood of being allergic to one or more allergens, although they probably do not have an inherited tendency to be allergic to any specific allergens. Children are much more likely to develop allergies if their parents have allergies, even if only one parent is allergic. Exposure to allergens at certain times when the body's defenses are lowered or weakened, such as after a viral infection or during pregnancy, seems to contribute to the development of allergies.

What Is an Allergic Reaction?

Normally, the immune system functions as the body's defense against invading agents such as bacteria and viruses. In most allergic reactions, however, the immune system is responding to a false alarm. When an allergic person first comes into contact with an allergen, the immune system treats the allergen as an invader and mobilizes to attack. The immune system does this by generating large amounts of a type of antibody (a disease-fighting protein) called immunoglobin E, or IgE. Each IgE antibody is specific for one particular allergenic (allergy-producing) substance. In the case of pollen allergy, the antibody is specific for each type of pollen: one type of antibody may be produced to react against oak pollen and another against ragweed pollen, for example.

These IgE molecules are special because IgE is the only class of antibody that attaches tightly to the body's mast cells, which are tissue cells, and to basophils, which are blood cells. When the allergen next encounters its specific IgE, it attaches to the antibody like a key fitting into a lock, signaling the cell to which the IgE is attached to release (and in some cases to produce) powerful inflammatory chemicals like histamine, cytokines, and leukotrienes. These chemicals act on tissues in various parts of the body, such as the respiratory system, and cause the symptoms of allergy.

Some children with allergy develop asthma. The symptoms of asthma include coughing, wheezing, and shortness of breath due to a narrowing of the bronchial passages (airways) in the lungs, and to excess mucus production and inflammation. Asthma can be disabling and sometimes can be fatal. If wheezing and shortness of breath accompany allergy symptoms, it is a signal that the bronchial tubes also have become involved, indicating the need for medical attention.

Symptoms of Allergies to Airborne Substances

The signs and symptoms are familiar to many:

- sneezing often accompanied by a runny or clogged nose
- coughing and postnasal drip
- itching eyes, nose, and throat
- allergic shiners (dark circles under the eyes caused by increased blood flow near the sinuses)
- the "allergic salute" (in a child, persistent upward rubbing of the nose that causes a crease mark on the nose)
- watering eyes
- conjunctivitis (an inflammation of the membrane that lines the eyelids, causing red-rimmed, swollen eyes, and crusting of the eyelids).

In people who are not allergic, the mucus in the nasal passages simply moves foreign particles to the throat, where they are swallowed or coughed out. But something different happens to a person who is sensitive to airborne allergens.

As soon as the allergen lands on the mucous membranes lining the inside of the nose, a chain reaction occurs that leads the mast cells in these tissues to release histamine and other chemicals. These powerful chemicals contract certain cells that line some small blood vessels in the nose. This allows fluids to escape, which causes the nasal passages to swell, resulting in nasal congestion.

Histamine also can cause sneezing, itching, irritation, and excess mucus production, which can result in allergic rhinitis (runny nose). Other chemicals made and released by mast cells, including cytokines and leukotrienes, also contribute to allergic symptoms.

Pollen Allergy

Each spring, summer, and fall, tiny particles are released from trees, weeds, and grasses. These particles, known as pollen, hitch rides on currents of air. Although their mission is to fertilize parts of other plants, many never reach their targets. Instead, they enter human noses and throats, triggering a type of seasonal allergic rhinitis called pollen allergy, which many people know as hay fever or rose fever (depending on the season in which the symptoms occur). Of all the things that can cause an allergy, pollen is one of the most widespread. Many of the foods, drugs, or animals that cause allergies can be avoided to a great extent; even insects and household dust are escapable. Short of staying indoors when the pollen count is high—and even that may not help—there is no easy way to evade windborne pollen.

People with pollen allergies often develop sensitivities to other troublemakers that are present all year, such as dust mites. For these allergy sufferers, the "sneezin' season" has no limit. Year-round airborne allergens cause perennial allergic rhinitis, as distinguished from seasonal allergic rhinitis.

What Is Pollen?

Plants produce microscopic round or oval pollen grains to reproduce. In some species, the plant uses the pollen from its own flowers to fertilize itself. Other types must be cross-pollinated; that is, in order for fertilization to take place and seeds to form, pollen must be transferred from the flower of one plant to that of another plant of the same species. Insects do this job for certain flowering plants, while other plants rely on wind transport.

The types of pollen that most commonly cause allergic reactions are produced by the plain-looking plants (trees, grasses, and weeds) that do not have showy flowers. These plants manufacture small, light, dry pollen granules that are custom-made for wind transport. Samples of ragweed pollen have been collected 400 miles out at sea and 2 miles high in the air. Because airborne pollen is carried for long distances, it does little good to rid an area of an offending plant—the pollen can drift in from many miles away. In addition, most allergenic pollen comes from plants that produce it in huge quantities. A single ragweed plant can generate a million grains of pollen a day.

The chemical makeup of pollen is the basic factor that determines whether it is likely to cause hay fever. For example, pine tree pollen is produced in large amounts by a common tree, which would make it a good candidate for causing allergy. The chemical composition of pine pollen, however, appears to make it less allergenic than other types. Because pine pollen is heavy, it tends to fall straight down and does not scatter. Therefore, it rarely reaches human noses.

Among North American plants, weeds are the most prolific producers of allergenic pollen. Ragweed is the major culprit, but others of importance are sagebrush, redroot pigweed, lamb's quarters, Russian thistle (tumbleweed), and English plantain.

Grasses and trees, too, are important sources of allergenic pollens. Although more than 1,000 species of grass grow in North America, only a few produce highly allergenic pollen. These include timothy grass, Kentucky bluegrass, Johnson grass, Bermuda grass, redtop grass, orchard grass, and sweet vernal grass. Trees that produce allergenic pollen include oak, ash, elm, hickory, pecan, box elder, and mountain cedar.

It is common to hear people say that they are allergic to colorful or scented flowers like roses. In fact, only florists, gardeners, and others who have prolonged, close contact with flowers are likely to become sensitized to pollen from these plants. Most people have little contact with the large, heavy, waxy pollen grains of many flowering plants because this type of pollen is not carried by wind but by insects such as butterflies and bees.

When Do Plants Make Pollen?

One of the most obvious features of pollen allergy is its seasonal nature—people experience it symptoms only when the pollen grains to which they are allergic are in the air. Each plant has a pollinating period that is more or less the same from year to year. Exactly when a plant starts to pollinate seems to depend on the relative length of night and day—and therefore on geographical location—rather than on the weather. (On the other hand, weather conditions during pollination can affect the amount of pollen produced and distributed in a specific year.) Thus, the farther north you go, the later the pollinating period and the later the allergy season.

A pollen count, which is familiar to many people from local weather reports, is a measure of how much pollen is in the air. This count represents the concentration of all the pollen (or of one particular type, like ragweed) in the air in a certain area at a specific time. It is expressed in grains of pollen per square meter of air collected over 24 hours. Pollen counts tend to be highest early in the morning on warm, dry, breezy days and lowest during chilly, wet periods. Although a pollen count is an approximate and fluctuating measure, it is useful as a general guide for when it is advisable to stay indoors and avoid contact with the pollen.

Mold Allergy

Along with pollens from trees, grasses, and weeds, molds are an important cause of seasonal allergic rhinitis. People allergic to molds may have symptoms from spring to late fall. The mold season often peaks from July to late summer. Unlike pollens, molds may persist after the first killing frost. Some can grow at sub-freezing temperatures, but most become dormant. Snow cover lowers the outdoor mold count dramatically but does not kill molds. After the spring thaw, molds thrive on the vegetation that has been killed by the winter cold.

In the warmest areas of the United States, however, molds thrive all year and can cause year-round (perennial) allergic problems. In addition, molds growing indoors can cause perennial allergic rhinitis even in the coldest climates.

What Is Mold?

There are thousands of types of molds and yeast, the two groups of plants in the fungus family. Yeasts are single cells that divide to form clusters. Molds consist of many cells that grow as branching threads called hyphae. Although both groups can probably cause allergic reactions, only a small number of molds are widely recognized offenders.

The seeds or reproductive particles of fungi are called spores. They differ in size, shape, and color among species. Each spore that germinates can give rise to new mold growth, which in turn can produce millions of spores.

What Is Mold Allergy?

When inhaled, microscopic fungal spores or, sometimes, fragments of fungi may cause allergic rhinitis. Because they are so small, mold spores may evade the protective mechanisms of the nose and upper respiratory tract to reach the lungs.

In a small number of people, symptoms of mold allergy may be brought on or worsened by eating certain foods, such as cheeses, processed with fungi. Occasionally, mushrooms, dried fruits, and foods containing yeast, soy sauce, or vinegar will produce allergic symptoms. There is no known relationship, however, between a respiratory allergy to the mold *Penicillium* and an allergy to the drug penicillin, made from the mold.

Where Do Molds Grow?

Molds can be found wherever there is moisture, oxygen, and a source of the few other chemicals they need. In the fall they grow on rotting logs and fallen leaves, especially in moist, shady areas. In gardens, they can be found in compost piles and on certain grasses and weeds. Some molds attach to grains such as wheat, oats, barley, and corn, making farms, grain bins, and silos likely places to find mold.

Hot spots of mold growth in the home include damp basements and closets, bathrooms (especially shower stalls), places where fresh food is stored, refrigerator drip trays, house plants, air conditioners, humidifiers, garbage pails, mattresses, upholstered furniture, and old foam rubber pillows.

Bakeries, breweries, barns, dairies, and greenhouses are favorite places for molds to grow. Loggers, mill workers, carpenters, furniture repairers, and upholsterers often work in moldy environments.

Which Molds Are Allergenic?

Like pollens, mold spores are important airborne allergens only if they are abundant, easily carried by air currents, and allergenic in their chemical makeup. Found almost everywhere, mold spores in some areas are so numerous they often outnumber the pollens in the air. Fortunately, however, only a few dozen different types are significant allergens.

In general, *Alternaria* and *Cladosporium* (*Hormodendrum*) are the molds most commonly found both indoors and outdoors throughout the United States. *Aspergillus, Penicillium, Helminthosporium, Epiccoccum, Fusarium, Mucor, Rhizopus,* and *Aureobasidium* (*Pullularia*) are also common.

Are Mold Counts Helpful?

Similar to pollen counts, mold counts may suggest the types and relative quantities of fungi present at a certain time and place. For several reasons, however, these counts probably cannot be used as a constant guide for daily activities. One reason is that the number and types of spores actually present in the mold count may have changed considerably in 24 hours because weather and spore dispersal are directly related. Many of the common allergenic molds are of the dry spore type—they release their spores during dry, windy weather. Other fungi need high humidity, fog, or dew to release their spores. Although rain washes many larger spores out of the air, it also causes some smaller spores to be shot into the air.

In addition to the effect of day-to-day weather changes on mold counts, spore populations may also differ between day and night. Day favors dispersal by dry spore types and night favors wet spore types.

Are There Other Mold-Related Disorders?

Fungi or microorganisms related to them may cause other health problems similar to allergic diseases. Some kinds of *Aspergillus* may cause several different illnesses, including both infections and allergy. These fungi may lodge in the airways or a distant part of the lung and grow until they form a compact sphere known as a "fungus ball." In people with lung damage or serious underlying illnesses, *Aspergillus* may grasp the opportunity to invade the lungs or the whole body.

In some individuals, exposure to these fungi also can lead to asthma or to a lung disease resembling severe inflammatory asthma called allergic bronchopulmonary aspergillosis. This latter condition, which occurs only in a minority of people with asthma, is characterized by wheezing, low-grade fever, and coughing up of brown-flecked masses or mucus plugs. Skin testing, blood tests, X-rays, and examination of the sputum for fungi can help establish the diagnosis. Corticosteroid drugs are usually effective in treating this reaction; immunotherapy (allergy shots) is not helpful.

Dust Mite Allergy

Dust mite allergy is an allergy to a microscopic organism that lives in the dust that is found in all dwellings and workplaces. Dust mites are perhaps the most common cause of perennial allergic rhinitis. Dust mite allergy usually produces symptoms similar to pollen allergy and also can produce symptoms of asthma.

What Is House Dust?

Rather than a single substance, so-called house dust is a varied mixture of potentially allergenic materials. It may contain fibers from different types of fabrics; cotton lint, feathers, and other stuffing materials; dander from cats, dogs, and other animals; bacteria; mold and fungus spores (especially in damp areas); food particles; bits of plants and insects; and other allergens peculiar to an individual home.

House dust also contains microscopic mites. These mites, which live in bedding, upholstered furniture, and carpets, thrive in summer and die in winter. In a warm, humid house, however, they continue to thrive even in the coldest months. The particles seen floating in a shaft of sunlight include dead dust mites and their waste products. These waste products, which are proteins, actually provoke the allergic reaction.

Waste products of cockroaches are also an important cause of allergy symptoms from household allergens, particularly in some urban areas of the United States.

Animal Allergy

Household pets are the most common source of allergic reactions to animals. Many people think that pet allergy is provoked by the fur of cats and dogs. But researchers have found that the major allergens are proteins secreted by oil glands in the animals' skin and shed in dander as well as proteins in the saliva, which sticks to the fur when the animal licks itself. Urine is also a source of allergy-causing proteins. When the substance carrying the proteins dries, the proteins can then float into the air. Cats may be more likely than dogs to cause allergic reactions because they lick themselves more and may be held more and spend more time in the house, close to humans.

Some rodents, such as guinea pigs and gerbils, have become increasingly popular as household pets. They, too, can cause allergic reactions in some people, as can mice and rats. Urine is the major source of allergens from these animals.

Allergies to animals can take two years or more to develop and may not subside until six months or more after ending contact with the animal. Carpet and furniture are a reservoir for pet allergens, and the allergens can remain in them for four to six weeks. In addition, these allergens can stay in household air for months after the animal has been removed. Therefore, it is wise for people with an animal allergy to check with the landlord or previous owner to find out if furry pets had lived previously on the premises.

Chemical Sensitivity

Some people report that they react to chemicals in their environment and that these allergy-like reactions appear to result from exposure to a wide variety of synthetic and natural substances, such as those found in paints, carpeting, plastics, perfumes, cigarette smoke, and plants. Although the symptoms may resemble some of the manifestations of allergies, sensitivity to chemicals does not represent a true allergic reaction involving IgE and the release of histamine or other chemicals.

Diagnosing Allergic Diseases

People with allergy symptoms, such as the runny nose of allergic rhinitis, may at first suspect they have a cold—but the "cold" lingers on. It is important to see a doctor about any respiratory illness that lasts longer than a week or two. When it appears that the symptoms are caused by an allergy, the patient should see a physician who understands the diagnosis and treatment of allergies. If the patient's medical history indicates that the symptoms recur at the same time each year, the physician will work under the theory that a seasonal allergen (like pollen) is involved. Properly trained specialists recognize the patterns of potential allergens common during local seasons and the association between these patterns and symptoms. The medical history suggests which allergens are the likely culprits. The doctor also will examine the mucous membranes, which often appear swollen and pale or bluish in persons with allergic conditions.

Skin Tests

Doctors use skin tests to determine whether a patient has IgE antibodies in the skin that react to a specific allergen. The doctor will use diluted extracts from allergens such as dust mites, pollens, or molds commonly found in the local area. The extract of each kind of allergen is injected under the patient's skin or is applied to a tiny scratch or puncture made on the patient's arm or back.

Skin tests are one way of measuring the level of IgE antibody in a patient. With a positive reaction, a small, raised, reddened area (called a wheal) with a surrounding flush (called a flare) will appear at the test site. The size of the wheal can give the physician an important diagnostic clue, but a positive reaction does not prove that a particular pollen is the cause of a patient's symptoms. Although such a reaction indicates that IgE antibody to a specific allergen is present in the skin, respiratory symptoms do not necessarily result.

Blood Tests

Although skin testing is the most sensitive and least costly way to identify allergies in patients, some patients such as those with widespread skin conditions like eczema should not be tested using that method. There are other diagnostic tests that use a blood sample from the patient to detect levels of IgE antibody to a particular allergen. One such blood test is called the RAST (radioallergosorbent test), which can be performed when eczema is present or if a patient has taken medications that interfere with skin testing.

Treating People with Allergic Diseases

Doctors use three general approaches to helping people with allergies: advise them on ways to avoid the allergen as much as possible, prescribe medication to relieve symptoms, and give a series of allergy shots. Although there is no cure for allergies, one of these strategies or a combination of them can provide varying degrees of relief from allergy symptoms.

Avoidance

Complete avoidance of allergenic pollen or mold means moving to a place where the offending substance does not grow and where it is not present in the air. But even this extreme solution may offer only temporary relief since a person who is sensitive to a specific pollen or mold may subsequently develop allergies to new allergens after repeated exposure. For example, people allergic to ragweed may leave their ragweed-ridden communities and relocate to areas where ragweed does not grow, only to develop allergies to other weeds or even to grasses or trees in their new surroundings. Because relocating is not a reliable solution, allergy specialists do not encourage this approach.

There are other ways to evade the offending pollen: remaining indoors in the morning, for example, when the outdoor pollen levels are highest. Sunny, windy days can be especially troublesome. If individuals with pollen allergy must work outdoors, they can wear face masks designed to filter pollen out of the air and keep it from reaching their nasal passages. As another approach, some people take their vacations at the height of the expected pollinating period and choose a location where such exposure would be minimal. The seashore, for example, may be an effective retreat for many with pollen allergies.

Mold allergens can be difficult to avoid, but some steps can be taken to at least reduce exposure to them. First, the allergy sufferer should avoid those hot spots mentioned earlier where molds tend to be concentrated. The lawn should be mowed and leaves should be raked up, but someone other than the allergic person should do these chores. If such work cannot be delegated, wearing a tightly fitting dust mask can greatly reduce exposure and resulting symptoms. Travel in the country, especially on dry, windy days or while crops are being harvested, should be avoided as should walks through tall vegetation. A summer cabin closed up all winter is probably full of molds and should be aired out and cleaned before a mold-sensitive person stays there.

Around the home, a dehumidifier will help dry out the basement, but the water extracted from the air must be removed frequently to prevent mold growth in the machine.

Those with dust mite allergy should pay careful attention to dust-proofing their bedrooms. The worst things to have in the bedroom are wall-to-wall carpets, venetian blinds, down-filled blankets, feather pillows, heating vents with forced hot air, dogs, cats, and closets full of clothing. Shades are preferred over Venetian blinds because they do not trap dust. Curtains can be used if they are washed periodically in hot water to kill the dust mites. Most important, bedding should be encased in a zippered, plastic, airtight, and dust-proof cover.

Although shag carpets are the worst type for the dust mite-sensitive person, all carpets trap dust and make dust control impossible. In addition, vacuuming can contribute to the amount of dust, unless the vacuum is equipped with a special high-efficiency particulate air (HEPA) filter. Wall-to-wall carpets should be replaced with washable throw rugs over hardwood, tile, or linoleum floors. Rugs on concrete floors encourage dust mite growth and should be avoided.

Reducing the amount of dust mites in a home may require new cleaning techniques as well as some changes in furnishings to eliminate dust collectors. Water is often the secret to effective dust removal. Washable items should be washed often using water hotter then 130 (degrees) Fahrenheit. Lower temperatures will not kill dust mites. If the water temperature must be set at a lower value, items can be washed at a commercial establishment that uses high wash temperatures. Dusting with a damp cloth or oiled mop should be done frequently.

The best way for a person allergic to pets, especially cats, to avoid allergic reactions is to find another home for the animal. There are, however, some suggestions that help lower the levels of cat allergens in the air: bathe the cat weekly and brush it more frequently (ideally, this should be done by someone other than the allergic person), remove carpets and soft furnishings, and use a vacuum cleaner with a high-efficiency filter and a room air cleaner (see section below). Wearing a face mask while house and cat cleaning and keeping the cat out of the bedroom are other methods that allow many people to live more happily with their pets.

Irritants such as chemicals can worsen airborne allergy symptoms and should be avoided as much as possible. For example, during periods of high pollen levels, people with pollen allergy should try to avoid unnecessary exposure to irritants such as insect sprays, tobacco smoke, air pollution, and fresh tar or paint.

Air Conditioners and Filters

When possible, an allergic person should use air conditioners inside the home or in a car to help prevent pollen and mold allergens from entering. Various types of air-filtering devices made with fiberglass or electrically charged plates may help reduce allergens produced in the home. These can be added to the heating and cooling systems. In addition, portable devices that can be used in individual rooms are especially helpful in reducing animal allergens.

An allergy specialist can suggest which kind of filter is best for the home of a particular patient. Before buying a filtering device, the patient should rent one and use it in a closed room (the bedroom, for instance) for a month or two to see whether allergy symptoms diminish. The airflow should be sufficient to exchange the air in the room five or six times per hour; therefore, the size and efficiency of the filtering device should be determined in part by the size of the room.

Persons with allergies should be wary of exaggerated claims for appliances that cannot really clean the air. Very small air cleaners cannot remove dust and pollen—and no air purifier can prevent viral or bacterial diseases such as influenza, pneumonia, or tuberculosis. Buyers of electrostatic precipitators should compare the machine's ozone output with Federal standards. Ozone can irritate the nose and airways of persons with allergies, especially those with asthma, and can increase the allergy symptoms. Other kinds of air filters such as HEPA (High Efficiency Particulate Air) filters do not release ozone into the air. HEPA filters, however, require adequate air flow to force air through them.

Medications

For people who find they cannot adequately avoid airborne allergens, the symptoms often can be controlled with medications. Effective medications that can be prescribed by a physician include antihistamines and topical nasal steroids—either of which can be used alone or in combination. Many effective antihistamines and decongestants also are available without a prescription.

Antihistamines. As the name indicates, an antihistamine counters the effects of histamine, which is released by the mast cells in the body's tissues and contributes to allergy symptoms. For many years, antihistamines have proven useful in relieving sneezing and itching in the nose, throat, and eyes, and in reducing nasal swelling and drainage.

Many people who take antihistamines experience some distressing side effects: drowsiness and loss of alertness and coordination. In children, such reactions can be misinterpreted as behavior problems. During the last few years, however, antihistamines that cause fewer of these side effects have become available by prescription. These non-sedating antihistamines are as effective as other antihistamines in preventing histamine-induced symptoms, but do so without causing sleepiness. Some of these non-sedating antihistamines, however, can have serious side effects, particularly if they are taken with certain other drugs. A patient should always let the doctor know what other medications he/she is taking.

Topical nasal steroids. This medication should not be confused with anabolic steroids, which are sometimes used by athletes to enlarge muscle mass and can have serious side effects. Topical nasal steroids are anti-inflammatory drugs that stop the allergic reaction. In addition to other beneficial actions, they reduce the number of mast cells in the nose and reduce mucus secretion and nasal swelling. The combination of antihistamines and nasal steroids is a very effective way to treat allergic rhinitis, especially in people with moderate or severe allergic rhinitis. Although topical nasal steroids can have side effects, they are safe when used at recommended doses. Some of the newer agents are even safer than older ones.

Cromolyn sodium. Cromolyn sodium for allergic rhinitis is a nasal spray that in some people helps to prevent allergic reactions from starting. When administered as a nasal spray, it can safely inhibit the release of chemicals like histamine from the mast cell. It has few side effects when used as directed, and significantly helps some patients with allergies.

Decongestants. Sometimes re-establishing drainage of the nasal passages will help to relieve symptoms such as congestion, swelling, excess secretions, and discomfort in the sinus areas that can be caused by nasal allergies. (These sinus areas are hollow air spaces located within the bones of the skull surrounding the nose.) The doctor may recommend using oral or nasal decongestants to reduce congestion along with an antihistamine to control allergic symptoms. Over-the-counter and prescription decongestant nose drops and sprays, however, should not be used for more than a few days. When used for longer periods, these drugs can lead to even more congestion and swelling of the nasal passages.

Immunotherapy

Immunotherapy, or a series of allergy shots, is the only available treatment that has a chance of reducing the allergy symptoms over a longer period of time. Patients receive subcutaneous (under the skin) injections of increasing concentrations of the allergen(s) to which they are sensitive. These injections reduce the amount of IgE antibodies in the blood and cause the body to make a protective antibody called IgG. Many patients with allergic rhinitis will have a significant reduction in their hay fever symptoms and in their need for medication within 12 months of starting immunotherapy. Patients who benefit from immunotherapy may continue it for three years and then consider stopping. Although many patients are able to stop the injections with good, long-term results, some do get worse after immunotherapy is stopped. As better allergens for immunotherapy are produced, this technique will become an even more effective treatment.

Chapter 79

Insect Allergies

Each year, many Americans are stung by insects. For most of those unfortunate enough to be stung, these stings mean pain and discomfort generally lasting only a few hours. Symptoms may include redness, swelling, and itching at the site of the sting.

However, some people are allergic to insect stings. This means that their immune systems overreact to the venom injected by a stinging insect. After the first sting, the allergic person's body produces an allergic substance called Immunoglobulin E (IgE) antibody, which reacts with the insect venom. The individual does not usually experience a severe allergic reaction from that first sting—but if he or she is stung again by an insect of the same or similar species, the insect venom interacts with the IgE antibody produced in response to the earlier sting. This triggers the release of histamine and other chemicals that cause allergic symptoms.

Symptoms of Severe Reactions

For a small number of people with severe venom allergy, stings may be life-threatening. Severe allergic reactions to insect stings can involve many body organs and may develop rapidly. This reaction is called anaphylaxis. Symptoms of anaphylaxis may include itching and hives over large areas of the body, swelling in the throat or tongue,

"Tips to Remember: Stinging Insect Allergy," © 1999 American Academy of Allergy, Asthma and Immunology; reprinted with permission. Available online at http://www.aaaai.org/patients/publicedmat/tips/stinginginsect.stm.

difficulty breathing, dizziness, stomach cramps, nausea, or diarrhea. In severe cases, a rapid fall in blood pressure may result in shock and loss of consciousness. Anaphylaxis is a medical emergency, and may be fatal. If you or anyone else experiences any of these symptoms after an insect sting, obtain emergency medical treatment immediately. After your symptoms are treated in the emergency room, you should also obtain referral to an allergist to learn about treatment options.

Identifying Stinging Insects

To avoid stinging insects, it's important to learn what they look like and where they live. Most sting reactions are caused by five types of insects: yellow jackets, honeybees, paper wasps, hornets, and fire ants.

Yellow jackets are black with yellow markings, and are found in various climates. Their nests, which are made of a papier-mâché material, are usually located underground, but can sometimes be found in the walls of frame buildings, cracks in masonry, or woodpiles.

Honeybees have a rounded, fuzzy body with dark brown coloring and yellow markings. Upon stinging, the honeybee usually leaves its barbed stinger in its victim; the bee dies as a result. Honeybees are nonaggressive and will only sting when provoked. However, Africanized honeybees, or so-called killer bees found in the southwestern United States and South and Central America, are more aggressive and may sting in swarms. Domesticated honeybees live in man-made hives, while wild honeybees live in colonies or honeycombs in hollow trees or cavities of buildings. Africanized honeybees may nest in holes in house frames, between fence posts, in old tires or holes in the ground, or other partially protected sites.

Paper wasps' slender, elongated bodies are black, brown, or red with yellow markings. Their nests are also made of a paper-like material that forms a circular comb of cells which opens downward. The nests are often located under eaves, behind shutters, or in shrubs or woodpiles.

Hornets are black or brown with white, orange, or yellow markings and are usually larger than yellow jackets. Their nests are gray or brown, football-shaped, and made of a paper material similar to that of yellow jackets' nests. Hornets' nests are usually found high above ground on branches of trees, in shrubbery, on gables or in tree hollows.

Fire ants are reddish brown stinging insects related to bees and wasps. Their prominent mounds, common in warmer climates, may measure up to three feet in diameter and 18 inches in height, and can contain up to 250,000 ants. Fire ants may attack with little warning: after firmly grasping the victim's skin with its jaws, the fire ant arches its back as it inserts its rear stinger into the skin. It then pivots at the head and typically inflicts about eight stings in a circular pattern. Fire ant venom has a high concentration of toxins, which cause burning pain.

Preventing Stings

Stay out of the territory of the stinging insects' nests. These insects are social and will sting if their homes are disturbed, so it is important to have hives and nests around your home destroyed. Since this activity can be dangerous, a trained exterminator should be hired.

If you encounter any flying stinging insects, remain calm and quiet, and move slowly. Many stinging insects are searching for nectar, so don't look or smell like a flower—avoid brightly colored clothing and perfume when outdoors. Because the smell of food attracts insects, be careful when cooking, eating, or drinking sweet drinks like soda or juice outdoors. Keep food covered until eaten. Wear closed-toe shoes outdoors and avoid going barefoot. Also, avoid loose-fitting garments that can trap insects between material and skin.

Treating Stings

If you are stung by a honeybee that has left its stinger (and attached venom sac) in your skin, remove the stinger within 30 seconds to avoid receiving more venom. A quick scrape of a fingernail removes the stinger and sac. Avoid squeezing the sac—this forces more venom through the stinger and into the skin. Hornets, wasps, and yellow jackets do not usually leave their stingers. Try to remain calm, and brush these insects from the skin promptly with deliberate movements to prevent additional stings. Then, quietly and immediately leave the area.

If you are stung by fire ants, carefully brush them off to prevent repeated stings, and leave the area. Fire ant stings cause a reaction in almost all their victims. An itchy, localized hive at the sting site forms and then usually subsides within 30 to 60 minutes. Within four hours, a small blister forms at the site of each sting; a sterile sore with pus forms in eight to 24 hours. This sore then ruptures and scars in

48 to 72 hours. Stings must be monitored for secondary bacterial infection. Diabetics and others with circulatory disorders, including varicose veins and phlebitis, can be particularly at risk for complications and should see a physician to monitor their condition after being stung. Up to 50% of patients develop large local reactions at the site of fire ant stings—swelling may last for several days and may be accompanied by itching, redness, and pain.

Taking the following steps can help in treating local reactions to insect stings:

- Elevate the affected arm or leg and apply ice or a cold compress to reduce swelling and pain.

- Gently clean blisters with soap and water to prevent secondary infections; do not break blisters.

- Use topical steroid ointments or oral antihistamines to relieve itching.

- See your doctor if swelling progresses or if the sting site seems infected.

If you are severely insect-allergic and have had prior reactions, try to avoid being outdoors alone in insect weather in case you require prompt emergency treatment. Carry an auto-injectable epinephrine (adrenalin) device, a short-term treatment for severe allergic reactions. Learn how to self-administer the epinephrine according to your allergist's instructions, and replace the device before the labeled expiration date.

Remember that injectable epinephrine is rescue medication only, and you must still have someone take you to an emergency room immediately if you are stung. Additional medical treatment may be necessary. Those with severe allergies may want to consider wearing a special bracelet or necklace that identifies the wearer as having severe allergies and supplies other important medical information.

Consulting Your Allergist

Anyone who has had a serious adverse reaction to an insect sting should be evaluated by an allergist, who will take a thorough history, perform an examination and recommend testing to determine whether you have an allergy, and which type of stinging insect caused the reaction. Skin or blood (RAST) testing for insect allergy is used to detect the presence of significant amounts of IgE antibody.

Your allergist will help you determine the best form of treatment. Those who have severe allergies to insect venom should consider receiving insect venom immunotherapy, a highly effective vaccination program that actually prevents future allergic sting reactions in 97% of treated patients. During immunotherapy, the allergist administers gradually stronger doses of venom extract every few weeks over a period of three to five years. This helps the patient's immune system to become more and more resistant to future insect stings.

If you have questions about venom immunotherapy or other treatments for stinging insect allergy, be sure to ask your allergist. Patients who receive appropriate treatment such as immunotherapy and who practice careful avoidance measures can participate in regular outdoor activities.

Chapter 80

Food Allergies

Chapter Contents

Section 80.1

Food Allergy and Food Intolerances

Excerpted from "Food Allergy and Intolerances," National Institute of Allergy and Infectious Diseases (NIAID), National Institutes of Health (NIH), http://www.niaid.nih.gov/factsheets/food.htm, June 2001.

Introduction

Food allergies or food intolerances affect nearly everyone at some point. People often have an unpleasant reaction to something they ate and wonder if they have a food allergy. One out of three people either say that they have a food allergy or that they modify the family diet because a family member is suspected of having a food allergy. But only about three percent of children have clinically proven allergic reactions to foods. In adults, the prevalence of food allergy drops to about one percent of the total population.

This difference between the clinically proven prevalence of food allergy and the public perception of the problem is in part due to reactions called "food intolerances" rather than food allergies. A food allergy, or hypersensitivity, is an abnormal response to a food that is triggered by the immune system. The immune system is not responsible for the symptoms of a food intolerance, even though these symptoms can resemble those of a food allergy.

It is extremely important for people who have true food allergies to identify them and prevent allergic reactions to food because these reactions can cause devastating illness and, in some cases, be fatal.

How Allergic Reactions Work

An allergic reaction involves two features of the human immune response. One is the production of immunoglobulin E (IgE), a type of protein called an antibody that circulates through the blood. The other is the mast cell, a specific cell that occurs in all body tissues but is especially common in areas of the body that are typical sites of allergic reactions, including the nose and throat, lungs, skin, and gastrointestinal tract.

The ability of a given individual to form IgE against something as benign as food is an inherited predisposition. Generally, such people come from families in which allergies are common not necessarily food allergies but perhaps hay fever, asthma, or hives. Someone with two allergic parents is more likely to develop food allergies than someone with one allergic parent.

Before an allergic reaction can occur, a person who is predisposed to form IgE to foods first has to be exposed to the food. As this food is digested, it triggers certain cells to produce specific IgE in large amounts. The IgE is then released and attaches to the surface of mast cells. The next time the person eats that food, it interacts with specific IgE on the surface of the mast cells and triggers the cells to release chemicals such as histamine. Depending upon the tissue in which they are released, these chemicals will cause a person to have various symptoms of food allergy. If the mast cells release chemicals in the ears, nose, and throat, a person may feel an itching in the mouth and may have trouble breathing or swallowing. If the affected mast cells are in the gastrointestinal tract, the person may have abdominal pain or diarrhea. The chemicals released by skin mast cells, in contrast, can prompt hives.

Food allergens (the food fragments responsible for an allergic reaction) are proteins within the food that usually are not broken down by the heat of cooking or by stomach acids or enzymes that digest food. As a result, they survive to cross the gastrointestinal lining, enter the bloodstream, and go to target organs, causing allergic reactions throughout the body.

The complex process of digestion affects the timing and the location of a reaction. If people are allergic to a particular food, for example, they may first experience itching in the mouth as they start to eat the food. After the food is digested in the stomach, abdominal symptoms such as vomiting, diarrhea, or pain may start. When the food allergens enter and travel through the bloodstream, they can cause a drop in blood pressure. As the allergens reach the skin, they can induce hives or eczema, or when they reach the lungs, they may cause asthma. All of this takes place within a few minutes to an hour.

Common Food Allergies

The most common food allergens that cause problems in children are eggs, milk, and peanuts. Adults usually do not lose their allergies, but children can sometimes outgrow them. Children are more likely to outgrow allergies to milk or soy than allergies to peanuts, fish, or shrimp.

The foods that adults or children react to are those foods they eat often. In Japan, for example, rice allergy is more frequent. In Scandinavia, codfish allergy is more common.

Cross Reactivity

If someone has a life-threatening reaction to a certain food, the doctor will counsel the patient to avoid similar foods that might trigger this reaction. For example, if someone has a history of allergy to shrimp, testing will usually show that the person is not only allergic to shrimp but also to crab, lobster, and crayfish as well. This is called cross-reactivity.

Another interesting example of cross-reactivity occurs in people who are highly sensitive to ragweed. During ragweed pollination season, these people sometimes find that when they try to eat melons, particularly cantaloupe, they have itching in their mouth and they simply cannot eat the melon. Similarly, people who have severe birch pollen allergy also may react to the peel of apples. This is called the "oral allergy syndrome."

Differential Diagnoses

A differential diagnosis means distinguishing food allergy from food intolerance or other illnesses. If a patient goes to the doctor's office and says, "I think I have a food allergy," the doctor has to consider the list of other possibilities that may lead to symptoms that could be confused with food allergy.

One possibility is the contamination of foods with microorganisms, such as bacteria, and their products, such as toxins. Contaminated meat sometimes mimics a food reaction when it is really a type of food poisoning.

There are also natural substances, such as histamine, that can occur in foods and stimulate a reaction similar to an allergic reaction. For example, histamine can reach high levels in cheese, some wines, and in certain kinds of fish, particularly tuna and mackerel. In fish, histamine is believed to stem from bacterial contamination, particularly in fish that hasn't been refrigerated properly. If someone eats one of these foods with a high level of histamine, that person may have a reaction that strongly resembles an allergic reaction to food. This reaction is called histamine toxicity.

Another cause of food intolerance that is often confused with a food allergy is lactase deficiency. This most common food intolerance affects at least one out of ten people. Lactase is an enzyme that is in the lining of the gut. This enzyme degrades lactose, which is in milk. If a person does not have enough lactase, the body cannot digest the lactose in most milk products. Instead, the lactose is used by bacteria, gas is formed, and the person experiences bloating, abdominal pain, and sometimes diarrhea. There are a couple of diagnostic tests in which the patient ingests a specific amount of lactose and then the doctor measures the body's response by analyzing a blood sample.

Another type of food intolerance is an adverse reaction to certain products that are added to food to enhance taste, provide color, or protect against the growth of microorganisms. Compounds that are most frequently tied to adverse reactions that can be confused with food allergy are yellow dye number 5, monosodium glutamate, and sulfites. Yellow dye number 5 can cause hives, although rarely. Monosodium glutamate (MSG) is a flavor enhancer, and, when consumed in large amounts, can cause flushing, sensations of warmth, headache, facial pressure, chest pain, or feelings of detachment in some people. These transient reactions occur rapidly after eating large amounts of food to which MSG has been added.

Sulfites can occur naturally in foods or are added to enhance crispness or prevent mold growth. Sulfites in high concentrations sometimes pose problems for people with severe asthma. Sulfites can give off a gas called sulfur dioxide, which the asthmatic inhales while eating the sulfited food. This irritates the lungs and can send an asthmatic into severe bronchospasm, a constriction of the lungs. Such reactions led the U.S. Food and Drug Administration (FDA) to ban sulfites as spray-on preservatives in fresh fruits and vegetables. But they are still used in some foods and are made naturally during the fermentation of wine, for example.

There are several other diseases that share symptoms with food allergies including ulcers and cancers of the gastrointestinal tract. These disorders can be associated with vomiting, diarrhea, or cramping abdominal pain exacerbated by eating.

Gluten intolerance is associated with the disease called gluten-sensitive enteropathy or celiac disease. It is caused by an abnormal immune response to gluten, which is a component of wheat and some other grains.

Some people may have a food intolerance that has a psychological trigger. In selected cases, a careful psychiatric evaluation may identify an unpleasant event in that person's life, often during childhood, tied to eating a particular food. The eating of that food years later, even as an adult, is associated with a rush of unpleasant sensations that can resemble an allergic reaction to food.

Diagnosis

To diagnose food allergy a doctor must first determine if the patient is having an adverse reaction to specific foods. This assessment is made with the help of a detailed patient history, the patient's diet diary, or an elimination diet.

The first of these techniques is the most valuable. The physician sits down with the person or parent of a child suspected of having a food allergy and takes a history to determine if the facts are consistent with a food allergy. The doctor asks such questions as:

- What was the timing of the reaction? Did the reaction come on quickly, usually within an hour after eating the food?

- Was allergy treatment successful? (Antihistamines should relieve hives, for example, if they stem from a food allergy.)

- Is the reaction always associated with a certain food?

- Did anyone else get sick? For example, if the person has eaten fish contaminated with histamine, everyone who ate the fish should be sick. In an allergic reaction, however, only the person allergic to the fish becomes ill.

- How much did the patient eat before experiencing a reaction? The severity of the patient's reaction is sometimes related to the amount of food the patient ate.

- How was the food prepared? Some people will have a violent allergic reaction only to raw or undercooked fish. Complete cooking of the fish destroys those allergens in the fish to which they react. If the fish is cooked thoroughly, they can eat it with no allergic reaction.

- Were other foods ingested at the same time of the allergic reaction? Some foods may delay digestion and thus delay the onset of the allergic reaction.

Sometimes a diagnosis cannot be made solely on the basis of history. In that case, the doctor may ask the patient or the patient's parent to go back and keep a record of the contents of each meal and whether he or she had a reaction. This gives more detail from which the doctor and the patient can determine if there is consistency in the reactions.

The next step some doctors use is an elimination diet. Under the doctor's direction, the patient does not eat a food suspected of causing the allergy, like eggs, and substitutes another food, in this case, another source of protein. If the patient removes the food and the symptoms go away, the doctor can almost always make a diagnosis. If the patient then eats the food (under the doctor's direction) and the symptoms come back, then the diagnosis is confirmed. This technique cannot be used, however, if the reactions are severe (in which case the patient should not resume eating the food) or infrequent.

If the patient's history, diet diary, or elimination diet suggests a specific food allergy is likely, the doctor will then use tests that can more objectively measure an allergic response to food. One of these is a scratch skin test, during which a dilute extract of the food is placed on the skin of the forearm or back. This portion of the skin is then scratched with a needle and observed for swelling or redness that would indicate a local allergic reaction. If the scratch test is positive, the patient has IgE on the skin's mast cells that is specific to the food being tested.

Skin tests are rapid, simple, and relatively safe. But a patient can have a positive skin test to a food allergen without experiencing allergic reactions to that food. A doctor diagnoses a food allergy only when a patient has a positive skin test to a specific allergen and the history of these reactions suggests an allergy to the same food.

In some extremely allergic patients who have severe anaphylactic reactions, skin testing cannot be used because it could evoke a dangerous reaction. Skin testing also cannot be done on patients with extensive eczema.

For these patients a doctor may use blood tests that measure the presence of food-specific IgE in the blood of patients. These tests may cost more than skin tests, and results are not available immediately. As with skin testing, positive tests do not necessarily make the diagnosis.

The final method used to objectively diagnose food allergy is double-blind food challenge. This testing has come to be the "gold standard" of allergy testing. Various foods, some of which are suspected of inducing an allergic reaction, are each placed in individual opaque capsules. The patient is asked to swallow a capsule and is then watched to see if a reaction occurs. This process is repeated until all the capsules have been swallowed. In a true double-blind test, the doctor is also "blinded" (the capsules having been made up by some other medical person) so that neither the patient nor the doctor knows which capsule contains the allergen.

The advantage of such a challenge is that if the patient has a reaction only to suspected foods and not to other foods tested, it confirms the diagnosis. Someone with a history of severe reactions, however, cannot be tested this way. In addition, this testing is expensive because it takes a lot of time to perform and multiple food allergies are difficult to evaluate with this procedure.

Consequently, double-blind food challenges are done infrequently. This type of testing is most commonly used when the doctor believes that the reaction a person is describing is not due to a specific food and the doctor wishes to obtain evidence to support this judgment so that additional efforts may be directed at finding the real cause of the reaction.

Exercise-Induced Food Allergy

At least one situation may require more than the simple ingestion of a food allergen to provoke a reaction: exercise-induced food allergy. People who experience this reaction eat a specific food before exercising. As they exercise and their body temperature goes up, they begin to itch, get light-headed, and soon have allergic reactions such as hives or even anaphylaxis. The cure for exercised-induced food allergy is simple—not eating for a couple of hours before exercising.

Treatment

Food allergy is treated by dietary avoidance. Once a patient and the patient's doctor have identified the food to which the patient is sensitive, the food must be removed from the patient's diet. To do this, patients or parents must read lengthy, detailed ingredient lists on each food they are considering eating. Many allergy-producing foods such as peanuts, eggs, and milk, appear in foods one normally would not associate them with. Peanuts, for example, are often used as a protein source and eggs are used in some salad dressings. The FDA requires ingredients in a food to appear on its label. People can avoid most of the things to which they are sensitive if they read food labels carefully and avoid restaurant-prepared foods that might have ingredients to which they are allergic.

In highly allergic people even minuscule amounts of a food allergen (for example, 1/44,000 of a peanut kernel) can prompt an allergic reaction. Other less sensitive people may be able to tolerate small amounts of a food to which they are allergic.

Patients with severe food allergies must be prepared to treat an inadvertent exposure. Even people who know a lot about what they are sensitive to occasionally make a mistake. To protect themselves, people who have had anaphylactic reactions to a food should wear medical alert bracelets or necklaces stating that they have a food allergy and that they are subject to severe reactions. Such people should always carry a syringe of adrenaline (epinephrine), obtained by prescription from their doctors, and be prepared to self-administer it if they think they are getting a food allergic reaction. They should then immediately seek medical help by either calling the rescue squad or by having themselves transported to an emergency room. Anaphylactic allergic reactions can be fatal even when they start off with mild symptoms such as a tingling in the mouth and throat or gastrointestinal discomfort.

Special precautions are warranted with children. Parents and caregivers must know how to protect children from foods to which the children are allergic and how to manage the children if they consume a food to which they are allergic, including the administration of epinephrine. Schools must have plans in place to address any emergency.

There are several medications that a patient can take to relieve food allergy symptoms that are not part of an anaphylactic reaction. These include antihistamines to relieve gastrointestinal symptoms, hives, or sneezing and a runny nose. Bronchodilators can relieve asthma symptoms. These medications are taken after people have inadvertently ingested a food to which they are allergic but are not effective in preventing an allergic reaction when taken prior to eating the food. No medication in any form can be taken before eating a certain food that will reliably prevent an allergic reaction to that food.

There are a few non-approved treatments for food allergies. One involves injections containing small quantities of the food extracts to which the patient is allergic. These shots are given on a regular basis for a long period of time with the aim of "desensitizing" the patient to the food allergen. Researchers have not yet proven that allergy shots relieve food allergies.

Infants and Children

Milk and soy allergies are particularly common in infants and young children. These allergies sometimes do not involve hives and asthma, but rather lead to colic, and perhaps blood in the stool or poor growth. Infants and children are thought to be particularly susceptible to this allergic syndrome because of the immaturity of their immune and digestive systems. Milk or soy allergies in infants can develop within days to months of birth. Sometimes there is a family history of allergies or feeding problems. The clinical picture is one of a very unhappy colicky child who may not sleep well at night. The doctor diagnoses food allergy partly by changing the child's diet. Rarely, food challenge is used.

If the baby is on cow's milk, the doctor may suggest a change to soy formula or exclusive breast milk, if possible. If soy formula causes an allergic reaction, the baby may be placed on an elemental formula. These formulas are processed proteins (basically sugars and amino acids). There are few if any allergens within these materials. The doctor will sometimes prescribe corticosteroids to treat infants with severe food allergies. Fortunately, time usually heals this particular gastrointestinal disease. It tends to resolve within the first few years of life.

Exclusive breast feeding (excluding all other foods) of infants for the first 6 to 12 months of life is often suggested to avoid milk or soy allergies from developing within that time frame. Such breast feeding often allows parents to avoid infant-feeding problems, especially if the parents are allergic (and the infant therefore is likely to be allergic). There are some children who are so sensitive to a certain food, however, that if the food is eaten by the mother, sufficient quantities enter the breast milk to cause a food reaction in the child. Mothers sometimes must themselves avoid eating those foods to which the baby is allergic.

There is no conclusive evidence that breast feeding prevents the development of allergies later in life. It does, however, delay the onset of food allergies by delaying the infant's exposure to those foods that can prompt allergies, and it may avoid altogether those feeding problems seen in infants. By delaying the introduction of solid foods until the infant is 6 months old or older, parents can also prolong the child's allergy-free period.

Controversial Issues

Some people believe hyperactivity in children is caused by food allergies. But researchers have found that this behavioral disorder in children is only occasionally associated with food additives, and then only when such additives are consumed in large amounts. There is no evidence that a true food allergy can affect a child's activity except for the proviso that if a child itches and sneezes and wheezes a lot, the child may be miserable and therefore more difficult to guide. Also, children who are on antiallergy medicines that can cause drowsiness may get sleepy in school or at home.

Section 80.2

Lactose Intolerance

Excerpted from "Lactose Intolerance," National Institute of Diabetes and Digestive and Kidney Diseases (NIDDK), NIH Pub. No. 02-2751, May 2002. Available online at http://www.niddk.nih.gov/health/digest/pubs/lactose/lactose.htm.

What Is Lactose Intolerance?

Lactose intolerance is the inability to digest significant amounts of lactose, the predominant sugar of milk. This inability results from a shortage of the enzyme lactase, which is normally produced by the cells that line the small intestine. Lactase breaks down milk sugar into simpler forms that can then be absorbed into the bloodstream. When there is not enough lactase to digest the amount of lactose consumed, the results, although not usually dangerous, may be very distressing. While not all persons deficient in lactase have symptoms, those who do are considered to be lactose intolerant.

Common symptoms include nausea, cramps, bloating, gas, and diarrhea, which begin about 30 minutes to 2 hours after eating or drinking foods containing lactose. The severity of symptoms varies depending on the amount of lactose each individual can tolerate.

Some causes of lactose intolerance are well known. For instance, certain digestive diseases and injuries to the small intestine can reduce the amount of enzymes produced. In rare cases, children are born without the ability to produce lactase. For most people, though, lactase deficiency is a condition that develops naturally over time. After about the age of 2 years, the body begins to produce less lactase. However, many people may not experience symptoms until they are much older.

Between 30 and 50 million Americans are lactose intolerant. Certain ethnic and racial populations are more widely affected than others. As many as 75 percent of all African Americans and American Indians, and 90 percent of Asian Americans are lactose intolerant. The condition is least common among persons of northern European descent.

557

How Is Lactose Intolerance Diagnosed?

The most common tests used to measure the absorption of lactose in the digestive system are the lactose tolerance test, the hydrogen breath test, and the stool acidity test. These tests are performed on an outpatient basis at a hospital, clinic, or doctor's office.

The lactose tolerance test begins with the individual fasting (not eating) before the test and then drinking a liquid that contains lactose. Several blood samples are taken over a 2-hour period to measure the person's blood glucose (blood sugar) level, which indicates how well the body is able to digest lactose.

Normally, when lactose reaches the digestive system, the lactase enzyme breaks down lactose into glucose and galactose. The liver then changes the galactose into glucose, which enters the bloodstream and raises the person's blood glucose level. If lactose is incompletely broken down, the blood glucose level does not rise and a diagnosis of lactose intolerance is confirmed.

The hydrogen breath test measures the amount of hydrogen in the breath. Normally, very little hydrogen is detectable in the breath. However, undigested lactose in the colon is fermented by bacteria, and various gases, including hydrogen, are produced. The hydrogen is absorbed from the intestines, carried through the bloodstream to the lungs, and exhaled. In the test, the patient drinks a lactose-loaded beverage, and the breath is analyzed at regular intervals. Raised levels of hydrogen in the breath indicate improper digestion of lactose. Certain foods, medications, and cigarettes can affect the test's accuracy and should be avoided before taking the test. This test is available for children and adults.

The lactose tolerance and hydrogen breath tests are not given to infants and very young children who are suspected of having lactose intolerance. A large lactose load may be dangerous for very young individuals because they are more prone to dehydration that can result from diarrhea caused by the lactose. If a baby or young child is experiencing symptoms of lactose intolerance, many pediatricians simply recommend changing from cow's milk to soy formula and waiting for symptoms to abate.

If necessary, a stool acidity test, which measures the amount of acid in the stool, may be given to infants and young children. Undigested lactose fermented by bacteria in the colon creates lactic acid and other short-chain fatty acids that can be detected in a stool sample. In addition, glucose may be present in the sample as a result of unabsorbed lactose in the colon.

How Is Lactose Intolerance Treated?

Fortunately, lactose intolerance is relatively easy to treat. No treatment exists to improve the body's ability to produce lactase, but symptoms can be controlled through diet.

Young children with lactase deficiency should not eat any foods containing lactose. Most older children and adults need not avoid lactose completely, but individuals differ in the amounts and types of foods they can handle. For example, one person may suffer symptoms after drinking a small glass of milk, while another can drink one glass but not two. Others may be able to manage ice cream and aged cheeses, such as cheddar and Swiss, but not other dairy products. Dietary control of lactose intolerance depends on each person's learning through trial and error how much lactose he or she can handle.

For those who react to very small amounts of lactose or have trouble limiting their intake of foods that contain lactose, lactase enzymes are available without a prescription. Lactase enzyme tablets are available to help people digest foods that contain lactose. The tablets are taken with the first bite of dairy food. Lactase enzyme is also available as a liquid. Adding a few drops of the enzyme will convert the lactose in milk or cream, making it more digestible for people with lactose intolerance.

Lactose-reduced milk and other products are available at most supermarkets. The milk contains all of the nutrients found in regular milk and remains fresh for about the same length of time, or longer if it is super-pasteurized.

How Is Nutrition Balanced?

Milk and other dairy products are a major source of nutrients in the American diet. The most important of these nutrients is calcium. Calcium is essential for the growth and repair of bones throughout life. In the middle and later years, a shortage of calcium may lead to thin, fragile bones that break easily, a condition called osteoporosis. A concern, then, for both children and adults with lactose intolerance, is getting enough calcium in a diet that includes little or no milk.

In 1997, the Institute of Medicine released a report recommending new requirements for daily calcium intake. How much calcium a person needs to maintain good health varies by age group. Recommendations from the report are listed in Table 80.1.

Table 80.1. Requirements for daily calcium intake.

Age group	Amount of calcium to consume daily in milligrams (mg)
0–6 months	210 mg
6–12 months	270 mg
1–3 years	500 mg
4–8 years	800 mg
9–18 years	1,300 mg
19–50 years	1,000 mg
51–70+ years	1,200 mg
Pregnant and nursing women under 19	1,300 mg
Pregnant and nursing women over 19	1,000 mg

In planning meals, making sure that each day's diet includes enough calcium is important, even if the diet does not contain dairy products. Many nondairy foods are high in calcium. Green vegetables, such as broccoli and kale, and fish with soft, edible bones, such as salmon and sardines, are excellent sources of calcium. To help in planning a high-calcium and low-lactose diet, the following chart lists some common foods that are good sources of dietary calcium and shows about how much lactose the foods contain.

Recent research shows that yogurt with active cultures may be a good source of calcium for many people with lactose intolerance, even though it is fairly high in lactose. Evidence shows that the bacterial cultures used in making yogurt produce some of the lactase enzyme required for proper digestion.

Many foods can provide the calcium and other nutrients the body needs, even when intake of milk and dairy products is limited. However, factors other than calcium and lactose content should be kept in mind when planning a diet. Some vegetables that are high in calcium (Swiss chard, spinach, and rhubarb, for instance) are not good sources of calcium because the body cannot use their calcium content. They contain substances called oxalates, which stop calcium absorption. Calcium is absorbed and used only when there is enough vitamin D in the body. A balanced diet should provide an adequate supply of vitamin D. Sources of vitamin D include eggs and liver. However,

Table 80.2. Calcium and lactose in common foods. Adapted from *Manual of Clinical Dietetics*. 6th ed. American Dietetic Association, 2000; and "Soy Dairy Alternatives." Available at: www.soyfoods.org. Accessed March 5, 2002.

	Calcium Content	Lactose Content
Calcium-fortified orange juice, 1 cup	308–344 mg	0
Sardines, with edible bones, 3 oz.	270 mg	0
Soymilk, fortified, 1 cup	200 mg	0
Salmon, canned, with edible bones, 3 oz.	205 mg	0
Broccoli (raw), 1 cup	90 mg	0
Pinto beans, ½ cup	40 mg	0
Orange, 1 medium	50 mg	0
Tuna, canned, 3 oz.	10 mg	0
Lettuce greens, ½ cup	10 mg	0
Dairy Products		
Yogurt, plain, low-fat, 1 cup	415 mg	5 g
Milk, reduced fat, 1 cup	295 mg	11 g
Swiss cheese, 1 oz.	270 mg	1 g
Ice cream, ½ cup	85 mg	6 g
Cottage cheese, ½ cup	75 mg	2–3 g

sunlight helps the body naturally absorb or synthesize vitamin D, and with enough exposure to the sun, food sources may not be necessary.

Some people with lactose intolerance may think they are not getting enough calcium and vitamin D in their diet. Consultation with a doctor or dietitian may be helpful in deciding whether any dietary supplements are needed. Taking vitamins or minerals of the wrong kind or in the wrong amounts can be harmful. A dietitian can help in planning meals that will provide the most nutrients with the least chance of causing discomfort.

What Is Hidden Lactose?

Although milk and foods made from milk are the only natural sources, lactose is often added to prepared foods. People with very low tolerance for lactose should know about the many food products that may contain lactose, even in small amounts. Food products that may contain lactose include

- bread and other baked goods
- processed breakfast cereals
- instant potatoes, soups, and breakfast drinks
- margarine
- lunch meats (other than kosher)
- salad dressings
- candies and other snacks
- mixes for pancakes, biscuits, and cookies

Some products labeled nondairy, such as powdered coffee creamer and whipped toppings, may also include ingredients that are derived from milk and therefore contain lactose.

Smart shoppers learn to read food labels with care, looking not only for milk and lactose among the contents but also for such words as whey, curds, milk by-products, dry milk solids, and nonfat dry milk powder. If any of these are listed on a label, the product contains lactose.

In addition, lactose is used as the base for more than 20 percent of prescription drugs and about 6 percent of over-the-counter medicines. Many types of birth control pills, for example, contain lactose, as do some tablets for stomach acid and gas. However, these products typically affect only people with severe lactose intolerance.

Summary

Even though lactose intolerance is widespread, it need not pose a serious threat to good health. People who have trouble digesting lactose can learn which dairy products and other foods they can eat without discomfort and which ones they should avoid. Many will be able to enjoy milk, ice cream, and other such products if they take them in small amounts or eat other food at the same time. Others can use lactase liquid or tablets to help digest the lactose. Even older women at risk for osteoporosis and growing children who must avoid milk and foods made with milk can meet most of their special dietary needs by eating greens, fish, and other calcium-rich foods that are free of lactose. A carefully chosen diet, with calcium supplements if the doctor or dietitian recommends them, is the key to reducing symptoms and protecting future health.

Section 80.3

Peanut Allergy: What You Need to Know

This information is reprinted from "Peanut Allergy in a Nutshell," produced by Public Health Dietitian/Nutritionists in Ontario, 1996, and distributed by the Community Health Services Department of the County of Lambton, Ontario, Canada. Updated in September 2002 by Dr. David A. Cooke, MD, Diplomate, American Board of Internal Medicine.

So your child is allergic to peanuts... You are not alone.

Peanut allergies have always been a common food allergy. In recent years, allergists have noted an increase in the number of people with allergies to peanuts.

Can Peanut Allergy Be Prevented?

No one knows exactly causes a given child to develop peanut allergy. There doesn't appear to be any single cause.

Genetic factors do seem to play a role. If a child has relatives with peanut allergy, there is a greater chance that he/she will have peanut allergy, too. Still, the chances for any given child developing the allergy are still quite small.

Exposure to nuts at a young age may also be an issue. Some experts recommend that pregnant and nursing mothers do not eat peanuts, and that children not be exposed to peanuts until at least three years of age. No one knows whether this can prevent development of the peanut allergy, however.

There is nothing that a parent can do wrong that will cause their child to develop peanut allergy. While certain precautions sometimes make sense, don't blame yourself if you child has peanut allergy. It probably would have happened, no matter what you did differently.

Is There a Cure for Peanut Allergy?

No. The only treatment is to avoid all products containing the peanut allergen.

Here are some tips to help when shopping...

- Read lists of ingredients every time you shop. Ingredients often change without warning—a product that was safe last week may not be safe this week.

- Words on a list of ingredients that could indicate the presence of peanut protein include: peanuts, mixed nuts, ground nuts, man-delonas, peanut butter, peanut oil, goober nuts, goober peas, beer nuts and peanut flour, artificial nuts, hydrolyzed peanut protein.

- Foods that may contain peanuts include: cookies, chocolate bars, chili, egg rolls, Thai dishes, Satay sauces, prepared soup (espe-cially dried packaged soup mixes), prepared and frozen desserts, hydrogenated oil, candy, baked goods, Chinese food, potato chips, fried foods, salad dressings, macaroons, icing paste, almond paste, vegetable burgers, vegetable oil, vegetable shortening, lard, margarine, chocolate from Europe and canned sardines

- Generally, the less processed a food, the less likely it is to con-tain peanut protein.

- Highly processed foods with many ingredients are more likely to have had peanut added to them.

- Avoid imported foods with foreign language ingredient lists. If you do not know what an ingredient word means, don't buy the food.

- Have a pad and pen with you when you shop. If you have a question about a product, write down the product name and the manufacturer's phone number or address. Contact the manufac-turer when you get home. Be direct. State that you have a food allergy, and need to know whether the product contains peanut protein.

- Avoid bulk bins. The scoop you use in the flour may have just come from the peanut bin.

- Beware of new nut products. New nut products contain peanuts that are deflavored, reflavored, pressed and sold as almonds, walnuts and other nuts.

Eating out

Always ask about the ingredients and the way food is prepared before you order. Even if the restaurant is part of a chain, there can be differences between restaurants. Ask. It is recommended that people with an allergy call a restaurant between meal hours and discuss the allergy with the chef.

Restaurants bearing an Allergy Aware sticker will have a senior staff member on each shift who can answer your questions about ingredients.

- Order simply prepared foods. Foods like baked potatoes, steamed vegetables, and broiled meat are less likely to create problems. Avoid added sauces and flavorings.

- Avoid buffets and salad bars. Often, persons will use the same spoon in different dishes.

- Asian, Thai, and African foods often contain peanuts. So do muffins and desserts.

- Peanut butter is sometimes used as a thickener, or even to hide a burnt taste in spaghetti sauce, chili or gravy. Peanuts may be used in pie crusts.

- Ask what oil is used. Most good Italian restaurants use olive oil but this should be checked out. Fondues and stir fries often use peanut oil because of its high smoking point.

Today, many fast food restaurants will have pamphlets with ingredient listings on request.

Will My Child Outgrow This Allergy?

It's possible. About one in five children will eventually outgrow peanut allergies. However, most do not. It is difficult to predict which children will outgrow this allergy. An allergy specialist may be able to perform tests to determine when it might be safe to try peanuts again. Because reactions can be so serious, *never* let a child with a history of peanut allergy eat peanuts except under direct medical supervision.

Peanut Oil May or May Not Be Safe

Usually, the process used to make commercial cooking oils gets rid of the protein present. Since it is the protein part of the peanut that causes allergic reaction, peanut oil treated in this way may be safe.

There are some exceptions, however. A different method is used in making cold pressed, expelled, or extruded peanut oils. These oils may contain peanut protein and are not safe. To be cautious, avoid peanut oil.

As well, safe oils may become unsafe when they have been used to fry a variety of foods which contain the peanut protein. In cooking, protein from peanut containing foods may leach out into the oil, making it unsafe.

Most allergic reactions are due to cross contamination. Safe foods become unsafe through contact with peanut. For example, a chopping board used to chop peanuts may later be used to chop onion; or a sandwich bag holding a peanut butter sandwich may later be used to hold a salmon sandwich. The onion and the salmon sandwich may both be contaminated with peanuts.

Buying soft ice cream can be tricky. If a previous customer had nuts on their ice cream, some could get stuck in the machine, and end up in your ice cream. Or, the same scoop that was used in a peanut-containing ice cream could be used in your ice cream.

Section 80.4

It's Probably Not a Food Allergy after All

Excerpted from "It's Probably Not a Food Allergy after All," April 1995, Pg. 13–15. From *Tufts University Diet & Nutrition Letter*, by Gershoff, Stanley N. Copyright 1995 by *Tufts Univ. Health & Nutrition Letter*. Reproduced with permission via Copyright Clearance Center. Reviewed in February 2001 by Dr. David A. Cooke, MD, Diplomate, American Board of Internal Medicine.

Introduction

The most common food allergies in children are milk, eggs, shellfish and nuts, but these allergies affect 1% of children. The diagnosis of an allergy should be made by a skin prick test done by a pediatric allergist because removing foods from the diet can cause health and development problems.

An Extreme Case

In trying to protect her, the girl's mother was literally starving her. Three months shy of her third birthday, the child had not yet reached three feet in height, and she weighed just 21 pounds—more or less the weight of the average nine-month-old. The reason?

When she was still an infant, she experienced some vomiting, which her mother attributed to food allergies. And in a well-meaning effort gone way out of control, the woman went on to remove more than 10 foods from her daughter's diet: beef, eggs, corn, chicken, soy, fish, chocolate, wheat, peanuts, white potatoes, fruits, and all fruit juices except for apple. It turns out the child wasn't allergic to any of them.

The case is an extreme one, but not as rare as you might think. Consider that out of 184 children evaluated in a national program, 11 had parents who removed an average of eight foods from their diets to "take care of" allergies. As a result, they experienced severely low rates of growth and weight gain, putting them at risk for brain damage and other developmental complications.

The irony here is that only two of the children, all of whom were under three years old, actually had any allergies to food. It's not surprising from a scientific perspective. While the common belief is that food allergies afflict large numbers of youngsters, the true figure is on the order of one in 100. And even then, it tends to be only one or two foods to which the child is allergic, not eight or more. The most common culprits: milk, eggs, shellfish, and nuts.

Still, "pediatricians say to us all the time that they have parents who unnecessarily remove foods from their children's diets because of false beliefs about food allergies," comments Thomas Roesler, M.D., a child psychiatrist at the National Jewish Center for Immunology and Respiratory Medicine in Denver, where the youngsters were evaluated. "Perhaps the children they're talking about didn't have their weight gain and growth rates slowed as much as those we examined," Dr. Roesler adds. "But there can be long-term complications even for a child with a milder decrease in his rate of development." Indeed, in a national survey of youngsters five to 11 years old in Great Britain, children seen by their parents as "food intolerant" were more than half an inch shorter than others; the more foods excluded from a child's diet, the shorter he or she was.

Mixed Signals at the Pediatrician's Office

Unfortunately, a pediatrician might unwittingly get sucked into a faulty belief system about food allergies in which a parent has become "stuck," says Dr. Roesler. "A mother or father may tell the child's doctor, 'Every time I give my kid tomatoes, he gets hives.' The pediatrician hasn't seen the hives, but he tells the parent to stop feeding the youngster tomatoes." From there, Dr. Roesler says, the parent might take it upon him or herself to remove more foods as he or she sees fit.

But a more collaborative approach with the pediatrician is called for, Dr. Roesler advises. For instance, if the parent describes only mild symptoms, the doctor may recommend taking the food out of the child's diet for three months and then feeding it again in his or her presence. That's because many symptoms of food allergies—runny nose, itchy skin rash, diarrhea, vomiting—are common to all kinds of childhood illnesses and usually have nothing to do with a particular food, which a little time usually makes clear.

In those rare cases that a food is indeed responsible for any unpleasant symptoms, it's usually worth reintroducing it to the diet after a time because studies show some 90 percent of symptoms commonly associated with food allergies disappear by age three. "Oftentimes after just three months," Dr. Roesler says, "the child will not react again."

Of course, if a parent tells a physician that a child suffered, say, breathing difficulties after eating a particular food, or has reactions to many different foods rather than just one, the pediatrician may feel a referral to a pediatric allergist is in order. Such an allergist, certified by the American Board of Allergy and Immunology, will take a detailed medical and diet history as well as conduct a skin-prick test. But even if the skin-prick test is positive, more tests may be necessary. That's because in nine out of 10 cases in which a child's skin reacts to a particular food, it won't be dangerous inside his body. Some small children, for instance, get a perfectly harmless redness on the skin around their lips when they eat tomatoes or oranges. More conclusive tests than skin pricks include feeding the food in the allergist's presence and having him or her examine the child for any untoward side effects.

Chapter 81

Drug Allergies

In general, adverse reactions to drugs are not uncommon, and almost any drug can cause an adverse reaction. Reactions range from irritating or mild side effects (such as nausea and vomiting), to allergic response including life-threatening anaphylaxis. Some drug reactions are idiosyncratic (unusual effects of the medication). For example, aspirin can cause non-allergic hives (no antibodies formed), or it may trigger asthma. Only a small proportion of these reactions are allergic in nature. Many individuals may confuse an uncomfortable but not serious side effect of a medicine, such as nausea, with a drug allergy, which can be life-threatening.

True drug allergies occur when there is an allergic reaction to a medication. This is caused by hypersensitivity of the immune system, leading to a misdirected response against a substance that does not cause a response in most people. The body becomes sensitized (the immune system is triggered) by the first exposure to the medication. The second or subsequent exposure causes an immune response, including the production of antibodies and release of histamine.

Most drug allergies cause minor skin rashes and hives. However, other symptoms occasionally develop and life-threatening acute allergic reaction involving the whole body (anaphylaxis) can occur. Serum sickness is a delayed type of drug allergy that occurs a week or more after exposure to a medication or vaccine.

Penicillin and related antibiotics are the most common cause of drug allergies. Other common allergy-causing drugs include sulfa drugs, barbiturates, anticonvulsants, insulin preparations (particularly animal sources of insulin), local anesthetics such as Novocain, and iodine (found in many X-ray contrast dyes).

Prevention

There is no known way to prevent development of a drug allergy. In people who have a known drug allergy, avoiding the medication is the best means to prevent an allergic reaction. In some cases, the medication may be given safely after pre-treatment with corticosteroids (such as prednisone) and antihistamines (such as diphenhydramine).

Symptoms

- hives (common)
- skin rash (common)
- itching of the skin or eyes (common)
- wheezing
- swelling of the lips, tongue, and/or face
- anaphylaxis, or severe allergic reaction (see below)

Symptoms of anaphylaxis include:

- difficulty breathing with wheeze or hoarse voice
- hives over different parts of the body
- fainting, light-headedness
- dizziness
- confusion
- rapid pulse
- sensation of feeling the heart beat (palpitations)
- nausea, vomiting
- diarrhea
- abdominal pain or cramping

Signs and Tests

An examination of the skin and face may show hives, rash, or angioedema (swelling of the lips, face, and/or tongue). Decreased blood pressure, wheezing, and other signs may indicate an anaphylactic reaction.

Skin testing may confirm allergy to penicillin-type medications. Testing may be ineffective (or in some cases, dangerous) for other medications. A history of allergic-type reaction after use of a medication is often considered adequately diagnostic for drug allergy. (No further testing is required to demonstrate the allergy.) The same applies to other substances that are not considered drugs but are used in hospitals, such as X-ray contrast dyes.

Treatment

The treatment goal is relief of symptoms and prevent consequences of a severe reaction, if present.

Antihistamines usually relieve mild symptoms (rash, hives, itching). Topical (applied to a localized area of the skin) corticosteroids may also be recommended. Bronchodilators such as albuterol may be prescribed to reduce asthma-like symptoms (moderate wheezing or cough). Epinephrine by injection may be necessary to treat anaphylaxis.

The offending medication should be avoided. Health care providers (including dentists, hospital personnel, etc.) should be advised of drug allergies before treating the allergic patient. Identifying jewelry or cards (such as Medic-Alert or others) may be advised.

Occasionally a penicillin allergy responds to desensitization (immunotherapy) in which increasing doses (each dose of the drug is slightly larger than the previous dose) are given to improve tolerance of the drug.

Prognosis

Most drug allergies respond readily to treatment. A few cases cause severe asthma or anaphylaxis.

Complications

- discomfort
- asthma
- anaphylaxis (life-threatening)

Call your health care provider if you are taking a medication and develop symptoms indicating drug allergy.

Go to the emergency room or call the local emergency number (such as 911) if you have difficulty breathing or develop other symptoms of severe asthma or anaphylaxis (see above); these are emergency conditions!

Part Nine

Additional Help
and Information

Chapter 82

Glossary of Terms Related to Childhood Diseases

acetaminophen: An antipyretic (a drug that reduces fevers) and analgesic (pain reliever), with potency similar to aspirin.

allergic salute: A characteristic wiping or rubbing of the nose with a transverse or upward movement of the hand, as seen in children with allergic rhinitis.

antibiotic: A soluble substance derived from a mold or bacterium that inhibits the growth of other microorganisms.

autism: A mental disorder characterized by severely abnormal development of social interaction and verbal and nonverbal communication skills. Affected individuals may adhere to inflexible, nonfunctional rituals or routine. They may become upset with even trivial changes in their environment. They often have a limited range of interests but may become preoccupied with a narrow range of subjects or activities. They appear unable to understand others' feelings and often have poor eye contact with others. Unpredictable mood swings may occur. Many demonstrate stereotypical motor mannerisms such as hand or finger flapping, body rocking, or dipping. The disorder is probably caused by organically based central nervous system dysfunction, especially in the ability to process social or emotional information or language.

---

bacterium (plural, bacteria): A microorganism that usually multiplies by cell division and has a cell wall that provides a constancy of form.

Candida: A genus of yeastlike fungi commonly found in nature; a few species are isolated from the skin, feces, and vaginal and pharyngeal tissue, but the gastrointestinal tract is the source of the single most important species, *Candida albicans.*

childhood tuberculosis: Initial (primary) infection with *Mycobacterium tuberculosis*, characterized by pneumonic lesions in the middle parts of the lungs, with rapid spread to lymph nodes; more often seen in childhood, but the pattern is not limited to children.

computed tomography (CT): Imaging anatomic information from a cross-sectional plane of the body, each image generated by a computer synthesis of x-ray transmission data obtained in many different directions in a given plane.

congenital: Existing at birth, referring to certain mental or physical traits, anomalies, malformations, diseases, etc. which may be either hereditary or due to an influence occurring during gestation up to the moment of birth.

constipation: A condition in which bowel movements are infrequent or incomplete.

croup: 1. Acute obstruction of upper airway in infants and children characterized by a barking cough with difficult and noisy respiration. 2. Laryngotracheobronchitis in infants and young children caused by parainfluenza viruses 1 and 2.

cystic fibrosis: A congenital metabolic disorder in which secretions of exocrine glands are abnormal; excessively viscid mucus causes obstruction of passageways (including pancreatic and bile ducts, intestines, and bronchi), and the sodium and chloride content of sweat are increased throughout the patient's life; symptoms usually appear in childhood and include meconium ileus, poor growth despite good appetite, malabsorption and foul bulky stools, chronic bronchitis with cough, recurrent pneumonia, bronchiectasis, emphysema, clubbing of the fingers, and salt depletion in hot weather.

drug resistance: The capacity of disease-causing microorganisms to withstand drugs previously toxic to them; achieved by spontaneous mutation or through selective pressure after exposure to the drug in question. Usually an organism that has acquired resistance to a given antibiotic is resistant to others in the same chemical class. Drug resistance is a growing problem worldwide. Many strains of bacteria, fungi, and parasites have developed resistance, including pneumococci, gonococci, salmonellae, *Mycobacterium tuberculosis*, *Tinea tonsurans*, and *Plasmodium falciparum*. In some parts of the U.S., 40% of pneumococcal isolates and 90% of staphylococci are resistant to penicillin. Factors favoring development of antibiotic resistance include inappropriate prescribing of antibiotics (for example, to treat viral infections); indiscriminate use of newly developed, extended-spectrum agents; empiric and broad-spectrum treatment of infections in certain populations (for example, children, the elderly, and residents of long-term care facilities); prescribing of sublethal doses; and failure of patients to complete courses of antibiotic treatment. The Centers for Disease Control and Prevention estimates that U.S. physicians write 50 million unnecessary antibiotic prescriptions annually, including 17 million to treat the common cold. Infectious disease experts and public health authorities have called for restraint by primary care physicians in prescribing antibiotics, particularly for children and for uncomplicated upper respiratory infections, acute bronchitis (nearly always viral), and acute sinusitis and otitis media (in neither of which have reliable diagnostic criteria for bacterial infection been established). They have also stressed the importance of public education, since inappropriate expectations of patients or their parents have been a driving factor in antibiotic overuse by physicians.

Duchenne dystrophy: The most common childhood muscular dystrophy, with onset usually before age 6. Characterized by symmetric weakness and wasting of first the pelvic and crural (leg and thigh) muscles and then the chest and proximal upper extremity muscles; an increase in size of non-functioning tissue of some muscles, especially the calf; heart involvement; sometimes mild mental retardation; progressive course and early death, usually in adolescence. X-linked inheritance (affects males and transmitted by females).

encopresis: The repeated, generally involuntary passage of feces into inappropriate places (for example, in clothing).

enuresis: Involuntary discharge or leakage of urine.

erythema infectiosum: A mild skin rash of childhood characterized by red lesions, resulting in a lacelike facial rash or "slapped cheek" appearance. Fever and arthritis may also accompany infection; caused by Parvovirus B 19.

fungus: A general term used to encompass the diverse structural forms of yeasts and molds.

growing pains: Aching pains, frequently felt at night, in the limbs of children; cause is unclear, but the condition is benign.

Haemophilus influenzae: A bacterial species found in the respiratory tract that causes acute respiratory infections, including pneumonia, acute conjunctivitis, otitis, and purulent meningitis in children (rarely in adults in whom it contributes to sinusitis and chronic bronchitis).

hand-and-foot syndrome: Recurrent painful swelling of the hands and feet occurring in infants and young children with sickle cell anemia.

hand-foot-and-mouth disease: A skin rash in small children usually consisting of small, pearl-gray vesicles of the fingers, toes, palms, and soles, accompanied by often painful vesicles and ulceration of the buccal (cheek) mucous membrane and the tongue and by slight fever; the disease lasts 4–7 days, and is usually caused by coxsackie virus type A-16, but other types have been identified.

hemolytic uremic syndrome: Hemolytic anemia (a type of anemia caused by the destruction of blood cells) and thrombocytopenia (a condition where there are too few platelets in the blood) occurring with acute renal (kidney) failure; in children, characterized by sudden onset of gastrointestinal bleeding, blood in the urine, the production of very little urine, and microangiopathic hemolytic anemia; often caused by infection with *Escherichia coli.*

ibuprofen: A propionic acid-derived, nonsteroidal analgesic and anti-inflammatory agent.

immunization: Vaccination; protection of susceptible individuals from communicable diseases by administration of a living modified agent (such as, yellow fever vaccine), a suspension of killed organisms (such as, pertussis vaccine), or an inactivated toxin (such as, tetanus vaccine).

impetigo: A contagious superficial skin infection, caused by *Staphylococcus aureus* and/or group A streptococci, that begins with a superficial flaccid vesicle that ruptures and forms a thick yellowish crust, most commonly occurring in children.

incontinence: Inability to prevent the discharge of any of the excretions, especially of urine or feces.

infection: Invasion of the body with organisms that have the potential to cause disease.

inflammation: A fundamental pathologic process consisting of a dynamic complex of cellular and chemical reactions that occur in the affected blood vessels and adjacent tissues in response to an injury or abnormal stimulation caused by a physical, chemical, or biologic agent, including: 1) the local reactions and resulting changes, 2) the destruction or removal of the injurious material, 3) the responses that lead to repair and healing. The so-called "cardinal signs" of inflammation are: rubor, redness; calor, heat (or warmth); tumor, swelling; and dolor, pain; a fifth sign, *functio laesa*, inhibited or lost function, is sometimes added. All of the signs may be observed in certain instances, but no one of them is necessarily always present.

juvenile arthritis: Chronic arthritis beginning in childhood, most cases of which affect few joints. Several patterns of illness have been identified: in one subset, primarily affecting girls, iritis is common and antinuclear antibody is usually present; another subset, primarily affecting boys, frequently includes spinal arthritis resembling ankylosing spondylitis; some cases are true rheumatoid arthritis beginning in childhood and characterized by the presence of rheumatoid factor and destructive deforming joint changes, often undergoing remission at puberty.

juvenile diabetes: Type 1 diabetes mellitus. Diabetes mellitus appearing in a child or adolescent; often fatal before the discovery of insulin, usually of abrupt onset during first or second decades of life; characterized by excessive urine production, excessive thirst, weight loss; usually severe, insulin dependent, and prone to periods of ketoacidosis; can be familial, follow a viral infection such as mumps; thought to be due to virus-induced or immune destruction of pancreatic islets.

Kawasaki disease: A systemic inflammation of blood vessels of unknown origin that occurs primarily in children under 8 years of age. Symptoms include a fever lasting more than 5 days, rashes, dry, cracking lips; conjunctival injection, swelling of the hands and feet, irritability, and enlarged lymph nodes. Approximately 20% of untreated patients may develop coronary artery aneurysms. As the child recovers from the illness, an increased number of blood platelets circulate in the blood and peeling of the fingertips occurs.

lead poisoning: Acute or chronic intoxication by lead or any of its salts; symptoms of acute lead poisoning usually are those of acute gastroenteritis in adults or a brain disorder in children; chronic lead poisoning is manifested chiefly by anemia, constipation, colicky abdominal pain, a nerve disorder with paralysis with wrist-drop involving the muscles of the forearm, bluish lead line of the gums, and kidney inflammation; saturnine gout, convulsions, and coma may occur.

Lyme disease: A subacute inflammatory disorder caused by infection with *Borrelia burgdorferi*, a type of organism that does not cause pus-forming lesions transmitted by *Ixodes scapularis*, the deer tick, in the eastern U.S. and *I. pacificus*, the western black-legged tick, in the western U.S.; the characteristic skin lesion, a round red rash, is usually preceded or accompanied by fever, malaise, fatigue, headache, and stiff neck; neurologic, cardiac, or articular manifestations may occur weeks to months later.

magnetic resonance imaging (MRI): A type of diagnostic tool, using a strong magnetic field. Signals, which vary in intensity according to nuclear abundance and molecular chemical environment, are converted into sets of images.

meningococcal meningitis: An acute infectious disease of children and young adults, caused by *Neisseria meningitidis* characterized by fever, headache, photophobia, vomiting, nuchal rigidity, seizures, coma, and a purpuric eruption; even in the absence of meningitis, meningococcemia can induce toxic phenomena such as vasculitis, disseminated intravascular coagulation, shock, and Waterhouse-Friderichsen syndrome due to adrenal hemorrhage; late complications include paralysis, mental retardation, and gangrene of extremities. Approximately 2,500 cases of invasive meningococcal disease occur annually in the U.S., with a case fatality rate of 10–15%. The incidence of endemic meningococcal disease peaks between late winter and early spring.

night terrors: A disorder occurring in children, in which the child awakes screaming with fright, the distress persisting for a time during a state of semiconsciousness.

parasite: An organism that lives on or in another and draws its nourishment therefrom.

Parvovirus B19: A single-stranded DNA virus belonging to the family *Parvoviridae*; the cause of erythema infectiosum (fifth disease) and aplastic crises. Parvovirus B19 (B19V) was first isolated in 1975 from a specimen of healthy donor blood. In 1983 it was linked to erythema infectiosum, also called fifth disease, a generally benign febrile exanthem of children. B19V infection occurs worldwide and can attack persons of any age. It is most often contracted in childhood.

pediatrician: A specialist in pediatrics.

pediatrics: The medical specialty concerned with the study and treatment of children in health and disease during development from birth through adolescence.

pediculosis capitis: The presence of lice on the scalp, seen especially in children, with nits attached to hairs.

Reye syndrome: An acquired brain disorder of young children that follows an acute febrile illness, usually influenza or varicella infection; characterized by recurrent vomiting, agitation, and lethargy, which may lead to coma with intracranial hypertension; ammonia and serum transaminases are elevated; death may result from edema of the brain and resulting cerebral herniation.

rheumatic fever: A subacute febrile syndrome occurring after group A streptococcal infection (usually pharyngitis) and mediated by an immune response to the organism; most often seen in children and young adults; features include fever, inflammation of heart muscles (causing rapid heart beat and sometimes acute cardiac failure), inflammation inside the heart (with valvular incompetence, followed after healing by scarring), and joint inflammation; less often, skin and movement disorders; relapses can occur after reinfection with streptococci.

rubella: An acute but mild disease with a skin rash caused by rubella virus (Rubivirus family *Togaviridae*), with enlargement of lymph nodes, but usually with little fever or constitutional reaction; a high incidence of birth defects in children results from maternal infection during the first trimester of fetal life (congenital rubella syndrome).

stool: The matter discharged at one movement of the bowels.

tinea capitis: A common form of fungus infection of the scalp caused by various species of *Microsporum* and *Trichophyton* on or within hair shafts, occurring most commonly in children and characterized by irregularly placed and variously sized patches of apparent baldness because of hairs breaking off at the surface of the scalp, scaling, black dots, and occasionally rashes.

Tourette syndrome: A tic disorder appearing in childhood, characterized by multiple motor tics and vocal tics present for more than 1 year. Obsessive-compulsive behavior, attention-deficit disorder, and other psychiatric disorders may be associated; coprolalia (saying obscenities) and echolalia (excessive repetition of words) rarely occur; autosomal dominant inheritance.

varicella: Chickenpox. An acute contagious disease, usually occurring in children, caused by the varicella-zoster virus genus, *Varicellovirus*, a member of the family *Herpesviridae*, and marked by a sparse eruption of papules, which become vesicles and then pustules, like that of smallpox although less severe and varying in stages, usually with mild constitutional symptoms; incubation period is about 14–17 days.

virus: Specifically, a term for a group of infectious agents, which with few exceptions are capable of passing through fine filters that retain most bacteria, are usually not visible through the light microscope, lack independent metabolism, and are incapable of growth or reproduction apart from living cells. The complete particle usually contains either DNA or RNA, not both, and is usually covered by a protein shell or capsid that protects the nucleic acid.

Chapter 83

References and Additional Reading

This chapter provides a sampling of books, brochures, pamphlets, articles, and websites that contain additional information about the topics in this *Sourcebook*. The lists do not represent all material available. They are intended only to serve as starting points for gathering additional information. Inclusion does not constitute endorsement.

Books

The following books, which may be available from your local library or bookstore, are listed alphabetically by title to make the topics more readily apparent.

American Dietetic Association Guide to Healthy Eating for Kids: How Your Children Can Eat Smart from 5 to 12
Written by the American Dietetic Association (ADA), Mary Catherine Mullen, Jo Ellen Shield, and Jodie Shield
Published by Wiley, John and Sons, Inc., August 2002

The American Medical Association Family Medical Guide, Revised Edition
Edited by Charles R. Clayman
Published bu Random House, Inc., August 1994

Anxiety Disorders in Children and Adolescents: Epidemiology, Risk Factors and Treatment
Edited by Cecilia A. Essau and Franz Petermann
Published by Brunner-Routledge, March 2002

Atlas of Pediatric Physical Diagnosis, 4th Edition
Edited by Basil J. Zitelli and Holly W. Davis
Published by Mosby-Year Book, Inc., July 2002

The Bipolar Child: The Definitive and Reassuring Guide to Childhood's Most Misunderstood Disorder, Revised and Expanded Edition
Written by Demitri F. Papolos and Janice Papolos
Published by Broadway Books, September 2002

Caring for Your Baby and Young Child: Birth to Age 5
Edited by the American Academy of Pediatrics, Steven P. Shelov, and Robert E. Hannemann
Published by Bantam Books, Inc., June 1998

Childhood and Adolescent Diabetes
Edited by Simon Court and Bill Lamb
Published by John Wiley and Son Ltd., July 1997

Childhood Asthma and Other Wheezing Disorders, 2nd Edition
Written by Michael Silverman
Published by Arnold, 2002

Childhood Cancer: A Parent's Guide to Solid Tumor Cancers, 2nd Edition
Written by Honna Janes-Hodder, Nancy Keene, and Garrett M. Brodeur
Published by O'Reilly and Associates, July 2002

Childhood Cancer Survivors: A Practical Guide to Your Future
Written by Nancy Keene, Kathy Ruccione, and Wendy L. Hobbie
Published by Patient-Centered Guides, April 2000

Childhood Emergencies: What to Do—A Quick Reference Guide, Revised Edition
Edited by the Marin Child Care Council
Published by Bull Publishing Company, 2000

The Clinical Handbook of Pediatric Infectious Disease
Written by Russell W. Steele
Published by CRC Press-Parthenon Publishers, August 1994

The Caring for Your School-Age Child Ages 5 to 12, Revised Edition
Edited by the American Academy of Pediatrics and Edward L. Schor
Published by Bantam Books, Inc., July 1999

Columbia University Children's Medical Guide, Revised Edition
Edited by Steve Z. Miller and Bernard Valman
Published by DK Publishing, Inc., October 2002

Dictionary of Childhood Health Problems, 2nd Edition
Written by Patricia Gilbert
Published by Fitzroy, 2000

Guide to Your Child's Asthma and Allergies: Breathing Easy and Bringing up Healthy, Active Children
Edited by the American Academy of Pediatrics
Published by Random House, Inc., June 2000

Guide to Your Child's Nutrition
Edited by the American Academy of Pediatrics, William H. Dietz, and Lorraine Stern
Published by Random House Adult Trade Publishing Group, December 1999

Guide to Your Child's Sleep: Birth through Adolescence
Written by George J. Cohen
Published by David Mckay, December 1999

Guide to Your Child's Symptoms: The Official, Complete Home Reference, Birth through Adolescence
Edited by the American Academy of Pediatrics, Donald Schiff, and Steven P. Shelov
Published by Random House Adult Trade Publishing Group, December 1998

Handbook of Pediatric Urology
Edited by Laurence S. Baskin, Barry A. Kogan, and John W. Duckett
Published by Lippincott Williams and Wilkins Publishers, January 1997

Health and Behavior in Childhood and Adolescence
Edited by Laura Lucia Hayman, Margaret M. Mahon, and J. Rick Turner
Published by Springer Publishing, 2002

The Heart of a Child: What Families Need to Know about Heart Disorders in Children, 2nd Edition
Edited by Edward B. Clark, Carleen Clark, and Catherine A. Neill
Published by Johns Hopkins University Press, June 2001

Homeopathy for Children: A Parent's Guide to the Treatment of Common Childhood Illnesses, Revised Edition
Written by Gabrielle Pinto and Murray Feldman
Published by C.W. Daniel, 2000

Hospice Care for Children, 2nd Edition
Edited by Ann Armstrong-Dailey and Sarah Zarbock
Published by Oxford University Press, August 2001

The KidsHealth Guide for Parents
Written by Steven Dowshen, Neil Izenberg, and Elizabeth Bass
Published by The McGraw-Hill Companies, December 2001

Living with Childhood Cancer: A Practical Guide to Help Families Cope
Written by Leigh A. Woznick and Carol D. Goodheart
Published by the American Psychological Association, January 2002

Medical Emergencies and Childhood Illnesses
Written by Penny A Shore and William Sears, M.D.
Published by Parent Kit Corporation, 2002

The Parent's Guide to Children's Congenital Heart Defects
Written by Gerri Freid Kramer and Shari Maurer
Published by Three Rivers Press, 2001

The Parent's Guide to Food Allergies: Clear and Complete Advice from the Experts on Raising Your Food Allergic Child
Written by Marianne S. Barber and Maryanne Bartoszek Scott
Published by Henry Holt and Company, Inc., March 2001

Primary and Secondary Preventive Nutrition
Edited by Adrianne Bendich and Richard J. Deckelbaum
Published by Humana Press, 2001

Primary Care of the Child with a Chronic Condition, 3rd Edition
Edited by Patricia Ludder Jackson
Published by Mosby, Inc., January 2000

Promoting Adherence to Medical Treatment in Chronic Childhood Illness
Edited by Dennis Drotar
Published by Erlbaum Associates, 2000

Salt in Your Sock and Other Tried-and-True Home Remedies
Written by Lillian M. Beard and Linda Lee Small
Published by Three Rivers Press, 2003

Seizures and Epilepsy in Childhood: A Guide for Parents, 2nd Edition
Written by John M. Freeman, Eileen P. G. Vining, and Diana J. Pillas
Published by Johns Hopkins University Press, January 1997

Shelter from the Storm: Caring for a Child with a Life-Threatening Condition
Written by Joanne Hilden, Karen Lindsey, and Daniel R. Tobin
Published by Perseus Publishing, November 2002

Straight Talk about Psychiatric Medications for Kids
Written by Timothy E. Wilens
Published by Guilford Publications, Inc., October 1998

Taking Care of Your Child: A Parent's Guide to Complete Medical Care, 6th Edition
Written by Robert H. Pantell, James Fries, and Donald Vickery
Published by Perseus Publishing, February 2002

Your Child's Health: A Medical Record Book
Edited by Richard J. Sagall
Published by Publications International, Ltd., May 1997

Your Child's Health: The Parents' Guide to Symptoms, Emergencies, Common Illnesses, Behavior, and School Problems, Revised Edition
Written by Barton D. Schmitt
Published by Bantam Books, Inc., July 1991

Your Child's Medical Journal
Written by Sharon Larsen
Published by Crown Publishing Group, January 1999

Additional Reading on the Internet

American Academy of Family Physicians
http://familydoctor.org

American Academy of Pediatrics
http://www.aap.org

Cincinnati Children's Hospital Medical Center
Your Child's Health
http://www.cincinnatichildrens.org/Health_Topics/
Your_Childs_Health/Default.htm

Dr. Alan Greene
Dr. Greene's HouseCalls
http://www.drgreene.com

Health on the Net Foundation
Common Childhood Diseases
http://www.hon.ch/Dossier/MotherChild/childhood_diseases/
childhood_diseases.html

Healthology
Select Topic: Children's Health
http://www.healthology.com

Immunization Action Coalition
http://www.immunize.org

KidsHealth
Nemours Foundation
http://www.kidshealth.com

National Center for Infectious Diseases
http://www.cdc.gov/ncidod

National Immunization Program
http://www.cdc.gov/nip/default.htm

National Institute of Child Health and Human Development
http://www.nichd.nih.gov

NOAH (New York Online Access to Health)
Child Health Issues
http://www.noah-health.org/english/wellness/healthyliving/
childhealth.html

Suite 101.com
Childhood Diseases Archives
http://www.suite101.com/welcome.cfm/childhood_diseases

Virtual Children's Hospital
http://www.vh.org/pediatric/index.html

Brochures and Articles

The following articles and brochures are listed alphabetically by title. To make topics more readily apparent, key words are shown in **bold**.

"Acyclovir Is Useful in Treating **Chickenpox** in Children," by R. Sadovsky. *American Family Physician*, March 1, 2002; 65(5)967.

"Addressing Spasticity-Related Pain in Children with Spastic **Cerebral Palsy**," by C.I. Roscigno. *Journal of Neuroscience Nursing*, June 2002; 34(3):123–33.

"Adventures in **Parenting**," National Institute of Child Health and Human Development (NICHD). 2001. Available at the NICHD Clearinghouse. Call toll-free: 800-370-2943.

"Alarming Increase in Children with Type 2 **Diabetes** Is a Wake-Up Call," *Obesity, Fitness and Wellness Week*, July 13, 2002; 13.

"Are Antibiotics Effective for Adults and Children with Acute **Sore Throats**?" by C.B. Del Mar, P.P. Glasziou, and A.B. Spinks. *The Western Journal of Medicine*, February 2001; 174(2):112.

"**Autism** and Genes—Autism Research at the NICHD," National Institute of Child Health and Human Development (NICHD), 2001. Available at the NICHD Clearinghouse. Call toll-free: 800-370-2943.

"**Autism** and the MMR Vaccine—Autism Research at the NICHD," National Institute of Child Health and Human Development (NICHD), 2001. Available at the NICHD Clearinghouse. Call toll-free: 800-370-2943.

"Backpacks and Musculoskeletal Pain: Do Children with Idiopathic **Scoliosis** Face a Greater Risk?" by S.R. Iyer. *Journal of School Health*, September 2002; 72(7)270–71.

"Bacteremic **Urinary Tract Infection** in Children," by R. Sadovsky, *American Family Physician*, January 15, 2001; 63(2):361.

"Behavioral Issues in Pediatric **Epilepsy**," D.W. Dunn. *Psychiatric Times*, September 1, 2002; 25.

"Breathing Easy: Solutions in Pediatric **Asthma**," The National Center for Education in Maternal and Child Health (NCEMCH), 2000.

"Bug Off! [**Lice**]," C. Costas. *Parents Magazine*, September 2000; 75(9)83–85).

"Can Urine Clarity Exclude the Diagnosis of **Urinary Tract Infection**?" by B. Bulloch, J.C. Bausher, W.J. Pomerantz, J.M. Connors, M. Mahabee-Gittens and M.D. Dowd. *Pediatrics*, November 2000; 106(5):1127.

"Care of the Child with **Sickle Cell Disease**: Acute Complications," by L.D. Jakubik and M. Thompson. *Pediatric Nursing*, July 2000; 26(4):373.

"**Cerebral Palsy**: Not Always What It Seems," R. Gupta and R.E. Appleton. *Archives of Disease in Childhood*, November 2001; 85(5): 356–60.

"The Childhood **Muscular Dystrophies**: Making Order out of Chaos," *Seminars in Neurology*. 1999; 19(1):9–23.

"Childhood **Vaccines**–United States, 1995-1999," by the Centers for Disease Control and Prevention. *JAMA, The Journal of the American Medical Association*, December 26, 2001; 286(24):3073–74.

"Children and Microbial **Foodborne Illness**," J.C. Buzby. *Food Review*, May-August 2001; 24(2):32–7.

"Childrens' and Adolescents' Use of Diaries for **Sickle Cell Pain**," V.E. Maikler, M.E. Broome, P. Bailey and G. Lea. *Journal of the Society of Pediatric Nurses*, October-December 2001; 6(4): 161–69.

"Chronic **Constipation** in Children: Rational Management," by J.A. DiPalma and D.A. Gremse. *Consultant*, November 2001; 41(13): 1723–8.

"**Chronically Ill** Kids Subdue Their Emotions," *Health and Medicine Week*, April 15, 2002; 6.

"**Colds** (Upper **Respiratory Infections**, or URIs)," by B.D. Schmitt. *Clinical Reference Systems*, 2001; 446.

"Comparative Study of Cefuroxime Axetil Versus Amoxicillin in Children with Early **Lyme Disease**," by S.C. Eppes and J.A. Childs. *Pediatrics*, June 2002, 109(6):1173–77.

"Comparison of Child-Only Versus Mother/Child Sample Collection in **Fragile X** Testing," by K.M. Murphy and M.E. Nunes. *American Journal of Human Genetics*, October 2000; 67(4):248.

"Consider Benign Action for Some **Skin Conditions**," by J.M. Wang. *Pediatric News*, July 2001; 35(7)28.

"Control of **Hepatitis A** through Routine Vaccination of Children," by F. Averhoff, C.N. Shapiro, B.P. Bell, I. Hyams, L. Burd, A. Deladisma, E.P. Simard, D. Nalin, B. Kuter, C. Ward, M. Lundberg, N. Smith, H.S. Margolis. *JAMA, The Journal of the American Medical Association*, December 19, 2001; 286(23)2968–73.

"Daily Coping Practice Predicts Treatment Effects in Children with **Sickle Cell Disease**," by C.L. Grus. *Journal of Developmental and Behavioral Pediatrics*, October 2001; 22(5):340.

"**Diabetes**: Is Your Child at Risk?" J. Sheehan. *Parents Magazine*, July 2002; 77(7):79–83.

"Distinguishing Illness Severity from Tic Severity in Children and Adolescents with **Tourette's Disorder**," B.J. Coffey, J. Biederman, D.A. Geller, T.J. Spencer, G.S. Kim, C.A. Bellordre, J.A. Frazier, K. Cradock, and M. Magovcevic. *Journal of the American Academy of Child and Adolescent Psychiatry*, May 2000; 39(5):556

"Do Hair Care Practices Affect the Acquisition of **Tinea Capitis**? A Case-Control Study," by V. Sharma, N.B. Silverberg, R. Howard, C.T. Tran, T.A. Laude, and I.J. Frieden. *Archives of Pediatrics and Adolescent Medicine*, July 2001; 155(7):818.

"Do Parents Understand **Immunizations**? A National Telephone Survey," by B.G. Gellin, E.W. Maibach, and E.K. Marcuse. *Pediatrics*, November 2000; 106(5):1097.

"**Down Syndrome**," by C. Finesilver. *RN*, November 2002; 65(11):43–48.

"**Duchenne Muscular Dystrophy**," by T. Metules. *RN*, October 2002; 65(10):39–45.

"Dysfunctional Eating Patterns Symptoms of Pica in Children and Adolescents with **Sickle Cell Disease**," by K.L. Lemanek, R.T. Brown, F.D. Armstrong, C. Hood, C. Pegelow and G. Woods. *Clinical Pediatrics*, September 2002; 41(7):493–500.

"The Early Origins of **Autism**," by P.M. Rodier. *Scientific American*. February 2000; 38–45.

"Effect of Infection Control Measures on the Frequency of Upper **Respiratory Infection** in Child Care: A Randomized, Controlled Trial," by L. Roberts, W. Smith, L. Jorm, M. Patel, R.M. Douglas, and C. McGilchrist. *Pediatrics*, April 2000; 105(4):738.

"The Effectiveness of Casts, Orthoses, and Splints for Children with **Neurological Disorders**," by R. Teplicky, M. Law, and D. Russell. *Infants and Young Children*, July 2002; 15(1):42–50.

"Effects of a Functional Therapy Program on Motor Abilities of Children with **Cerebral Palsy**," by M. Ketelaar, A. Vermeer, H. Hart, E. van Petegem-van Beek, and P.J.M. Helders. *Physical Therapy*, September 2001; 81(9)1534–45.

"The Effects of Early Motor Intervention on Children with **Down Syndrome** or **Cerebral Palsy**: A Field-Based Study," G. Mahoney, C. Robinson, and R.R. Fewell. *Journal of Developmental and Behavioral Pediatrics*, June 2001; 22(3):153.

"**Enuresis** [Urinary **Incontinence**]," by S.E. Cossio. *Southern Medical Journal*, February 2002; 95(2) 183–8.

"Establishing **Sun Protective Behaviors** in Children," by K.E. Miller. *American Family Physician*, May 15, 2002; 65(10):2147.

"Ethical Issues with **Genetic Testing** in Pediatrics," *Pediatrics*, June 2001; 107(6):1451.

"Experimental Drug Shortens **Sickle Cell** Crises," M.A. Moon. *Pediatric News*, April 2002; 36(4):9.

"Facts about **McCune-Albright Syndrome**," National Institute of Child Health and Human Development (NICHD), 1993. Available at the NICHD Clearinghouse. Call toll-free: 800-370-2943.

"**Food Allergies**: Keeping Kids Safe," by H. Putman. *RN*, June 2002; 65(6):26–30.

"**Food-Allergic Reactions** in Schools and Preschools," by A. Nowak-Wegrzyn, M.K. Conover-Walker, and R.A. Wood. *Archives of Pediatrics and Adolescent Medicine*, July 2001; 155(7):790.

"Genes and **Addiction**," by E.J. Nestler. *Nature Genetics*, 2000; 26:277–281.

"Genetics of **Bipolar Disorder**," by N. Craddock and I. Jones. *Journal of Medical Genetics*, 1999; 36(8): 585–594.

"A Guide to Early Detection of **Scoliosis**," by K.R. Chin, J.S. Price, and S. Zimbler. *Contemporary Pediatrics*, September 2001; 18(9):77.

"**Head Lice**," by B.L. Frankowski and L.B. Weiner. *Pediatrics*, September 2002; 110(3)638–41.

"**Headaches** in Children and Adolescents," by D.W. LEWIS. *American Family Physician*, February 15, 2002; 65(4):625.

"Health Issues in Survivors of Childhood **Cancer**," by S. Castellino and M.M. Hudson. *Southern Medical Journal*, September 2002; 95(9):977–84.

"Health Supervision for Children with **Down Syndrome**," by the Committee on Genetics, American Academy of Pediatrics, *Pediatrics*, February 2001; 107(2):442–49.

"Health Tips for Kids Coping with **Asthma** and **Allergies**," *Immunotherapy Weekly*, November 7, 2001; 27.

"***Helicobacter Pylori*** Infection May Cause **Iron Deficiency** in Children," *TB and Outbreaks Week*, October 15, 2002; 17.

"**Hepatitis A**: Should My Child Get the Vaccine?" R.M. Brayden. *Clinical Reference Systems*, 2001; 1000.

"**Hormone-Associated Conditions** in Children," A.K.C. Leung and C.P. Kao. *Consultant*, September 2000; 40(10):1838.

"In Harm's Way: **Toxic Threats** to Child Development," by J. Stein, T. Schettler, D. Wallinga and M. Valenti. *Journal of Developmental and Behavioral Pediatrics*, February 2002; 23:S13–23.

"Infections of the **Central Nervous System**," by G.C. Townsend and W.M. Scheld. *Advances in Internal Medicine*, 1998; 43:403–44.

"Infections of the **Nervous System**," by A.A. Pruitt. *Neurology Clinics* 1998; 16(2):419–44.

"Influence of Attendance at Day Care on the **Common Cold** from Birth through 13 Years of Age," by T.M. Ball, C.J. Holberg, M.B. Aldous, F.D. Martinez, and A.L. Wright. *Archives of Pediatrics and Adolescent Medicine*, February 2002; 156(2):121–26.

"Inherited **Skeletal Muscle Disorders**," by N.G. Laing and F.L. Mastaglia. *Annals of Human Biology*. 1999; 26(6):507–25.

"**Intolerance [Lactose]** to Cow's Milk and **Constipation** in Children," by J.T. Kirchner. *American Family Physician*, February 15, 1999; 1021.

"**Iron Deficiency** Anemia," *CareNotes*, December 2001.

"**Iron**: Helping Your Child Get Enough," by Ellyn Satter. *Clinical Reference Systems*, 2001; 1142.

"The Ketogenic Diet [for **Epilepsy**]: A 3- to 6-Year Follow-Up of 150 Children Enrolled Prospectively," C. Hemingway, J.M. Freeman, D.J. Pillas, and P.L. Pyzik. *Pediatrics*, October 2001; 108(4):898.

"Laparoscopic Exploration for the Clinically Undetected **Hernia** in Infancy and Childhood," by D.P. Geisler, S. Jegathesan, M.C. Parmley, J.M. McGee, M.G. Nolen and T.A. Broughan. *American Journal of Surgery*, December 2001; 182(6)693–96.

"**Lice**, Nits, and School Policy," L.K. Williams, A. Reichert, W.R. MacKenzie, A.W. Hightower, and P.A. Blake. *Pediatrics*, May 2001; 107(5):1011.

"**Lyme Disease**: Are Your Kids at Risk?" A.L. Kelly. *Parents Magazine*, May 2001; 76(5):65–69.

"Managing **Constipation**: Evidence Put to Practice," S. Nurko, S.S. Baker, R.B. Colletti, J.M. Croffie, C. Di Lorenzo, W. Ector and G.S. Liptak. *Contemporary Pediatrics*, December 2001; 18(12)56–66).

"Managing **Incontinence**: Helping Children Learn about and Overcome the Challenges," by G. Jurasek. *The Exceptional Parent*, September 2000; 30(9):100.

"Manifestations of **Food Allergy**: Evaluation and Management," S.H. Sicherer. *American Family Physician*, January 15, 1999; 59(2):415.

"The Many Causes of Childhood **Stridor**," by M.F. Conar. *Physician Assistant*, September 2001; 25(9):35.

"Mommy, My **Ear** Hurts!" by K.M. Heins. *Better Homes and Gardens*, January 2000; 78:52.

"National Action Plan for Childhood **Cancer**: Report of the National Summit Meetings on Childhood Cancer," by R. Arceci, A. Ettinger, E. Forman, G.M. Haase, D. Hammond, R. Hoffman, M.J. Kupst, M.P. Link, C.P. Lustig and D.S. Traynor. *Ca*, November-December 2002, 52(6): 377–79.

"Neurologic Disorders after **Measles-Mumps-Rubella Vaccination**," by A. Makela, J.P. Nuorti, and H. Peltola. *Pediatrics*, November 2002; 110(5)957–64.

"**Neuromuscular** Rehabilitation and Electrodiagnosis," by D.P. Moore D.P. and K.J. Kowalske. *Archives of Physical Medicine and Rehabilitation*. March 2000; 81(3 Suppl 1):S32–5; quiz S36–44.

"New Centers to Investigate Impact of **Environment** on Childhood Disorders," *The Brown University Child and Adolescent Behavior Letter*, December 2001; 17(2):3.

"Parent Advice on MMR [**Measles, Mumps** and **Rubella**] **Vaccination**," J. Gray. *Practice Nurse*, June 8, 2001; 22(1):16.

"Parental Expectations of **Antibiotic Treatment** in Children," by K.E. Miller. *American Family Physician*, February 1, 2002; 65(3):498.

"**Peanut Allergy**: An Increasing Health Risk for Children," by P.L. Jackson. *Pediatric Nursing*, September-October 2002; 28(5):496–99.

"A Population-Based Study of **Measles, Mumps**, and **Rubella Vaccination** and **Autism**," K.M. Madsen, A. Hviid, M. Vestergaard, D. Schendel, J. Wohlfahrt, P. Thorsen, J. Olsen and M. Melbye. *The New England Journal of Medicine*, November 7, 2002; 347(19):1477–82.

"Predictive Factors for Short-Term Symptom Persistence in Children after Emergency Department Evaluation for **Constipation**," by H. Patel, A. Law, and S. Gouin. *Archives of Pediatrics and Adolescent Medicine*, December 2000; 154(12):1204.

"Putting a Dent in **Iron Deficiency**," L. Lesperance, A.C. Wu, and H. Bernstein. *Contemporary Pediatrics*, July 2002; 19(7):60–73

"Save Your Child from **Skin Cancer**," by D. Debrovner. *Parents Magazine*, May 2002; 77(5):109–12.

"**Scoliosis** and Spinal Conditions in Children," *GP*, September 23, 2002; 53.

"Simultaneous Administration of Varicella Vaccine and Other Recommended Childhood **Vaccines**–United States, 1995-1999," *Morbidity and Mortality Weekly Report*, November 30, 2001; 50(47):1058–61.

"**Soiling** (**Encopresis**) without Constipation," B.D. Schmitt. *Clinical Reference Systems*, 2001; 1801.

"Summary of **Notifiable Diseases**, United States, 2000," Centers for Disease Control and Prevention. *Morbidity and Mortality Weekly Report* 2000; 49(53).

"Symptoms and Suffering at the End of Life in Children with **Cancer**," J. Wolfe, H.E. Grier, N. Klar, S.B. Levin, J.M. Ellenbogen, S. Salem-Schatz, E.J. Emanuel and J.C. Weeks. *The New England Journal of Medicine*, February 3, 2000; 342(5):326–33.

"Talking about **Epilepsy**," by P. Crumrine. *The Exceptional Parent*, February 2001; 31(2):88.

"Therapies in **Muscular Dystrophy**: Current Concepts and Future Prospects," by J.A. Urtizberea. *European Neurology*. 2000;43(3):127–32.

"Timeliness of Childhood **Immunizations**," by E.T. Luman, M.M. McCauley, S. Stokley, S.Y. Chu and L.K. Pickering. *Pediatrics*, November 2002; 110(5):935–40.

"**Tonsil** and **Adenoid** Surgery: Discharge Instructions," by G. Mills. *Clinical Reference Systems*, 2001; 2032.

"**Tonsillectomy** and **Adenotonsillectomy** for Recurrent Throat Infection in Moderately Affected Children," by J.L. Paradise, C.D. Bluestone, D.K. Colborn, B.S. Bernard, H.E. Rockette, and M. Kurs-Lasky. *Pediatrics*, July 2002; 110(1):7–16.

"Tough **Seizures**: When the First Anticonvulsant Fails," by E.H. Kossoff. *Contemporary Pediatrics*, September 2002; 19(9):85–94.

"Toxicity of Cough and Cold **Medications** in Children," by G.B. Huffman. *American Family Physician*, March 15, 2002; 65(6):1195.

"Treatment of URIs [Upper **Respiratory Tract Infections**] in Children," by A.D. Walling. *American Family Physician*, November 15, 2000; 62(10):2344.

"**Tummy Ache**," by J. Collins. *The Times*, March 21, 2000; S15.

"Uncertainty in the Management of Viral Lower **Respiratory Tract Disease**," by H.C. Meissner. *Pediatrics*, October 2001; 108(4):1000.

"Use of **Sunscreen**, Sunburning Rates, and Tanning Bed Use Among More Than 10,000 U.S. Children and Adolescents," by A.C. Geller, G. Colditz, S. Oliveria, K. Emmons, C. Jorgensen, G.N. Aweh and A.L. Frazier. *Pediatrics*, June 2002; 109(6):1009–14.

"The Usefulness of Children's Drawings in the Diagnosis of **Headache**," by C.E. Stafstrom, K. Rostasy, and A. Minster. *Pediatrics*, March 2002; 109(3):460–73.

"UTI [**Urinary Tract Infection**]: Diagnosis and Evaluation in Symptomatic Pediatric Patients," by F.J. Heldrich, M.A. Barone, and E. Spiegler. *Clinical Pediatrics*, August 2000; 39(8):461–72.

"Viral (Aseptic) **Meningitis**," Centers for Disease Control and Prevention (www.cdc.gov), August 20, 2001.

"Viral **Respiratory Infection** in Schoolchildren: Effects on Middle **Ear** Pressure," by B. Winther, F.G. Hayden, E. Arruda, R. Dutkowski, P. Ward and J.O. Hendley. *Pediatrics*, May 2002; 109(5):826–32.

"What Environmental Modifications Improve Pediatric **Asthma**?" by T. Dudley and J. Nashelsky. *Journal of Family Practice*, July 2002; 51(7):618–19.

"What Parents Don't Know about Chickenpox," by J.A. Goodkin. *Contemporary Pediatrics*, October 2001; 18(10)15.

"What's in a Name? **Muscular Dystrophy** Revisited," by V. Dubowitz. *European Journal of Paediatric Neurology*. 1998; 2(6):279–84.

"When **Earaches** and **Sore Throats** Are More Than a Pain in the Neck," by S. Skoda-Smith and D.J. Barrett. *Contemporary Pediatrics*, March 2000; 17(3):156.

"When Your Child Is Diagnosed: Your Child's **Diabetes** Can Cause a Tidal Wave of Emotions," by C.E. Watkins. *Diabetes Forecast*, September 2002; 55(9):82–86.

"Why We Must Do a Better Job Controlling **Asthma**," by D.P. Skoner. *Contemporary Pediatrics*, August 2001; 18(8):49.

"Younger Age at Vaccination May Increase Risk of Varicella [**Chicken-pox**] Vaccine Failure," by K. Galil, E. Fair, N. Mountcastle, P. Britz and J. Seward. *Journal of Infectious Diseases*, July 1, 2002; 186(1): 102–04.

Chapter 84

Resources for Information about Childhood Diseases

This chapter lists contact information for government agencies, professional organizations, websites, and publications related to childhood diseases and ailments. Information is listed according to the organization of the sections in this *Sourcebook*.

Introduction to Child Health

Administration for Children and Families
U.S. Department of Health and Human Services
Mail Stop: HHH 300F
370 L'Enfant Promenade SW
Washington, DC 20447
Phone: 202-690-6590
Website: http://www.acf.dhhs.gov

Agency for Healthcare Research and Quality
2101 E. Jefferson St., Suite 501
Rockville, MD 20852
Phone: 301-594-1364
Website: http://www.ahrq.gov
E-mail: info@ahrq.gov

American Academy of Family Physicians
11400 Tomahawk Creek Parkway
Leawood, KS 66211-2672
Toll-Free: 800-274-2237
Phone: 913-906-6000
Website: http://www.aafp.org
E-mail: fp@aafp.org

The resources listed in this section were compiled from a wide variety of sources deemed accurate. Contact information was verified and updated between October 2002 and January 2003. Inclusion does not constitute endorsement.

American Academy of Pediatrics
141 Northwest Point Boulevard
Elk Grove Village, IL
60007-1098
Phone: 847-434-4000
Fax: 847-434-8000
Website: http://www.aap.org
E-mail: kidsdocs@aap.org

Association of State and Territorial Directors of Health Promotion and Public Health Education
1101 15ᵗʰ Street, NW, Suite 601
Washington, DC 20005
Phone: 202-659-2230
Fax: 202-659-2339
Website: http://
www.astdhpphe.org
E-mail: director@astdhpphe.org

American Association of Poison Control Centers
3201 New Mexico Avenue
Suite 310
Washington, DC 20016
Toll-Free: 800-222-1222 (For Poisoning Emergency)
Phone: 202-362-7217
Website: http://www.aapcc.org
E-mail: aapcc@poison.org

Canadian Paediatric Society
100-2204 Walkley Rd.
Ottawa, ON K1G 4G8
Canada
Phone: 613-526-9397
Fax: 613-526-3332
Website: http://
www.caringforkids.cps.ca
E-mail: info@cps.ca

Cincinnati Children's Hospital Medical Center
3333 Burnet Avenue
Cincinnati, OH 45229-3039
Toll-Free: 800-344-2462
Phone: 513-636-4200
Website: http://
cincinnatichildrens.org

Cleveland Clinic
9500 Euclid Avenue
Cleveland, OH 44195
Toll-Free: 800-223-2273
Phone: 216-444-2200
TTY: 216-444-0261
Website: http://
www.clevelandclinic.org

Lucile Packard Children's Hospital
725 Welch Road
Palo Alto, CA 94304
Toll-Free: 800-690-2282 (Parent Information Referral Center)
Phone: 650-497-8000
Website: http://
www.packardchildrenshospital.org

Mayo Clinic
Website: http://
www.mayohealth.org

Mayo Clinic—Arizona
13400 East Shea Blvd.
Scottsdale, AZ 85259
Phone: 480-301-8000
Fax: 480-301-7006

Mayo Clinic—Florida
4500 San Pablo Road
Jacksonville, FL 32224
Phone: 904-953-2000
Fax: 904-953-2300

Mayo Clinic—Minnesota
200 First St., SW
Rochester, MN 55905
Phone: 507-284-2511
Fax: 507-284-0161

Medical College of Wisconsin
MCW HealthLink
Office of Clinical Informatics
9200 West Wisconsin Ave.
Suite 2977
Milwaukee, Wisconsin 53226
Phone: 414-456-4700
Fax: 414-805-6337
Website: http://healthlink.mcw.edu
E-mail: healthlink@mcw.edu

National Institute of Child Health and Human Development
Bldg. 31, Room 2A32
MSC 2425
31 Center Drive
Bethesda, MD 20892-2425
Toll-Free: 800-370-2943
Phone: 301-496-5133
Website: http://www.nichd.nih.gov
E-mail: nichdwebmaster@mail.nih.gov

Nemours Foundation
KidsHealth
1600 Rockland Road
Wilmington, DE 19803
Phone: 302-651-4046
Website: http://www.kidshealth.org
E-mail: info@KidsHealth.org

U.S. Centers for Disease Control and Prevention
Mail Stop A-26
1600 Clifton Road, NE
Atlanta, GA 30333
Toll-Free: 888-232-3228
Website: http://www.cdc.gov
E-mail: pubfaq@cdc.gov

U.S. Food and Drug Administration
5600 Fishers Lane
Rockville, MD 20857
Toll-Free: 800-532-4440
Website: http://www.fda.gov

Virtual Children's Hospital
University of Iowa
200 Hawkins Drive
Iowa City, IA 52242
Toll-Free: 800-777-8442
Phone: 319-356-1616
TDD: 800-855-1155
Website: http://www.vh.org

World Health Organization
Avenue Appia 20
1211 Geneva 27
Switzerland
Phone: 011-41-22-791-2222
Website: http://www.who.int

Common Respiratory Tract Ailments

Allergy and Asthma Network/ Mothers of Asthmatics, Inc.
2751 Prosperity Avenue, Suite 150
Fairfax, VA 22031
Phone: 800-878-4403
Fax: 703-573-7794
Website: http://www.aanma.org

American College of Chest Physicians
3300 Dundee Rd.
Northbrook, IL 60062-2348
Toll-Free: 800-343-2227
Phone: 847-498-1400
Fax: 847-498-5460
Website: http://www.chestnet.org

American Lung Association
61 Broadway
6th Floor
New York, NY 10006
Phone: 212-315-8700
Toll-Free: 800-LUNG-USA
Website: http://www.lungusa.org

Cystic Fibrosis Foundation
6931 Arlington Road
Bethesda, MD 20814
Toll-Free: 800-344-4823
Phone: 301-951-4422
Fax: 301-951-6378
Website: http://www.cff.org
E-mail: info@cff.org

National Heart, Lung, and Blood Institute
Lung Information Center
P.O. Box 30105
Bethesda, MD 20824-0105
Phone: 301-592-8573
Fax: 301-592-8563
TTY: 240-629-3255
Website: http://
www.nhlbi.nih.gov/health/public/
lung/index.htm
E-mail:
nhlbiinfo@rover.nhlbi.nih.gov

National Jewish Medical and Research Center
1400 Jackson Street
Denver, CO 80206
Toll-Free: 800-222-LUNG (5864)
Phone: 303-388-4461
Website: http://www.njc.org
E-mail: lungline@njc.org

Ailments of the Head, Throat, and Mouth

American Academy of Audiology
8300 Greensboro Drive, Suite 750
McLean, VA 22102-3611
Toll-Free: 800-AAA-2336
Phone: 703-790-8466
Fax: 703-790-8631
Website: http://www.audiology.org

American Academy of Otolaryngology-Head and Neck Surgery
1 Prince Street
Alexandria, VA 22314
Phone: 703-836-4444
Website: http://www.entnet.org
E-mail: entinfo@aol.com

American Academy of Periodontology
737 North Michigan Avenue
Suite 800
Chicago, IL 60611-2690
Toll-Free: 800-282-4867
Phone: 312-787-5518
Fax: 312-573-3223
Website: http://www.perio.org

American Auditory Society
352 Sundial Ridge Circle
Dammeron Valley, UT 84783
Phone: 435-547-0062
Fax: 435-574-0063
Website: http://
www.amauditorysoc.org

American Council for Headache Education
19 Mantua Road
Mt. Royal, NJ 08061
Phone: 856-423-0258
Fax: 856-423-0082
Website: http://www.achenet.org
E-mail: achehq@talley.com

American Speech-Language-Hearing Association
10801 Rockville Pike
Rockville, MD 20852
Toll-Free: 800-638-8255
Phone/TTY: 301-897-5700
Fax: 301-571-0457
Website: http://www.asha.org
E-mail: actioncenter@asha.org

Bicycle Helmet Safety Institute
4611 Seventh Street South
Arlington, VA 22204-1419
Phone: 703-486-0100 (voice and fax)
Website: http://www.helmets.org
E-mail: info@helmets.org

Brain Injury Association
105 North Alfred Street
Alexandria, VA 22314
Toll-Free: 800-444-6443 (Family Helpline)
Website: http://www.biausa.org
E-mail: familyhelpline@biausa.org

Columbia Presbyterian Medical Center
Department of Otolaryngology/
Head and Neck Surgery
161 Fort Washington Ave.
5th Floor
New York, NY 10032
Phone: 212-305-8555
Website: http://
www.entcolumbia.org

House Ear Institute
2100 W. 3rd Street
Los Angeles, CA 90057
Phone: 213-483-4431
TDD: 213-484-2642
Fax: 213-483-8789
Website: http://www.hei.org
E-mail: webmaster@hei.org

National Headache Foundation
820 N. Orleans
Suite 217
Chicago, IL 60610
Toll-Free: 888-NHF-5552
Website: http://
www.headaches.org
E-mail: info@headaches.org

Digestive and Genitourinary Diseases and Disorders

American Dietetic Association
216 W. Jackson Boulevard
Chicago, IL 60606-6995
Toll-Free: 800-877-1600
Fax: 312-899-0040
Website: http://www.eatright.org
E-mail: ada@eatright.org

American Foundation for Urologic Disease
1128 North Charles Street
Baltimore, MD 21201
Toll-Free: 800-242-2383
Phone: 410-468-1800
Fax: 410-468-1808
Website: http://www.afud.org
E-mail: admin@afud.org

Cyclic Vomiting Association
3585 Cedar Hill Road, NW
Canal Winchester, OH 43110
Phone: 614-837-2586
(voice and fax)
Website: http://
www.cvsaonline.org/index.html

National Association for Continence
P.O. Box 8310
Spartanburg, SC 29305
Toll-Free: 1-800-BLADDER
Phone: 864-579-7900
Website: http://www.nafc.org
E-mail:
memberservices@nafc.org

National Kidney and Urologic Diseases Information Clearinghouse
3 Information Way
Bethesda, MD 20892-3580
Toll-Free: 800-891-5390
Phone: 301-654-4415
Fax: 301-907-8906
Website: http://
www.niddk.nih.gov/health/kidney/nkudic.htm
E-mail:
nkudic@info.niddk.nih.gov

National Kidney Foundation, Inc.
30 East 33rd Street
New York, NY 10016
Toll-Free: 800-622-9010
Phone: 212-889-2210
Fax: 212-689-9261
Website: http://www.kidney.org
E-mail: info@kidney.org

Pediatric/Adolescent Gastroesophageal Reflux Association (PAGER)
P.O. Box 1153
Germantown, MD 20875-1153
Phone: 301-601-9541
Website: www.reflux.org
E-mail: gergroup@aol.com

Simon Foundation for Continence
P.O. Box 835-F
Wilmette, IL 60091
Toll-Free: 800-23-SIMON
Phone: 847-864-3913
Fax: 847-864-9758
Website: http://
www.simonfoundation.org
E-mail:
simoninfo@simonfoundation.org

Society of Urologic Nurses and Associates (SUNA)
SUNA National Headquarters
East Holly Avenue, Box 56
Pitman, NJ 08071-0056
Toll-Free: 888-TAP-SUNA
Fax: 856-589-7463
Website: Website: http://
suna.inurse.com
E-mail: suna@inurse.com

U.S. Department of Agriculture

Food and Nutrition Information Center
10301 Baltimore Avenue
Beltsville, MD 30705-2351
Phone: 301-504-5719
Fax: 301-504-6409
TTY: 301-504-6856
Website: http://www.nalusda.gov/fnic/index.html
E-mail: fnic@nal.usda.gov

Skin and Scalp Ailments

American Academy of Dermatology

930 E. Woodfield Rd.
Schaumburg, IL 60173-4927
Toll-Free: 888-462-DERM
Website: http://www.aad.org

Eczema Association

6600 SW 92nd Ave., Suite 230
Portland, OR 97223-0704
Toll-Free: 800-818-7546
Phone: 503-228-4430
Fax: 503-224-3363
Website: Website: http://www.nationaleczema.org
E-mail: info@nationaleczema.org

National Arthritis, Musculoskeletal, and Skin Diseases Information Clearinghouse

One AMS Circle
Bethesda, MD 20892-3675
Phone: 301-495-4484
Website: http://www.nih.gov/niams

National Pediculosis Association

50 Kearney Road
Needham, MA 02494
Phone: 781-449-NITS
Fax: 781-449-8129
Website: http://www.headlice.org
E-mail: npa@headlice.org

Society for Pediatric Dermatology

5422 North Bernard
Chicago, IL 60625
Phone: 773-583-9780
Fax: 773-583-9765
Website: http://www.pedsderm.net

Infectious Diseases

All Kids Count

750 Commerce Drive
Suite 400
Decatur, GA 30030
Toll-Free: 800-874-4338
Fax: 800-765-7520
Website: http://www.allkidscount.org
E-mail: info@allkidscount.org

Hepatitis Foundation International

504 Blick Drive
Silver Spring, MD 20904-2901
Toll-Free: 800-891-0707
Phone: 301-622-4200
Website: http://www.hepfi.org
E-mail: hfi@Comcast.net

Immunization Action Coalition
1573 Selby Avenue
St. Paul, MN 55104
Phone: 651-647-9009
Fax: 651-647-9131
Website: http://
www.immunize.org
E-mail: admin@immunize.org

Immunization Education and Action Committee
National Healthy Mothers,
Healthy Babies Coalition
121 North Washington St.
Suite 300
Alexandria, VA 22314
Phone: 703-836-6110
Fax: 703-836-3470
Website: http://www.hmhb.org
E-mail: info@hmhb.org

Meningitis Foundation of America
6610 North Shadeland Avenue,
Suite 200
Indianapolis, IN 46220-4393
Toll-Free: 800-668-1129
Phone: 317-595-6383
Fax: 317-595-6370
Website: http://www.musa.org

National Immunization Program
Mailstop E-05
1600 Clifton Rd., NE
Atlanta, GA 30333
Toll-Free: 800-232-2522 (English)
Toll-Free: 800-232-0233 (Spanish)
Fax: 888-232-3299
Website: http://www.cdc.gov/nip
E-mail: NPINFO@cdc.gov

National Vaccine Injury Compensation Program
Parklawn Building
Room 16C-17
5600 Fishers Lane
Rockville, MD 20857
Toll-Free: 800-338-2382
Website: http://www.hrsa.gov/
vicp

Chronic Physical, Developmental, and Behavioral Conditions

Administration on Developmental Disabilities
U.S. Department of Health and Human Services
Mail Stop: HHH 300F
370 L'Enfant Promenade SW
Washington, DC 20447
Phone: 202-690-6590
Website: http://
www.acf.dhhs.gov/programs/add

American Academy of Child and Adolescent Psychiatry
3615 Wisconsin Ave., NW
Washington, DC 20016-3007
Phone: 202-966-7300
Fax: 202-966-2891
Website: http://www.aacap.org

American Cancer Society
National Headquarters
1599 Clifton Road, NE
Atlanta, GA 30329
Toll-Free: 800-ACS-2345
Website: http://www.cancer.org

American Diabetes Association
1701 North Beauregard Street
Alexandria, VA 22311
Toll-Free: 800-342-2383
Website: http://www.diabetes.org
E-mail: AskADA@diabetes.org

American Physical Therapy Association
111 North Fairfax Street
Alexandria, VA 22314-1488
Toll-Free: 800-999-2782
Phone: 703-684-2783
Fax: 703-684-7343
Website: http://www.apta.org

Association of Persons with Severe Handicaps (TASH)
29 West Susquehanna Avenue, Suite 210
Baltimore, MD 21204
Phone: 410-828-8274
Fax: 410-828-6706
Website: http://www.tash.org

American Sickle Cell Anemia Association
10300 Carnegie Avenue
Cleveland Clinic/East Office Building (EEb18)
Cleveland, OH 44106
Phone: 216-229-8600
Website: http://www.ascaa.org

Association of University Centers on Disabilities (AUCD)
8630 Fenton Street, Suite 410
Silver Spring, MD 20910
Phone: 301-588-8252
Fax: 301-588-2842
Website: http://www.aucd.org

The Autism National Committee
P.O. Box 6175
North Plymouth, MA 02362-6175
Toll-Free: 800-378-0386
Fax: 608-222-7670
Website: http://www.autcom.org

Autism Research Institute
4182 Adams Ave.
San Diego, CA 92116
Phone: 619-281-7165
Fax: 619-563-6840
Website: http://www.autism.com/ari

Autism Society of America, Inc.
7910 Woodmont Avenue
Suite 300
Bethesda, MD 20814-3067
Toll-Free: 800-3-AUTISM
Phone: 301-657-0881
Fax: 301-657-0869
Website: http://www.autism-society.org
E-mail: info@autism-society.org

Beach Center on Families and Disability
University of Kansas
Haworth Hall, Room 3136
1200 Sunnyside Ave.
Lawrence, KA 66045-7534
Phone: 785-864-7600
Fax: 785-864-7605
Website: http://www.beachcenter.org
E-mail: beach@dole.lsi.ukans.edu

Cancer Information Service
Office of Cancer Communications
National Cancer Institute
31 Center Drive MSC 2580
Building 31, Room 10A16
Bethesda, MD 20892-2580
Toll-Free: 1-800-4-CANCER
Website: http://oc.nci.nih.gov
E-mail: nciocomm-r@mail.nih.gov

Candlelighters Childhood Cancer Foundation
P.O. Box 498
Kensington, MD 20895-0498
Toll-Free: 800-366-CCCF
Phone: 301-962-3520
Fax: 301-962-3521
Website: http://
www.candlelighters.org
E-mail: info@candlelighters.org

Children's Blood Foundation
333 East 38th Street, Suite 830
New York, NY 10016
Phone: 212-297-4336
Fax: 212-297-4340
Website: http://
www.childrensbloodfoundation.org
E-mail:
info@childrensbloodfoundation.org

Children's Hospice International
901 North Washington Street
Suite 230
Alexandria, VA 22314
Toll-Free: 800-242-4453
Phone: 703-684-0330
Fax: 703-684-0226
Website: http://www.chionline.org
E-mail: chiorg@aol.com

Cooley's Anemia Foundation, Inc.
129-09 26th Avenue, #203
Flushing, NY 11354
Toll-Free: 800-522-7222
Phone: 718-321-2873
Fax: 718-321-3340
Website: http://
www.cooleysanemia.org
E-mail: info@cooleysanemia.org

Cornelia de Lange Syndrome Foundation
302 West Main Street, #100
Avon, CT 06001
Toll-Free: 800-223-8355
Phone: 860-676-8166
Fax: 860-676-8337
Website: http://www.cdlsusa.org
E-mail: info@cdlsusa.org

Council for Exceptional Children
1110 North Glebe Road
Suite 300
Arlington, VA 22201-5704
Toll-Free: 888-CEC-SPED
Phone: 703-620-3660
Fax: 703-264-9494
TTY: 703-264-9946
Website: http://www.cec.sped.org

Cure Autism Now (CAN)
5455 Wilshire Boulevard
Suite 715
Los Angeles, CA 90036
Toll-Free: 888-8-AUTISM
Phone: 323-549-0500
Website: http://
www.canfoundation.org
E-mail: info@cureautismnow.org

Division TEACCH (Treatment and Education of Autistic and Related Communication Handicapped Children)
Campus Box 7180
University of North Carolina
Chapel Hill, NC 27599-7180
Phone: 919-966-2173
Website: http://www.teach.com
E-mail: teacch@unc.edu

Easter Seals
230 West Monroe Street
Suite 1800
Chicago, IL 60606-4802
Toll-Free: 800-221-6827
Phone: 312-726-6200
Fax: 312-726-1494
TTY: 312-726-4258
Website: http://
www.easter-seals.org

Epilepsy Foundation
4351 Garden City Drive
Landover, MD 20785-7223
Toll-Free: 800-EFA-1000
Website: http://
www.epilepsyfoundation.org

Facioscapulohumeral Dystrophy (FSHD) Society
3 Westwood Road
Lexington, MA 02420
Phone: 781-860-0501
Fax: 781-860-0599
Website: http://
www.fshsociety.org
E-mail: info@fshsociety.org

Federation for Children with Special Needs
1135 Tremont Street, Suite 420
Boston, MA 02120
Toll-Free: 800-331-0688
Phone: 617-236-7210
Fax: 617-572-2094
Website: http://www.fcsn.org
E-mail: fcsninfo@fcsn.org

Federation of Families for Children's Mental Health
1101 King Street, Suite 420
Alexandria, VA 22314
Phone: 703-684-7710
Fax: 703-836-1040
Website: http://www.ffcmh.org
E-mail: ffcmh@ffcmh.org

FRAXA Research Foundation, Inc.
45 Pleasant Street
Newburyport, MA 01950
Phone: 978-462-1866
Fax: 978-463-9985
Website: http://www.fraxa.org
E-mail: info@fraxa.org

Indiana Resource Center on Autism
Institute for the Study of
Developmental Disabilities
Indiana University
2853 East Tenth Street
Bloomington, IN 47408-2696
Phone: 812-855-6508
Fax: 812-855-9630
TTY: 812-855-9396
Website: http://
www.idc.Indiana.edu/irca

International Dyslexia Association

Chester Building, Suite 382
8600 La Salle Road
Baltimore, MD 21286
Toll-Free: 800-ABCD123
Phone: 410-296-0232
Fax: 410-321-5069
Website: http://www.interdys.org

Iron Overload Diseases Association

433 Westwind Drive
North Palm Beach, FL 33408-5123
Phone: 561-840-8512
Fax: 561-842-9881
Website: http://www.ironoverload.org
E-mail: iod@ironoverload.org

Iron Disorders Institute

P.O. Box 2031
Greenville, SC 29602
Toll-Free: 888-565-IRON (4766)
Phone: 864-292-1175
Fax: 864-292-1878
Website: http://www.irondisorders.org
E-mail: irondis@aol.com

Joslin Diabetes Center

One Joslin Place
Boston, MA 02214
Phone: 617-732-2400
Website: http://www.joslin.org

Juvenile Diabetes Research Foundation

120 Wall Street
New York, NY 10005-4001
Toll-Free: 800-533-CURE (2873)
Fax: 212-785-9595
Website: http://www.jdrf.org
E-mail: info@jdrf.org

Klinefelter Syndrome and Associates

P.O. Box 119
Roseville, CA 95678-0119
Phone: 916-773-2999
Website: http://www.genetic.org/ks
E-mail: ksinfo@genetic.org

Learning Disabilities Association of America

4156 Library Road
Pittsburgh, PA 15234
Phone: 412-341-1515
Fax: 412-344-0224
Website: http://www.ldanatl.org
E-mail: info@ldaamerica.org

Leukemia and Lymphoma Society

1211 Mamaronek Avenue
White Plains, NY 10605
Phone: 914-949-5213
Fax: 914-949-6691
Website: http://www.leukemia.org

March of Dimes Birth Defects Foundation

1275 Mamaroneck Avenue
White Plains, NY 10605
Toll-Free: 888-MODIMES
Phone: 914-428-7100
Fax: 914-977-4537
Website: http://www.modimes.org

Maternal and Fetal Medicine

Genetics, Room 1988
4755 Ogletown-Stanton Road
P.O. Box 6001
Newark, DE 19718
Phone: 302-733-6732
Fax: 301-733-4339
Website: http://www.pitt.edu/
~marhgn

Muscular Dystrophy Association

3300 East Sunrise Drive
Tucson, AZ 85718-3208
Toll-Free: 800-572-1717
Website: http://www.mdausa.org
E-mail: mda@mdausa.org

Muscular Dystrophy Family Foundation

2330 North Meridian Street
Indianapolis, Indiana 46208-5730
Toll-Free: 800-544-1213
Phone: 317-632-6333
Website: http://www.mdff.org
E-mail: mdff@prodigy.net

National Alliance for Autism Research

99 Wall St.
Research Park
Princeton, NJ 08540
Toll-Free: 888-777-NAAR
Phone: 609-430-9160
Fax: 609-430-9163
Website: http://www.naar.org
E-mail: naar@naar.org

National Alliance for the Mentally Ill

Colonial Place Three
2107 Wilson Blvd.
Suite 300
Arlington, VA 22201
Toll-Free: 800-950-NAMI (6264)
Phone: 703-524-7600
TDD: 703-516-7227
Website: http://www.nami.org

National Cancer Institute

31 Center Drive, MSC 2580
Building 31, Room 10A16
Bethesda, MD 20892-2580
Website: http://oc.nci.nih.gov
E-mail: nciocomm-r@mail.nih.gov

National Down Syndrome Congress

7000 Peachtree-Dunwoody
Road, NE
Lake Ridge 400
Office Park
Building #5, Suite 100
Atlanta, GA 30328
Toll-Free: 800-232-6372
Phone: 770-604-9500
Website: http://
www.ndsccenter.org

National Down Syndrome Society

1370 Center Drive, Suite 102
Atlanta, GA 30338
Toll-Free: 800-232-NDSC
Phone: 770-604-9500
Website: http://www.ndss.org
E-mail: info@ndsccenter.org

National Fragile X Foundation
P.O. Box 190488
San Francisco, CA 94119
Toll-Free: 800-688-8765
Fax: 925-938-9315
Website: http://www.fraglex.org
E-mail: natlfx@fragilex.org

National Information Center for Children and Youth with Disabilities (NICHCY)
P.O. Box 1492
Washington, DC 20013-1492
Toll-Free: 800-695-0285
Fax: 202-884-8441
Website: http://www.nichcy.org
E-mail: nichcy@aed.org

National Institute of Mental Health (NIMH)
6001 Executive Boulevard
Room 8184, MSC 9663
Bethesda, MD 20892-9663
Phone: 301-443-4513
FAX: 301-443-4279
TTY: 301-443-8431
Website: http://
www.nimh.nih.gov
E-mail: nimhinfo@nh.gov

National Institute of Neurological Disorders and Stroke
P.O. Box 5801
Bethesda, MD 20824
Toll-Free: 800-352-9424
Phone: 301-496-5981
Website: http://
www.ninds.nih.gov

National Institute on Deafness and Other Communication Disorders
31 Center Drive
MSC 2320
Bethesda, MD 20892
Toll-Free: 800-241-1044
Phone: 301-496-7243
Website: http://
www.nidcd.nih.gov

National Scoliosis Foundation
5 Cabot Place
Stoughton, MA 02072
Toll-Free: 800-NSF-MYBACK
(800-673-6922)
Phone: 781-341-6333
Fax: 781-341-8333
Website: http://www.scoliosis.org
E-mail: NSF@scoliosis.org

National Society of Genetic Counselors
233 Canterbury Drive
Wallingford, PA 19086
Phone: 610-872-7608
Website: http://www.nsgc.org
E-mail: nsgc@nsgc.org

Parent Project for Muscular Dystrophy Research
1012 N. University Blvd.
Middletown OH 45042
Toll-Free: 800-714-KIDS
Phone: 513-424-0696
Fax: 513-425-9907
Website: http://
www.parentprojectmd.org
E-mail: ParentProject@aol.com

Ronald McDonald Houses

Ronald McDonald House
Coordinator
c/o McDonalds Corporation
1 Kroc Drive
Oak Brook, IL 60521
Phone: 312-836-7100

Scoliosis Association, Inc.

P.O. Box 811705
Boca Raton, FL 33481-1705
Toll-Free: 800-800-0669
Phone: 561-994-4435
Fax: 561-994-2455
Website: http://www.scoliosis-assoc.org

Scoliosis Research Society

611 East Wells Street
Milwaukee, WI 53202
Phone: 414-289-9107
Fax: 414-276-3349
Website: http://www.srs.org

Sickle Cell Disease Association of America

200 Corporate Pointe, Suite 495
Culver City, CA 90230-8727
Toll-Free: 800-421-8453
Phone: 310-216-6363
Fax: 310-215-3722
Website: http://sicklecelldisease.org
E-mail: scdaa@sicklecelldisease.org

Tourette Syndrome Association

42-40 Bell Boulevard
Bayside, NY 11361
Phone: 718-224-2999
Website: http://tsa-usa.org
E-mail: tsa@tsa-usa.org

United Cerebral Palsy Associations, Inc. and The United Cerebral Palsy Research and Educational Foundation

1660 L Street, NW
Suite 700
Washington, DC 20036
Toll-Free: 800-USA-5UCP
Website: http://www.ucpa.org

U.S. Department of Education

Office of Special Education
Programs
400 Maryland Ave., SW
Washington, DC 20202
Phone: 202-205-5507
Website: http://ed.gov/offices/OSERS/OSEP

Allergies

American Academy of Allergy, Asthma and Immunology

611 East Wells Street
Milwaukee, WI 53202
Toll-Free: 800-822-2762
Website: http://www.aaaai.org

American College of Allergy, Asthma and Immunology

85 W. Algonquin Road
Suite 550
Arlington Heights, IL 60005
Toll-Free: 800-842-7777
Website: http://allergy.mcg.edu

American Association of Immunologists
9650 Rockville Pike
Bethesda, MD 20814
Phone: 301-634-7178
Fax: 301-571-1816
Website: http://www.aai.org
E-mail: infoaai@aai.faseb.org

Asthma and Allergy Foundation of America
1125 15th Street, NW, Suite 502
Washington, DC 20036
Toll-Free: 800-7-ASTHMA
Website: http://www.aafa.org

Food Allergy Network
10400 Eaton Place, Suite 107
Fairfax, VA 22030
Toll-Free: 800-929-4040
Fax: 703-691-2713
Website: http://
www.foodallergy.org
E-mail: faan@foodallergy.org

National Foundation for the Chemically Hypersensitive
4407 Swinson Rd.
Rhodes, MI 48652
Phone: 989-689-6369
Website: http://
www.mcsrelief.com

National Institute of Allergy and Infectious Diseases
Building 31, Room 7A-50
31 Center Drive, MSC 2520
Bethesda, MD 20892-2520
Phone: 301-402-1663
Fax: 301-402-0120
Website: http://
www.niaid.nih.gov

Index

Index

617

W

walking pneumonia 98
warts 238–40, 265–68
"Warts" (American Academy of Dermatology) 265n
weight gain, cancer treatment 397
Weledniger, Richard M. 151n
"What Is Thalassemia?" (Cooley's Anemia Foundation) 415n
white blood cell count, described 20
WHO *see* World Health Organization
whooping cough *see* pertussis
Woolston, Chris 153n, 157
World Health Organization (WHO), contact information 601

X

X-linked interitance, described 577
XXY males 443–48

Y

Yersinia entercolitica 182–84
"*Yersinia Enterocolitica*" (CDC) 182n
yersiniosis 182–84
"Young People with Cancer, A Handbook for Parents" (NCI) 368n, 384n
"Your Child and Medication" (NIMH) 29n

Z

zafirlukast 47
zalcitabine (ddC) 406
Zamula, Evelyn 33n, 38
ZDV *see* zidovudine
Zerit (stavudine) 406
Ziagen (abacavir) 405
zidovudine (AZT; ZDV) 406–7
Zilactin 154
zileuton 47
zinc oxide 236
Zovirax (acyclovir) 287
Zyflo (zileuton) 47

Health Reference Series
COMPLETE CATALOG

Adolescent Health Sourcebook

Basic Consumer Health Information about Common Medical, Mental, and Emotional Concerns in Adolescents, Including Facts about Acne, Body Piercing, Mononucleosis, Nutrition, Eating Disorders, Stress, Depression, Behavior Problems, Peer Pressure, Violence, Gangs, Drug Use, Puberty, Sexuality, Pregnancy, Learning Disabilities, and More

Along with a Glossary of Terms and Other Resources for Further Help and Information

Edited by Chad T. Kimball. 658 pages. 2002. 0-7808-0248-9. $78.

"A good starting point for information related to common medical, mental, and emotional concerns of adolescents." — *School Library Journal, Nov '02*

"This book provides accurate information in an easy to access format. It addresses topics that parents and caregivers might not be aware of and provides practical, useable information." — *Doody's Health Sciences Book Review Journal, Sep-Oct '02*

"Recommended reference source."
— *Booklist, American Library Association, Sep '02*

—

AIDS Sourcebook, 1st Edition

Basic Information about AIDS and HIV Infection, Featuring Historical and Statistical Data, Current Research, Prevention, and Other Special Topics of Interest for Persons Living with AIDS

Along with Source Listings for Further Assistance

Edited by Karen Bellenir and Peter D. Dresser. 831 pages. 1995. 0-7808-0031-1. $78.

"One strength of this book is its practical emphasis. The intended audience is the lay reader . . . useful as an educational tool for health care providers who work with AIDS patients. Recommended for public libraries as well as hospital or academic libraries that collect consumer materials."
— *Bulletin of the Medical Library Association, Jan '96*

"This is the most comprehensive volume of its kind on an important medical topic. Highly recommended for all libraries." — *Reference Book Review, '96*

"Very useful reference for all libraries."
— *Choice, Association of College and Research Libraries, Oct '95*

"There is a wealth of information here that can provide much educational assistance. It is a must book for all libraries and should be on the desk of each and every congressional leader. Highly recommended."
— *AIDS Book Review Journal, Aug '95*

"Recommended for most collections."
— *Library Journal, Jul '95*

AIDS Sourcebook, 2nd Edition

Basic Consumer Health Information about Acquired Immune Deficiency Syndrome (AIDS) and Human Immunodeficiency Virus (HIV) Infection, Featuring Updated Statistical Data, Reports on Recent Research and Prevention Initiatives, and Other Special Topics of Interest for Persons Living with AIDS, Including New Antiretroviral Treatment Options, Strategies for Combating Opportunistic Infections, Information about Clinical Trials, and More

Along with a Glossary of Important Terms and Resource Listings for Further Help and Information

Edited by Karen Bellenir. 751 pages. 1999. 0-7808-0225-X. $78.

"Highly recommended."
— *American Reference Books Annual, 2000*

"Excellent sourcebook. This continues to be a highly recommended book. There is no other book that provides as much information as this book provides."
— *AIDS Book Review Journal, Dec-Jan 2000*

"Recommended reference source."
— *Booklist, American Library Association, Dec '99*

"A solid text for college-level health libraries."
— *The Bookwatch, Aug '99*

Cited in *Reference Sources for Small and Medium-Sized Libraries, American Library Association, 1999*

—

AIDS Sourcebook, 3rd Edition

Basic Consumer Health Information about Acquired Immune Deficiency Syndrome (AIDS) and Human Immunodeficiency Virus (HIV) Infection, Including Facts about Transmission, Prevention, Diagnosis, Treatment, Opportunistic Infections, and Other Complications, with a Section for Women and Children, Including Details about Associated Gynecological Concerns, Pregnancy, and Pediatric Care

Along with Updated Statistical Information, Reports on Current Research Initiatives, a Glossary, and Directories of Internet, Hotline, and Other Resources

Edited by Dawn D. Matthews. 664 pages. 2003. 0-7808-0631-X. $78.

—

Alcoholism Sourcebook

Basic Consumer Health Information about the Physical and Mental Consequences of Alcohol Abuse, Including Liver Disease, Pancreatitis, Wernicke-Korsakoff Syndrome (Alcoholic Dementia), Fetal Alcohol Syndrome, Heart Disease, Kidney Disorders, Gastrointestinal Problems, and Immune System Compromise and Featuring Facts about Addiction, Detoxification, Alcohol Withdrawal, Recovery, and the Maintenance of Sobriety

Along with a Glossary and Directories of Resources for Further Help and Information

Edited by Karen Bellenir. 613 pages. 2000. 0-7808-0325-6. $78.

"This title is one of the few reference works on alcoholism for general readers. For some readers this will be a welcome complement to the many self-help books on the market. Recommended for collections serving general readers and consumer health collections."
— E-Streams, Mar '01

"This book is an excellent choice for public and academic libraries."
— American Reference Books Annual, 2001

"Recommended reference source."
— Booklist, American Library Association, Dec '00

"Presents a wealth of information on alcohol use and abuse and its effects on the body and mind, treatment, and prevention." — SciTech Book News, Dec '00

"Important new health guide which packs in the latest consumer information about the problems of alcoholism." — Reviewer's Bookwatch, Nov '00

SEE ALSO Drug Abuse Sourcebook, Substance Abuse Sourcebook

Allergies Sourcebook, 1st Edition

Basic Information about Major Forms and Mechanisms of Common Allergic Reactions, Sensitivities, and Intolerances, Including Anaphylaxis, Asthma, Hives and Other Dermatologic Symptoms, Rhinitis, and Sinusitis Along with Their Usual Triggers Like Animal Fur, Chemicals, Drugs, Dust, Foods, Insects, Latex, Pollen, and Poison Ivy, Oak, and Sumac; Plus Information on Prevention, Identification, and Treatment

Edited by Allan R. Cook. 611 pages. 1997. 0-7808-0036-2. $78.

Allergies Sourcebook, 2nd Edition

Basic Consumer Health Information about Allergic Disorders, Triggers, Reactions, and Related Symptoms, Including Anaphylaxis, Rhinitis, Sinusitis, Asthma, Dermatitis, Conjunctivitis, and Multiple Chemical Sensitivity

Along with Tips on Diagnosis, Prevention, and Treatment, Statistical Data, a Glossary, and a Directory of Sources for Further Help and Information

Edited by Annemarie S. Muth. 598 pages. 2002. 0-7808-0376-0. $78.

"This second edition would be useful to laypersons with little or advanced knowledge of the subject matter. This book would also serve as a resource for nursing and other health care professions students. It would be useful in public, academic, and hospital libraries with consumer health collections." — E-Streams, Jul '02

Alternative Medicine Sourcebook, 1st Edition

Basic Consumer Health Information about Alternatives to Conventional Medicine, Including Acupressure, Acupuncture, Aromatherapy, Ayurveda, Bioelectromagnetics, Environmental Medicine, Essence Therapy, Food and Nutrition Therapy, Herbal Therapy, Homeopathy, Imaging, Massage, Naturopathy, Reflexology, Relaxation and Meditation, Sound Therapy, Vitamin and Mineral Therapy, and Yoga, and More

Edited by Allan R. Cook. 737 pages. 1999. 0-7808-0200-4. $78.

"Recommended reference source."
— Booklist, American Library Association, Feb '00

"A great addition to the reference collection of every type of library." — American Reference Books Annual, 2000

Alternative Medicine Sourcebook, 2nd Edition

Basic Consumer Health Information about Alternative and Complementary Medical Practices, Including Acupuncture, Chiropractic, Herbal Medicine, Homeopathy, Naturopathic Medicine, Mind-Body Interventions, Ayurveda, and Other Non-Western Medical Traditions

Along with Facts about such Specific Therapies as Massage Therapy, Aromatherapy, Qigong, Hypnosis, Prayer, Dance, and Art Therapies, a Glossary, and Resources for Further Information

Edited by Dawn D. Matthews. 618 pages. 2002. 0-7808-0605-0. $78.

"An important alternate health reference."
— MBR Bookwatch, Oct '02

Alzheimer's, Stroke & 29 Other Neurological Disorders Sourcebook, 1st Edition

Basic Information for the Layperson on 31 Diseases or Disorders Affecting the Brain and Nervous System, First Describing the Illness, Then Listing Symptoms, Diagnostic Methods, and Treatment Options, and Including Statistics on Incidences and Causes

Edited by Frank E. Bair. 579 pages. 1993. 1-55888-748-2. $78.

"Nontechnical reference book that provides reader-friendly information."
— Family Caregiver Alliance Update, Winter '96

"Should be included in any library's patient education section." — American Reference Books Annual, 1994

"Written in an approachable and accessible style. Recommended for patient education and consumer health collections in health science center and public libraries." — Academic Library Book Review, Dec '93

"It is very handy to have information on more than thirty neurological disorders under one cover, and there is no recent source like it." — *Reference Quarterly, American Library Association, Fall '93*

SEE ALSO Brain Disorders Sourcebook

Alzheimer's Disease Sourcebook, 2nd Edition

Basic Consumer Health Information about Alzheimer's Disease, Related Disorders, and Other Dementias, Including Multi-Infarct Dementia, AIDS-Related Dementia, Alcoholic Dementia, Huntington's Disease, Delirium, and Confusional States

Along with Reports Detailing Current Research Efforts in Prevention and Treatment, Long-Term Care Issues, and Listings of Sources for Additional Help and Information

Edited by Karen Bellenir. 524 pages. 1999. 0-7808-0223-3. $78.

"Provides a wealth of useful information not otherwise available in one place. This resource is recommended for all types of libraries."
— *American Reference Books Annual, 2000*

"Recommended reference source."
— *Booklist, American Library Association, Oct '99*

Arthritis Sourcebook

Basic Consumer Health Information about Specific Forms of Arthritis and Related Disorders, Including Rheumatoid Arthritis, Osteoarthritis, Gout, Polymyalgia Rheumatica, Psoriatic Arthritis, Spondyloarthropathies, Juvenile Rheumatoid Arthritis, and Juvenile Ankylosing Spondylitis

Along with Information about Medical, Surgical, and Alternative Treatment Options, and Including Strategies for Coping with Pain, Fatigue, and Stress

Edited by Allan R. Cook. 550 pages. 1998. 0-7808-0201-2. $78.

". . . accessible to the layperson."
— *Reference and Research Book News, Feb '99*

Asthma Sourcebook

Basic Consumer Health Information about Asthma, Including Symptoms, Traditional and Nontraditional Remedies, Treatment Advances, Quality-of-Life Aids, Medical Research Updates, and the Role of Allergies, Exercise, Age, the Environment, and Genetics in the Development of Asthma

Along with Statistical Data, a Glossary, and Directories of Support Groups, and Other Resources for Further Information

Edited by Annemarie S. Muth. 628 pages. 2000. 0-7808-0381-7. $78.

"A worthwhile reference acquisition for public libraries and academic medical libraries whose readers desire a quick introduction to the wide range of asthma information." — *Choice, Association of College & Research Libraries, Jun '01*

"Recommended reference source."
— *Booklist, American Library Association, Feb '01*

"Highly recommended." — *The Bookwatch, Jan '01*

"There is much good information for patients and their families who deal with asthma daily."
— *American Medical Writers Association Journal, Winter '01*

"This informative text is recommended for consumer health collections in public, secondary school, and community college libraries and the libraries of universities with a large undergraduate population."
— *American Reference Books Annual, 2001*

Attention Deficit Disorder Sourcebook

Basic Consumer Health Information about Attention Deficit/Hyperactivity Disorder in Children and Adults, Including Facts about Causes, Symptoms, Diagnostic Criteria, and Treatment Options Such as Medications, Behavior Therapy, Coaching, and Homeopathy

Along with Reports on Current Research Initiatives, Legal Issues, and Government Regulations, and Featuring a Glossary of Related Terms, Internet Resources, and a List of Additional Reading Material

Edited by Dawn D. Matthews. 470 pages. 2002. 0-7808-0624-7. $78.

Back & Neck Disorders Sourcebook

Basic Information about Disorders and Injuries of the Spinal Cord and Vertebrae, Including Facts on Chiropractic Treatment, Surgical Interventions, Paralysis, and Rehabilitation

Along with Advice for Preventing Back Trouble

Edited by Karen Bellenir. 548 pages. 1997. 0-7808-0202-0. $78.

"The strength of this work is its basic, easy-to-read format. Recommended."
— *Reference and User Services Quarterly, American Library Association, Winter '97*

Blood & Circulatory Disorders Sourcebook

Basic Information about Blood and Its Components, Anemias, Leukemias, Bleeding Disorders, and Circulatory Disorders, Including Aplastic Anemia, Thalassemia, Sickle-Cell Disease, Hemochromatosis, Hemophilia, Von Willebrand Disease, and Vascular Diseases

Along with a Special Section on Blood Transfusions and Blood Supply Safety, a Glossary, and Source Listings for Further Help and Information

Edited by Karen Bellenir and Linda M. Shin. 554 pages. 1998. 0-7808-0203-9. $78.

"Recommended reference source."
—*Booklist, American Library Association, Feb '99*

"An important reference sourcebook written in simple language for everyday, non-technical users. "
—*Reviewer's Bookwatch, Jan '99*

Brain Disorders Sourcebook

Basic Consumer Health Information about Strokes, Epilepsy, Amyotrophic Lateral Sclerosis (ALS/Lou Gehrig's Disease), Parkinson's Disease, Brain Tumors, Cerebral Palsy, Headache, Tourette Syndrome, and More

Along with Statistical Data, Treatment and Rehabilitation Options, Coping Strategies, Reports on Current Research Initiatives, a Glossary, and Resource Listings for Additional Help and Information

Edited by Karen Bellenir. 481 pages. 1999. 0-7808-0229-2. $78.

"Belongs on the shelves of any library with a consumer health collection."   —*E-Streams, Mar '00*

"Recommended reference source."
—*Booklist, American Library Association, Oct '99*

SEE ALSO Alzheimer's Disease Sourcebook, 2nd Edition

Breast Cancer Sourcebook

Basic Consumer Health Information about Breast Cancer, Including Diagnostic Methods, Treatment Options, Alternative Therapies, Self-Help Information, Related Health Concerns, Statistical and Demographic Data, and Facts for Men with Breast Cancer

Along with Reports on Current Research Initiatives, a Glossary of Related Medical Terms, and a Directory of Sources for Further Help and Information

Edited by Edward J. Prucha and Karen Bellenir. 580 pages. 2001. 0-7808-0244-6. $78.

"Recommended reference source."
—*Booklist, American Library Association, Jan '02*

"This reference source is highly recommended. It is quite informative, comprehensive and detailed in nature, and yet it offers practical advice in easy-to-read language. It could be thought of as the 'bible' of breast cancer for the consumer."   —*E-Streams, Jan '02*

"The broad range of topics covered in lay language make the *Breast Cancer Sourcebook* an excellent addition to public and consumer health library collections."
—*American Reference Books Annual 2002*

"From the pros and cons of different screening methods and results to treatment options, *Breast Cancer Sourcebook* provides the latest information on the subject."
—*Library Bookwatch, Dec '01*

"This thoroughgoing, very readable reference covers all aspects of breast health and cancer. . . . Readers will find much to consider here. Recommended for all public and patient health collections."
—*Library Journal, Sep '01*

SEE ALSO Cancer Sourcebook for Women, 1st and 2nd Editions, Women's Health Concerns Sourcebook

---

Breastfeeding Sourcebook

Basic Consumer Health Information about the Benefits of Breastmilk, Preparing to Breastfeed, Breastfeeding as a Baby Grows, Nutrition, and More, Including Information on Special Situations and Concerns Such as Mastitis, Illness, Medications, Allergies, Multiple Births, Prematurity, Special Needs, and Adoption

Along with a Glossary and Resources for Additional Help and Information

Edited by Jenni Lynn Colson. 388 pages. 2002. 0-7808-0332-9. $78.

SEE ALSO Pregnancy & Birth Sourcebook

Burns Sourcebook

Basic Consumer Health Information about Various Types of Burns and Scalds, Including Flame, Heat, Cold, Electrical, Chemical, and Sun Burns

Along with Information on Short-Term and Long-Term Treatments, Tissue Reconstruction, Plastic Surgery, Prevention Suggestions, and First Aid

Edited by Allan R. Cook. 604 pages. 1999. 0-7808-0204-7. $78.

"This is an exceptional addition to the series and is highly recommended for all consumer health collections, hospital libraries, and academic medical centers."
—*E-Streams, Mar '00*

"This key reference guide is an invaluable addition to all health care and public libraries in confronting this ongoing health issue."
—*American Reference Books Annual, 2000*

"Recommended reference source."
—*Booklist, American Library Association, Dec '99*

SEE ALSO Skin Disorders Sourcebook

Cancer Sourcebook, 1st Edition

Basic Information on Cancer Types, Symptoms, Diagnostic Methods, and Treatments, Including Statistics on Cancer Occurrences Worldwide and the Risks Associated with Known Carcinogens and Activities

Edited by Frank E. Bair. 932 pages. 1990. 1-55888-888-8. $78.

Cited in Reference Sources for Small and Medium-Sized Libraries, American Library Association, 1999

"Written in nontechnical language. Useful for patients, their families, medical professionals, and librarians."
—*Guide to Reference Books, 1996*

"Designed with the non-medical professional in mind. Libraries and medical facilities interested in patient education should certainly consider adding the *Cancer Sourcebook* to their holdings. This compact collection of reliable information . . . is an invaluable tool for helping patients and patients' families and friends to take the first steps in coping with the many difficulties of cancer."
— *Medical Reference Services Quarterly, Winter '91*

"Specifically created for the nontechnical reader . . . an important resource for the general reader trying to understand the complexities of cancer."
— *American Reference Books Annual, 1991*

"This publication's nontechnical nature and very comprehensive format make it useful for both the general public and undergraduate students."
— *Choice, Association of College and Research Libraries, Oct '90*

New Cancer Sourcebook, 2nd Edition

Basic Information about Major Forms and Stages of Cancer, Featuring Facts about Primary and Secondary Tumors of the Respiratory, Nervous, Lymphatic, Circulatory, Skeletal, and Gastrointestinal Systems; Specific Organs; Statistical and Demographic Data; Treatment Options; and Strategies for Coping

Edited by Allan R. Cook. 1,313 pages. 1996. 0-7808-0041-9. $78.

"An excellent resource for patients with newly diagnosed cancer and their families. The dialogue is simple, direct, and comprehensive. Highly recommended for patients and families to aid in their understanding of cancer and its treatment."
— *Booklist Health Sciences Supplement, American Library Association, Oct '97*

"The amount of factual and useful information is extensive. The writing is very clear, geared to general readers. Recommended for all levels." — *Choice, Association of College & Research Libraries, Jan '97*

Cancer Sourcebook, 3rd Edition

Basic Consumer Health Information about Major Forms and Stages of Cancer, Featuring Facts about Primary and Secondary Tumors of the Respiratory, Nervous, Lymphatic, Circulatory, Skeletal, and Gastrointestinal Systems, and Specific Organs

Along with Statistical and Demographic Data, Treatment Options, Strategies for Coping, a Glossary, and a Directory of Sources for Additional Help and Information

Edited by Edward J. Prucha. 1,069 pages. 2000. 0-7808-0227-6. $78.

"This title is recommended for health sciences and public libraries with consumer health collections."
— *E-Streams, Feb '01*

". . . can be effectively used by cancer patients and their families who are looking for answers in a language they can understand. Public and hospital libraries should have it on their shelves."
— *American Reference Books Annual, 2001*

"Recommended reference source."
— *Booklist, American Library Association, Dec '00*

Cancer Sourcebook, Fourth Edition

Basic Consumer Health Information about Major Forms and Stages of Cancer, Featuring Facts about Head and Neck Cancers, Lung Cancers, Gastrointestinal Cancers, Genitourinary Cancers, Lymphomas, Blood Cell Cancers, Endocrine Cancers, Skin Cancers, Bone Cancers, Sarcomas, and Others, and Including Information about Cancer Treatments and Therapies, Identifying and Reducing Cancer Risks, and Strategies for Coping with Cancer and the Side Effects of Treatment

Along with a Cancer Glossary, Statistical and Demographic Data, and a Directory of Sources for Additional Help and Information

Edited by Karen Bellenir. 966 pages. 2003. 0-7808-0633-6. $78.

Cancer Sourcebook for Women, 1st Edition

Basic Information about Specific Forms of Cancer That Affect Women, Featuring Facts about Breast Cancer, Cervical Cancer, Ovarian Cancer, Cancer of the Uterus and Uterine Sarcoma, Cancer of the Vagina, and Cancer of the Vulva; Statistical and Demographic Data; Treatments, Self-Help Management Suggestions, and Current Research Initiatives

Edited by Allan R. Cook and Peter D. Dresser. 524 pages. 1996. 0-7808-0076-1. $78.

". . . written in easily understandable, non-technical language. Recommended for public libraries or hospital and academic libraries that collect patient education or consumer health materials."
— *Medical Reference Services Quarterly, Spring '97*

"Would be of value in a consumer health library. . . . written with the health care consumer in mind. Medical jargon is at a minimum, and medical terms are explained in clear, understandable sentences."
— *Bulletin of the Medical Library Association, Oct '96*

"The availability under one cover of all these pertinent publications, grouped under cohesive headings, makes this certainly a most useful sourcebook." — *Choice, Association of College & Research Libraries, Jun '96*

"Presents a comprehensive knowledge base for general readers. Men and women both benefit from the gold mine of information nestled between the two covers of this book. Recommended."
— *Academic Library Book Review, Summer '96*

Cancer Sourcebook for Women, 2nd Edition

Basic Consumer Health Information about Gynecologic Cancers and Related Concerns, Including Cervical Cancer, Endometrial Cancer, Gestational Trophoblastic Tumor, Ovarian Cancer, Uterine Cancer, Vaginal Cancer, Vulvar Cancer, Breast Cancer, and Common Non-Cancerous Uterine Conditions, with Facts about Cancer Risk Factors, Screening and Prevention, Treatment Options, and Reports on Current Research Initiatives

Along with a Glossary of Cancer Terms and a Directory of Resources for Additional Help and Information

Edited by Karen Bellenir. 604 pages. 2002. 0-7808-0226-8. $78.

SEE ALSO *Breast Cancer Sourcebook, Women's Health Concerns Sourcebook*

Cardiovascular Diseases & Disorders Sourcebook, 1st Edition

Basic Information about Cardiovascular Diseases and Disorders, Featuring Facts about the Cardiovascular System, Demographic and Statistical Data, Descriptions of Pharmacological and Surgical Interventions, Lifestyle Modifications, and a Special Section Focusing on Heart Disorders in Children

Edited by Karen Bellenir and Peter D. Dresser. 683 pages. 1995. 0-7808-0032-X. $78.

SEE ALSO *Healthy Heart Sourcebook for Women, Heart Diseases & Disorders Sourcebook, 2nd Edition*

Caregiving Sourcebook

Basic Consumer Health Information for Caregivers, Including a Profile of Caregivers, Caregiving Responsibilities and Concerns, Tips for Specific Conditions, Care Environments, and the Effects of Caregiving

Along with Facts about Legal Issues, Financial Information, and Future Planning, a Glossary, and a Listing of Additional Resources

Edited by Joyce Brennfleck Shannon. 600 pages. 2001. 0-7808-0331-0. $78.

Childhood Diseases & Disorders Sourcebook

Basic Consumer Health Information about Medical Problems Often Encountered in Pre-Adolescent Children, Including Respiratory Tract Ailments, Ear Infections, Sore Throats, Disorders of the Skin and Scalp, Digestive and Genitourinary Diseases, Infectious Diseases, Inflammatory Disorders, Chronic Physical and Developmental Disorders, Allergies, and More

Along with Information about Diagnostic Tests, Common Childhood Surgeries, and Frequently Used Medications, with a Glossary of Important Terms and Resource Directory

Edited by Chad T. Kimball. 662 pages. 2003. 0-7808-0458-9. $78.

Colds, Flu & Other Common Ailments Sourcebook

Basic Consumer Health Information about Common Ailments and Injuries, Including Colds, Coughs, the Flu, Sinus Problems, Headaches, Fever, Nausea and Vomiting, Menstrual Cramps, Diarrhea, Constipation, Hemorrhoids, Back Pain, Dandruff, Dry and Itchy Skin, Cuts, Scrapes, Sprains, Bruises, and More

Along with Information about Prevention, Self-Care, Choosing a Doctor, Over-the-Counter Medications, Folk Remedies, and Alternative Therapies, and Including a Glossary of Important Terms and a Directory of Resources for Further Help and Information

Edited by Chad T. Kimball. 638 pages. 2001. 0-7808-0435-X. $78.

"Will prove valuable to any library seeking to maintain a current, comprehensive reference collection of health resources. . . . Excellent reference."
— *The Bookwatch, Aug '01*

"Recommended reference source."
— *Booklist, American Library Association, July '01*

Communication Disorders Sourcebook

Basic Information about Deafness and Hearing Loss, Speech and Language Disorders, Voice Disorders, Balance and Vestibular Disorders, and Disorders of Smell, Taste, and Touch

Edited by Linda M. Ross. 533 pages. 1996. 0-7808-0077-X. $78.

"This is skillfully edited and is a welcome resource for the layperson. It should be found in every public and medical library." — *Booklist Health Sciences Supplement, American Library Association, Oct '97*

Congenital Disorders Sourcebook

Basic Information about Disorders Acquired during Gestation, Including Spina Bifida, Hydrocephalus, Cerebral Palsy, Heart Defects, Craniofacial Abnormalities, Fetal Alcohol Syndrome, and More

Along with Current Treatment Options and Statistical Data

Edited by Karen Bellenir. 607 pages. 1997. 0-7808-0205-5. $78.

"Recommended reference source."
— *Booklist, American Library Association, Oct '97*

SEE ALSO Pregnancy & Birth Sourcebook

Consumer Issues in Health Care Sourcebook

Basic Information about Health Care Fundamentals and Related Consumer Issues, Including Exams and Screening Tests, Physician Specialties, Choosing a Doctor, Using Prescription and Over-the-Counter Medications Safely, Avoiding Health Scams, Managing Common Health Risks in the Home, Care Options for Chronically or Terminally Ill Patients, and a List of Resources for Obtaining Help and Further Information

Edited by Karen Bellenir. 618 pages. 1998. 0-7808-0221-7. $78.

"Both public and academic libraries will want to have a copy in their collection for readers who are interested in self-education on health issues."
— *American Reference Books Annual, 2000*

"The editor has researched the literature from government agencies and others, saving readers the time and effort of having to do the research themselves. Recommended for public libraries."
— *Reference and User Services Quarterly, American Library Association, Spring '99*

"Recommended reference source."
— *Booklist, American Library Association, Dec '98*

Contagious & Non-Contagious Infectious Diseases Sourcebook

Basic Information about Contagious Diseases like Measles, Polio, Hepatitis B, and Infectious Mononucleosis, and Non-Contagious Infectious Diseases like Tetanus and Toxic Shock Syndrome, and Diseases Occurring as Secondary Infections Such as Shingles and Reye Syndrome

Along with Vaccination, Prevention, and Treatment Information, and a Section Describing Emerging Infectious Disease Threats

Edited by Karen Bellenir and Peter D. Dresser. 566 pages. 1996. 0-7808-0075-3. $78.

Death & Dying Sourcebook

Basic Consumer Health Information for the Layperson about End-of-Life Care and Related Ethical and Legal Issues, Including Chief Causes of Death, Autopsies, Pain Management for the Terminally Ill, Life Support Systems, Insurance, Euthanasia, Assisted Suicide, Hospice Programs, Living Wills, Funeral Planning, Counseling, Mourning, Organ Donation, and Physician Training

Along with Statistical Data, a Glossary, and Listings of Sources for Further Help and Information

Edited by Annemarie S. Muth. 641 pages. 1999. 0-7808-0230-6. $78.

"Public libraries, medical libraries, and academic libraries will all find this sourcebook a useful addition to their collections."
— *American Reference Books Annual, 2001*

"An extremely useful resource for those concerned with death and dying in the United States."
— *Respiratory Care, Nov '00*

"Recommended reference source."
— *Booklist, American Library Association, Aug '00*

"This book is a definite must for all those involved in end-of-life care." — *Doody's Review Service, 2000*

Depression Sourcebook

Basic Consumer Health Information about Unipolar Depression, Bipolar Disorder, Postpartum Depression, Seasonal Affective Disorder, and Other Types of Depression in Children, Adolescents, Women, Men, the Elderly, and Other Selected Populations

Along with Facts about Causes, Risk Factors, Diagnostic Criteria, Treatment Options, Coping Strategies, Suicide Prevention, a Glossary, and a Directory of Sources for Additional Help and Information

Edited by Karen Belleni. 602 pages. 2002. 0-7808-0611-5. $78.

Diabetes Sourcebook, 1st Edition

Basic Information about Insulin-Dependent and Non-insulin-Dependent Diabetes Mellitus, Gestational Diabetes, and Diabetic Complications, Symptoms, Treatment, and Research Results, Including Statistics on Prevalence, Morbidity, and Mortality

Along with Source Listings for Further Help and Information

Edited by Karen Bellenir and Peter D. Dresser. 827 pages. 1994. 1-55888-751-2. $78.

". . . very informative and understandable for the layperson without being simplistic. It provides a comprehensive overview for laypersons who want a general understanding of the disease or who want to focus on various aspects of the disease."
— Bulletin of the Medical Library Association, Jan '96

Diabetes Sourcebook, 2nd Edition

Basic Consumer Health Information about Type 1 Diabetes (Insulin-Dependent or Juvenile-Onset Diabetes), Type 2 (Noninsulin-Dependent or Adult-Onset Diabetes), Gestational Diabetes, and Related Disorders, Including Diabetes Prevalence Data, Management Issues, the Role of Diet and Exercise in Controlling Diabetes, Insulin and Other Diabetes Medicines, and Complications of Diabetes Such as Eye Diseases, Periodontal Disease, Amputation, and End-Stage Renal Disease

Along with Reports on Current Research Initiatives, a Glossary, and Resource Listings for Further Help and Information

Edited by Karen Bellenir. 688 pages. 1998. 0-7808-0224-1. $78.

"An invaluable reference." — Library Journal, May '00

Selected as one of the 250 "Best Health Sciences Books of 1999." — Doody's Rating Service, Mar-Apr 2000

"This comprehensive book is an excellent addition for high school, academic, medical, and public libraries. This volume is highly recommended."
— American Reference Books Annual, 2000

"Provides useful information for the general public."
— Healthlines, University of Michigan Health Management Research Center, Sep/Oct '99

". . . provides reliable mainstream medical information . . . belongs on the shelves of any library with a consumer health collection." — E-Streams, Sep '99

"Recommended reference source."
— Booklist, American Library Association, Feb '99

Diabetes Sourcebook, 3rd Edition

Basic Consumer Health Information about Type 1 Diabetes (Insulin-Dependent or Juvenile-Onset Diabetes), Type 2 Diabetes (Noninsulin-Dependent or Adult-Onset Diabetes), Gestational Diabetes, Impaired Glucose Tolerance (IGT), and Related Complications, Such as Amputation, Eye Disease, Gum Disease, Nerve Damage, and End-Stage Renal Disease, Including Facts

about Insulin, Oral Diabetes Medications, Blood Sugar Testing, and the Role of Exercise and Nutrition in the Control of Diabetes

Along with a Glossary and Resources for Further Help and Information

Edited by Dawn D. Matthews. 622 pages. 2003. 0-7808-0629-8. $78.

Diet & Nutrition Sourcebook, 1st Edition

Basic Information about Nutrition, Including the Dietary Guidelines for Americans, the Food Guide Pyramid, and Their Applications in Daily Diet, Nutritional Advice for Specific Age Groups, Current Nutritional Issues and Controversies, the New Food Label and How to Use It to Promote Healthy Eating, and Recent Developments in Nutritional Research

Edited by Dan R. Harris. 662 pages. 1996. 0-7808-0084-2. $78.

"Useful reference as a food and nutrition sourcebook for the general consumer." — Booklist Health Sciences Supplement, American Library Association, Oct '97

"Recommended for public libraries and medical libraries that receive general information requests on nutrition. It is readable and will appeal to those interested in learning more about healthy dietary practices."
— Medical Reference Services Quarterly, Fall '97

"An abundance of medical and social statistics is translated into readable information geared toward the general reader." — Bookwatch, Mar '97

"With dozens of questionable diet books on the market, it is so refreshing to find a reliable and factual reference book. Recommended to aspiring professionals, librarians, and others seeking and giving reliable dietary advice. An excellent compilation." — Choice, Association of College and Research Libraries, Feb '97

SEE ALSO Digestive Diseases & Disorders Sourcebook, Gastrointestinal Diseases & Disorders Sourcebook

Diet & Nutrition Sourcebook, 2nd Edition

Basic Consumer Health Information about Dietary Guidelines, Recommended Daily Intake Values, Vitamins, Minerals, Fiber, Fat, Weight Control, Dietary Supplements, and Food Additives

Along with Special Sections on Nutrition Needs throughout Life and Nutrition for People with Such Specific Medical Concerns as Allergies, High Blood Cholesterol, Hypertension, Diabetes, Celiac Disease, Seizure Disorders, Phenylketonuria (PKU), Cancer, and Eating Disorders, and Including Reports on Current Nutrition Research and Source Listings for Additional Help and Information

Edited by Karen Bellenir. 650 pages. 1999. 0-7808-0228-4. $78.

"This book is an excellent source of basic diet and nutrition information." — *Booklist Health Sciences Supplement, American Library Association, Dec '00*

"This reference document should be in any public library, but it would be a very good guide for beginning students in the health sciences. If the other books in this publisher's series are as good as this, they should all be in the health sciences collections." —*American Reference Books Annual, 2000*

"This book is an excellent general nutrition reference for consumers who desire to take an active role in their health care for prevention. Consumers of all ages who select this book can feel confident they are receiving current and accurate information." — *Journal of Nutrition for the Elderly, Vol. 19, No. 4, '00*

"Recommended reference source." —*Booklist, American Library Association, Dec '99*

SEE ALSO *Digestive Diseases & Disorders Sourcebook, Gastrointestinal Diseases & Disorders Sourcebook*

Digestive Diseases & Disorders Sourcebook

Basic Consumer Health Information about Diseases and Disorders that Impact the Upper and Lower Digestive System, Including Celiac Disease, Constipation, Crohn's Disease, Cyclic Vomiting Syndrome, Diarrhea, Diverticulosis and Diverticulitis, Gallstones, Heartburn, Hemorrhoids, Hernias, Indigestion (Dyspepsia), Irritable Bowel Syndrome, Lactose Intolerance, Ulcers, and More

Along with Information about Medications and Other Treatments, Tips for Maintaining a Healthy Digestive Tract, a Glossary, and Directory of Digestive Diseases Organizations

Edited by Karen Bellenir. 335 pages. 2000. 0-7808-0327-2. $78.

"This title would be an excellent addition to all public or patient-research libraries." —*American Reference Books Annual, 2001*

"This title is recommended for public, hospital, and health sciences libraries with consumer health collections." — *E-Streams, Jul-Aug '00*

"Recommended reference source." —*Booklist, American Library Association, May '00*

SEE ALSO *Diet & Nutrition Sourcebook, 1st and 2nd Editions, Gastrointestinal Diseases & Disorders Sourcebook*

Disabilities Sourcebook

Basic Consumer Health Information about Physical and Psychiatric Disabilities, Including Descriptions of Major Causes of Disability, Assistive and Adaptive Aids, Workplace Issues, and Accessibility Concerns

Along with Information about the Americans with Disabilities Act, a Glossary, and Resources for Additional Help and Information

Edited by Dawn D. Matthews. 616 pages. 2000. 0-7808-0389-2. $78.

"It is a must for libraries with a consumer health section." — *American Reference Books Annual 2002*

"A much needed addition to the Omnigraphics *Health Reference Series*. A current reference work to provide people with disabilities, their families, caregivers or those who work with them, a broad range of information in one volume, has not been available until now. . . . It is recommended for all public and academic library reference collections." — *E-Streams, May '01*

"An excellent source book in easy-to-read format covering many current topics; highly recommended for all libraries." — *Choice, Association of College and Research Libraries, Jan '01*

"Recommended reference source." —*Booklist, American Library Association, Jul '00*

Domestic Violence & Child Abuse Sourcebook

Basic Consumer Health Information about Spousal/ Partner, Child, Sibling, Parent, and Elder Abuse, Covering Physical, Emotional, and Sexual Abuse, Teen Dating Violence, and Stalking; Includes Information about Hotlines, Safe Houses, Safety Plans, and Other Resources for Support and Assistance, Community Initiatives, and Reports on Current Directions in Research and Treatment

Along with a Glossary, Sources for Further Reading, and Governmental and Non-Governmental Organizations Contact Information

Edited by Helene Henderson. 1,064 pages. 2001. 0-7808-0235-7. $78.

"This is important information. The Web has many resources but this sourcebook fills an important societal need. I am not aware of any other resources of this type." — *Doody's Review Service, Sep '01*

"Recommended for all libraries, scholars, and practitioners." — *Choice, Association of College & Research Libraries, Jul '01*

"Recommended reference source." — *Booklist, American Library Association, Apr '01*

"Important pick for college-level health reference libraries." — *The Bookwatch, Mar '01*

"Because this problem is so widespread and because this book includes a lot of issues within one volume, this work is recommended for all public libraries." — *American Reference Books Annual, 2001*

Drug Abuse Sourcebook

Basic Consumer Health Information about Illicit Substances of Abuse and the Diversion of Prescription Medications, Including Depressants, Hallucinogens, Inhalants, Marijuana, Narcotics, Stimulants, and Anabolic Steroids

Along with Facts about Related Health Risks, Treatment Issues, and Substance Abuse Prevention Pro-

grams, a Glossary of Terms, Statistical Data, and Directories of Hotline Services, Self-Help Groups, and Organizations Able to Provide Further Information

Edited by Karen Bellenir. 629 pages. 2000. 0-7808-0242-X. $78.

"Containing a wealth of information .... This resource belongs in libraries that serve a lower-division undergraduate or community college clientele as well as the general public." —Choice, Association of College and Research Libraries, Jun '01

"Recommended reference source."
—Booklist, American Library Association, Feb '01

"Highly recommended." —The Bookwatch, Jan '01

"Even though there is a plethora of books on drug abuse, this volume is recommended for school, public, and college libraries."
—American Reference Books Annual, 2001

SEE ALSO Alcoholism Sourcebook, Substance Abuse Sourcebook

Ear, Nose & Throat Disorders Sourcebook

Basic Information about Disorders of the Ears, Nose, Sinus Cavities, Pharynx, and Larynx, Including Ear Infections, Tinnitus, Vestibular Disorders, Allergic and Non-Allergic Rhinitis, Sore Throats, Tonsillitis, and Cancers That Affect the Ears, Nose, Sinuses, and Throat

Along with Reports on Current Research Initiatives, a Glossary of Related Medical Terms, and a Directory of Sources for Further Help and Information

Edited by Karen Bellenir and Linda M. Shin. 576 pages. 1998. 0-7808-0206-3. $78.

"Overall, this sourcebook is helpful for the consumer seeking information on ENT issues. It is recommended for public libraries."
—American Reference Books Annual, 1999

"Recommended reference source."
—Booklist, American Library Association, Dec '98

Eating Disorders Sourcebook

Basic Consumer Health Information about Eating Disorders, Including Information about Anorexia Nervosa, Bulimia Nervosa, Binge Eating, Body Dysmorphic Disorder, Pica, Laxative Abuse, and Night Eating Syndrome

Along with Information about Causes, Adverse Effects, and Treatment and Prevention Issues, and Featuring a Section on Concerns Specific to Children and Adolescents, a Glossary, and Resources for Further Help and Information

Edited by Dawn D. Matthews. 322 pages. 2001. 0-7808-0335-3. $78.

"Recommended for health science libraries that are open to the public, as well as hospital libraries. This book is a good resource for the consumer who is concerned about eating disorders." —E-Streams, Mar '02

"This volume is another convenient collection of excerpted articles. Recommended for school and public library patrons; lower-division undergraduates; and two-year technical program students." —Choice, Association of College & Research Libraries, Jan '02

"Recommended reference source." —Booklist, American Library Association, Oct '01

Emergency Medical Services Sourcebook

Basic Consumer Health Information about Preventing, Preparing for, and Managing Emergency Situations, When and Who to Call for Help, What to Expect in the Emergency Room, the Emergency Medical Team, Patient Issues, and Current Topics in Emergency Medicine

Along with Statistical Data, a Glossary, and Sources of Additional Help and Information

Edited by Jenni Lynn Colson. 494 pages. 2002. 0-7808-0420-1. $78.

Endocrine & Metabolic Disorders Sourcebook

Basic Information for the Layperson about Pancreatic and Insulin-Related Disorders Such as Pancreatitis, Diabetes, and Hypoglycemia; Adrenal Gland Disorders Such as Cushing's Syndrome, Addison's Disease, and Congenital Adrenal Hyperplasia; Pituitary Gland Disorders Such as Growth Hormone Deficiency, Acromegaly, and Pituitary Tumors; Thyroid Disorders Such as Hypothyroidism, Graves' Disease, Hashimoto's Disease, and Goiter; Hyperparathyroidism; and Other Diseases and Syndromes of Hormone Imbalance or Metabolic Dysfunction

Along with Reports on Current Research Initiatives

Edited by Linda M. Shin. 574 pages. 1998. 0-7808-0207-1. $78.

"Omnigraphics has produced another needed resource for health information consumers."
—American Reference Books Annual, 2000

"Recommended reference source."
—Booklist, American Library Association, Dec '98

Environmentally Induced Disorders Sourcebook, 1st Edition

Basic Information about Diseases and Syndromes Linked to Exposure to Pollutants and Other Substances in Outdoor and Indoor Environments Such as Lead, Asbestos, Formaldehyde, Mercury, Emissions, Noise, and More

Edited by Allan R. Cook. 620 pages. 1997. 0-7808-0083-4. $78.

"Recommended reference source."
—Booklist, American Library Association, Sep '98

"This book will be a useful addition to anyone's library." — *Choice Health Sciences Supplement, Association of College and Research Libraries, May '98*

". . . a good survey of numerous environmentally induced physical disorders . . . a useful addition to anyone's library."
— *Doody's Health Sciences Book Reviews, Jan '98*

". . . provide[s] introductory information from the best authorities around. Since this volume covers topics that potentially affect everyone, it will surely be one of the most frequently consulted volumes in the *Health Reference Series.*" — *Rettig on Reference, Nov '97*

Ethnic Diseases Sourcebook

Basic Consumer Health Information for Ethnic and Racial Minority Groups in the United States, Including General Health Indicators and Behaviors, Ethnic Diseases, Genetic Testing, the Impact of Chronic Diseases, Women's Health, Mental Health Issues, and Preventive Health Care Services

Along with a Glossary and a Listing of Additional Resources

Edited by Joyce Brennfleck Shannon. 664 pages. 2001. 0-7808-0336-1. $78.

"Recommended for health sciences libraries where public health programs are a priority."
— *E-Streams, Jan '02*

"Not many books have been written on this topic to date, and the *Ethnic Diseases Sourcebook* is a strong addition to the list. It will be an important introductory resource for health consumers, students, health care personnel, and social scientists. It is recommended for public, academic, and large hospital libraries."
— *American Reference Books Annual 2002*

"Recommended reference source."
— *Booklist, American Library Association, Oct '01*

"Will prove valuable to any library seeking to maintain a current, comprehensive reference collection of health resources. . . . An excellent source of health information about genetic disorders which affect particular ethnic and racial minorities in the U.S."
— *The Bookwatch, Aug '01*

Eye Care Sourcebook, 2nd Edition

Basic Consumer Health Information about Eye Care and Eye Disorders, Including Facts about the Diagnosis, Prevention, and Treatment of Common Refractive Problems Such as Myopia, Hyperopia, Astigmatism, and Presbyopia, and Eye Diseases, Including Glaucoma, Cataract, Age-Related Macular Degeneration, and Diabetic Retinopathy

Along with a Section on Vision Correction and Refractive Surgeries, Including LASIK and LASEK, a Glossary, and Directories of Resources for Additional Help and Information

Edited by Amy L. Sutton. 543 pages. 2003. 0-7808-0635-2. $78.

Family Planning Sourcebook

Basic Consumer Health Information about Planning for Pregnancy and Contraception, Including Traditional Methods, Barrier Methods, Hormonal Methods, Permanent Methods, Future Methods, Emergency Contraception, and Birth Control Choices for Women at Each Stage of Life

Along with Statistics, a Glossary, and Sources of Additional Information

Edited by Amy Marcaccio Keyzer. 520 pages. 2001. 0-7808-0379-5. $78.

"Recommended for public, health, and undergraduate libraries as part of the circulating collection."
— *E-Streams, Mar '02*

"Information is presented in an unbiased, readable manner, and the sourcebook will certainly be a necessary addition to those public and high school libraries where Internet access is restricted or otherwise problematic." — *American Reference Books Annual 2002*

"Recommended reference source."
— *Booklist, American Library Association, Oct '01*

"Will prove valuable to any library seeking to maintain a current, comprehensive reference collection of health resources. . . . Excellent reference."
— *The Bookwatch, Aug '01*

SEE ALSO *Pregnancy & Birth Sourcebook*

Fitness & Exercise Sourcebook, 1st Edition

Basic Information on Fitness and Exercise, Including Fitness Activities for Specific Age Groups, Exercise for People with Specific Medical Conditions, How to Begin a Fitness Program in Running, Walking, Swimming, Cycling, and Other Athletic Activities, and Recent Research in Fitness and Exercise

Edited by Dan R. Harris. 663 pages. 1996. 0-7808-0186-5. $78.

"A good resource for general readers." — *Choice, Association of College and Research Libraries, Nov '97*

"The perennial popularity of the topic . . . make this an appealing selection for public libraries."
— *Rettig on Reference, Jun/Jul '97*

Fitness & Exercise Sourcebook, 2nd Edition

Basic Consumer Health Information about the Fundamentals of Fitness and Exercise, Including How to Begin and Maintain a Fitness Program, Fitness as a Lifestyle, the Link between Fitness and Diet, Advice for Specific Groups of People, Exercise as It Relates to Specific Medical Conditions, and Recent Research in Fitness and Exercise

Along with a Glossary of Important Terms and Resources for Additional Help and Information

Edited by Kristen M. Gledhill. 646 pages. 2001. 0-7808-0334-5. $78.

"This work is recommended for all general reference collections."
— *American Reference Books Annual 2002*

"Highly recommended for public, consumer, and school grades fourth through college."
— *E-Streams, Nov '01*

"Recommended reference source." — *Booklist, American Library Association, Oct '01*

"The information appears quite comprehensive and is considered reliable. . . . This second edition is a welcomed addition to the series."
— *Doody's Review Service, Sep '01*

"This reference is a valuable choice for those who desire a broad source of information on exercise, fitness, and chronic-disease prevention through a healthy lifestyle." — *American Medical Writers Association Journal, Fall '01*

"Will prove valuable to any library seeking to maintain a current, comprehensive reference collection of health resources. . . . Excellent reference."
— *The Bookwatch, Aug '01*

Food & Animal Borne Diseases Sourcebook

Basic Information about Diseases That Can Be Spread to Humans through the Ingestion of Contaminated Food or Water or by Contact with Infected Animals and Insects, Such as Botulism, E. Coli, Hepatitis A, Trichinosis, Lyme Disease, and Rabies

Along with Information Regarding Prevention and Treatment Methods, and Including a Special Section for International Travelers Describing Diseases Such as Cholera, Malaria, Travelers' Diarrhea, and Yellow Fever, and Offering Recommendations for Avoiding Illness

Edited by Karen Bellenir and Peter D. Dresser. 535 pages. 1995. 0-7808-0033-8. $78.

"Targeting general readers and providing them with a single, comprehensive source of information on selected topics, this book continues, with the excellent caliber of its predecessors, to catalog topical information on health matters of general interest. Readable and thorough, this valuable resource is highly recommended for all libraries."
— *Academic Library Book Review, Summer '96*

"A comprehensive collection of authoritative information." — *Emergency Medical Services, Oct '95*

Food Safety Sourcebook

Basic Consumer Health Information about the Safe Handling of Meat, Poultry, Seafood, Eggs, Fruit Juices, and Other Food Items, and Facts about Pesticides, Drinking Water, Food Safety Overseas, and the Onset, Duration, and Symptoms of Foodborne Illnesses, Including Types of Pathogenic Bacteria, Parasitic Protozoa, Worms, Viruses, and Natural Toxins

Along with the Role of the Consumer, the Food Handler, and the Government in Food Safety; a Glossary, and Resources for Additional Help and Information

Edited by Dawn D. Matthews. 339 pages. 1999. 0-7808-0326-4. $78.

"This book is recommended for public libraries and universities with home economic and food science programs." — *E-Streams, Nov '00*

"Recommended reference source."
— *Booklist, American Library Association, May '00*

"This book takes the complex issues of food safety and foodborne pathogens and presents them in an easily understood manner. [It does] an excellent job of covering a large and often confusing topic."
— *American Reference Books Annual, 2000*

Forensic Medicine Sourcebook

Basic Consumer Information for the Layperson about Forensic Medicine, Including Crime Scene Investigation, Evidence Collection and Analysis, Expert Testimony, Computer-Aided Criminal Identification, Digital Imaging in the Courtroom, DNA Profiling, Accident Reconstruction, Autopsies, Ballistics, Drugs and Explosives Detection, Latent Fingerprints, Product Tampering, and Questioned Document Examination

Along with Statistical Data, a Glossary of Forensics Terminology, and Listings of Sources for Further Help and Information

Edited by Annemarie S. Muth. 574 pages. 1999. 0-7808-0232-2. $78.

"Given the expected widespread interest in its content and its easy to read style, this book is recommended for most public and all college and university libraries."
— *E-Streams, Feb '01*

"Recommended for public libraries."
— *Reference & User Services Quarterly, American Library Association, Spring 2000*

"Recommended reference source."
— *Booklist, American Library Association, Feb '00*

"A wealth of information, useful statistics, references are up-to-date and extremely complete. This wonderful collection of data will help students who are interested in a career in any type of forensic field. It is a great resource for attorneys who need information about types of expert witnesses needed in a particular case. It also offers useful information for fiction and nonfiction writers whose work involves a crime. A fascinating compilation. All levels." — *Choice, Association of College and Research Libraries, Jan 2000*

"There are several items that make this book attractive to consumers who are seeking certain forensic data. . . . This is a useful current source for those seeking general forensic medical answers."
— *American Reference Books Annual, 2000*

Gastrointestinal Diseases & Disorders Sourcebook

Basic Information about Gastroesophageal Reflux Disease (Heartburn), Ulcers, Diverticulosis, Irritable

Bowel Syndrome, Crohn's Disease, Ulcerative Colitis, Diarrhea, Constipation, Lactose Intolerance, Hemorrhoids, Hepatitis, Cirrhosis, and Other Digestive Problems, Featuring Statistics, Descriptions of Symptoms, and Current Treatment Methods of Interest for Persons Living with Upper and Lower Gastrointestinal Maladies

Edited by Linda M. Ross. 413 pages. 1996. 0-7808-0078-8. $78.

". . . very readable form. The successful editorial work that brought this material together into a useful and understandable reference makes accessible to all readers information that can help them more effectively understand and obtain help for digestive tract problems."
—*Choice, Association of College & Research Libraries, Feb '97*

SEE ALSO *Diet & Nutrition Sourcebook, 1st and 2nd Editions, Digestive Diseases & Disorders*

■

Genetic Disorders Sourcebook, 1st Edition

Basic Information about Heritable Diseases and Disorders Such as Down Syndrome, PKU, Hemophilia, Von Willebrand Disease, Gaucher Disease, Tay-Sachs Disease, and Sickle-Cell Disease, Along with Information about Genetic Screening, Gene Therapy, Home Care, and Including Source Listings for Further Help and Information on More Than 300 Disorders

Edited by Karen Bellenir. 642 pages. 1996. 0-7808-0034-6. $78.

"Recommended for undergraduate libraries or libraries that serve the public."
—*Science & Technology Libraries, Vol. 18, No. 1, '99*

"Provides essential medical information to both the general public and those diagnosed with a serious or fatal genetic disease or disorder." —*Choice, Association of College and Research Libraries, Jan '97*

"Geared toward the lay public. It would be well placed in all public libraries and in those hospital and medical libraries in which access to genetic references is limited." —*Doody's Health Sciences Book Review, Oct '96*

■

Genetic Disorders Sourcebook, 2nd Edition

Basic Consumer Health Information about Hereditary Diseases and Disorders, Including Cystic Fibrosis, Down Syndrome, Hemophilia, Huntington's Disease, Sickle Cell Anemia, and More; Facts about Genes, Gene Research and Therapy, Genetic Screening, Ethics of Gene Testing, Genetic Counseling, and Advice on Coping and Caring

Along with a Glossary of Genetic Terminology and a Resource List for Help, Support, and Further Information

Edited by Kathy Massimini. 768 pages. 2001. 0-7808-0241-1. $78.

"Recommended for public libraries and medical and hospital libraries with consumer health collections."
—*E-Streams, May '01*

"Recommended reference source."
—*Booklist, American Library Association, Apr '01*

"Important pick for college-level health reference libraries." —*The Bookwatch, Mar '01*

■

Head Trauma Sourcebook

Basic Information for the Layperson about Open-Head and Closed-Head Injuries, Treatment Advances, Recovery, and Rehabilitation

Along with Reports on Current Research Initiatives

Edited by Karen Bellenir. 414 pages. 1997. 0-7808-0208-X. $78.

■

Headache Sourcebook

Basic Consumer Health Information about Migraine, Tension, Cluster, Rebound and Other Types of Headaches, with Facts about the Cause and Prevention of Headaches, the Effects of Stress and the Environment, Headaches during Pregnancy and Menopause, and Childhood Headaches

Along with a Glossary and Other Resources for Additional Help and Information

Edited by Dawn D. Matthews. 362 pages. 2002. 0-7808-0337-X. $78.

"Highly recommended for academic and medical reference collections." —*Library Bookwatch, Sep '02*

■

Health Insurance Sourcebook

Basic Information about Managed Care Organizations, Traditional Fee-for-Service Insurance, Insurance Portability and Pre-Existing Conditions Clauses, Medicare, Medicaid, Social Security, and Military Health Care

Along with Information about Insurance Fraud

Edited by Wendy Wilcox. 530 pages. 1997. 0-7808-0222-5. $78.

"Particularly useful because it brings much of this information together in one volume. This book will be a handy reference source in the health sciences library, hospital library, college and university library, and medium to large public library."
—*Medical Reference Services Quarterly, Fall '98*

Awarded "Books of the Year Award"
—*American Journal of Nursing, 1997*

"The layout of the book is particularly helpful as it provides easy access to reference material. A most useful addition to the vast amount of information about health insurance. The use of data from U.S. government agencies is most commendable. Useful in a library or learning center for healthcare professional students."
—*Doody's Health Sciences Book Reviews, Nov '97*

Health Reference Series Cumulative Index 1999

A Comprehensive Index to the Individual Volumes of the Health Reference Series, Including a Subject Index, Name Index, Organization Index, and Publication Index

Along with a Master List of Acronyms and Abbreviations

Edited by Edward J. Prucha, Anne Holmes, and Robert Rudnick. 990 pages. 2000. 0-7808-0382-5. $78.

"This volume will be most helpful in libraries that have a relatively complete collection of the Health Reference Series." —*American Reference Books Annual, 2001*

"Essential for collections that hold any of the numerous *Health Reference Series* titles." —*Choice, Association of College and Research Libraries, Nov '00*

Healthy Aging Sourcebook

Basic Consumer Health Information about Maintaining Health through the Aging Process, Including Advice on Nutrition, Exercise, and Sleep, Help in Making Decisions about Midlife Issues and Retirement, and Guidance Concerning Practical and Informed Choices in Health Consumerism

Along with Data Concerning the Theories of Aging, Different Experiences in Aging by Minority Groups, and Facts about Aging Now and Aging in the Future; and Featuring a Glossary, a Guide to Consumer Help, Additional Suggested Reading, and Practical Resource Directory

Edited by Jenifer Swanson. 536 pages. 1999. 0-7808-0390-6. $78.

"Recommended reference source." —*Booklist, American Library Association, Feb '00*

SEE ALSO *Physical & Mental Issues in Aging Sourcebook*

Healthy Heart Sourcebook for Women

Basic Consumer Health Information about Cardiac Issues Specific to Women, Including Facts about Major Risk Factors and Prevention, Treatment and Control Strategies, and Important Dietary Issues

Along with a Special Section Regarding the Pros and Cons of Hormone Replacement Therapy and Its Impact on Heart Health, and Additional Help, Including Recipes, a Glossary, and a Directory of Resources

Edited by Dawn D. Matthews. 336 pages. 2000. 0-7808-0329-9. $78.

"A good reference source and recommended for all public, academic, medical, and hospital libraries." —*Medical Reference Services Quarterly, Summer '01*

"Because of the lack of information specific to women on this topic, this book is recommended for public libraries and consumer libraries." —*American Reference Books Annual, 2001*

"Contains very important information about coronary artery disease that all women should know. The information is current and presented in an easy-to-read format. The book will make a good addition to any library." —*American Medical Writers Association Journal, Summer '00*

"Important, basic reference." —*Reviewer's Bookwatch, Jul '00*

SEE ALSO *Cardiovascular Diseases & Disorders Sourcebook, 1st Edition, Heart Diseases & Disorders Sourcebook, 2nd Edition, Women's Health Concerns Sourcebook*

Heart Diseases & Disorders Sourcebook, 2nd Edition

Basic Consumer Health Information about Heart Attacks, Angina, Rhythm Disorders, Heart Failure, Valve Disease, Congenital Heart Disorders, and More, Including Descriptions of Surgical Procedures and Other Interventions, Medications, Cardiac Rehabilitation, Risk Identification, and Prevention Tips

Along with Statistical Data, Reports on Current Research Initiatives, a Glossary of Cardiovascular Terms, and Resource Directory

Edited by Karen Bellenir. 612 pages. 2000. 0-7808-0238-1. $78.

"This work stands out as an imminently accessible resource for the general public. It is recommended for the reference and circulating shelves of school, public, and academic libraries." —*American Reference Books Annual, 2001*

"Recommended reference source." —*Booklist, American Library Association, Dec '00*

"Provides comprehensive coverage of matters related to the heart. This title is recommended for health sciences and public libraries with consumer health collections." —*E-Streams, Oct '00*

SEE ALSO *Cardiovascular Diseases & Disorders Sourcebook, 1st Edition; Healthy Heart Sourcebook for Women*

Household Safety Sourcebook

Basic Consumer Health Information about Household Safety, Including Information about Poisons, Chemicals, Fire, and Water Hazards in the Home

Along with Advice about the Safe Use of Home Maintenance Equipment, Choosing Toys and Nursery Furniture, Holiday and Recreation Safety, a Glossary, and Resources for Further Help and Information

Edited by Dawn D. Matthews. 606 pages. 2002. 0-7808-0338-8. $78.

"As a sourcebook on household safety this book meets its mark. It is encyclopedic in scope and covers a wide range of safety issues that are commonly seen in the home." —*E-Streams, Jul '02*

Immune System Disorders Sourcebook

Basic Information about Lupus, Multiple Sclerosis, Guillain-Barré Syndrome, Chronic Granulomatous Disease, and More

Along with Statistical and Demographic Data and Reports on Current Research Initiatives

Edited by Allan R. Cook. 608 pages. 1997. 0-7808-0209-8. $78.

Infant & Toddler Health Sourcebook

Basic Consumer Health Information about the Physical and Mental Development of Newborns, Infants, and Toddlers, Including Neonatal Concerns, Nutrition Recommendations, Immunization Schedules, Common Pediatric Disorders, Assessments and Milestones, Safety Tips, and Advice for Parents and Other Caregivers

Along with a Glossary of Terms and Resource Listings for Additional Help

Edited by Jenifer Swanson. 585 pages. 2000. 0-7808-0246-2. $78.

"As a reference for the general public, this would be useful in any library." — *E-Streams, May '01*

"Recommended reference source." — *Booklist, American Library Association, Feb '01*

"This is a good source for general use." — *American Reference Books Annual, 2001*

Injury & Trauma Sourcebook

Basic Consumer Health Information about the Impact of Injury, the Diagnosis and Treatment of Common and Traumatic Injuries, Emergency Care, and Specific Injuries Related to Home, Community, Workplace, Transportation, and Recreation

Along with Guidelines for Injury Prevention, a Glossary, and a Directory of Additional Resources

Edited by Joyce Brennfleck Shannon. 696 pages. 2002. 0-7808-0421-X. $78.

"Practitioners should be aware of guides such as this in order to facilitate their use by patients and their families." — *Doody's Health Sciences Book Review Journal, Sep-Oct '02*

"Recommended reference source." — *Booklist, American Library Association, Sep '02*

"Highly recommended for academic and medical reference collections." — *Library Bookwatch, Sep '02*

Kidney & Urinary Tract Diseases & Disorders Sourcebook

Basic Information about Kidney Stones, Urinary Incontinence, Bladder Disease, End Stage Renal Disease, Dialysis, and More

Along with Statistical and Demographic Data and Reports on Current Research Initiatives

Edited by Linda M. Ross. 602 pages. 1997. 0-7808-0079-6. $78.

Learning Disabilities Sourcebook, 1st Edition

Basic Information about Disorders Such as Dyslexia, Visual and Auditory Processing Deficits, Attention Deficit/Hyperactivity Disorder, and Autism

Along with Statistical and Demographic Data, Reports on Current Research Initiatives, an Explanation of the Assessment Process, and a Special Section for Adults with Learning Disabilities

Edited by Linda M. Shin. 579 pages. 1998. 0-7808-0210-1. $78.

Named "Outstanding Reference Book of 1999." — *New York Public Library, Feb 2000*

"An excellent candidate for inclusion in a public library reference section. It's a great source of information. Teachers will also find the book useful. Definitely worth reading." — *Journal of Adolescent & Adult Literacy, Feb 2000*

"Readable . . . provides a solid base of information regarding successful techniques used with individuals who have learning disabilities, as well as practical suggestions for educators and family members. Clear language, concise descriptions, and pertinent information for contacting multiple resources add to the strength of this book as a useful tool." — *Choice, Association of College and Research Libraries, Feb '99*

"Recommended reference source." — *Booklist, American Library Association, Sep '98*

"A useful resource for libraries and for those who don't have the time to identify and locate the individual publications." — *Disability Resources Monthly, Sep '98*

Learning Disabilities Sourcebook, 2nd Edition

Basic Consumer Health Information about Learning Disabilities, Including Dyslexia, Developmental Speech and Language Disabilities, Non-Verbal Learning Disorders, Developmental Arithmetic Disorder, Developmental Writing Disorder, and Other Conditions That Impede Learning Such as Attention Deficit/ Hyperactivity Disorder, Brain Injury, Hearing Impairment, Klinefelter Syndrome, Dyspraxia, and Tourette Syndrome

Along with Facts about Educational Issues and Assistive Technology, Coping Strategies, a Glossary of Related Terms, and Resources for Further Help and Information

Edited by Dawn D. Matthews. 621 pages. 2003. 0-7808-0626-3. $78.

Liver Disorders Sourcebook

Basic Consumer Health Information about the Liver and How It Works; Liver Diseases, Including Cancer, Cirrhosis, Hepatitis, and Toxic and Drug Related Diseases; Tips for Maintaining a Healthy Liver; Laboratory Tests, Radiology Tests, and Facts about Liver Transplantation

Along with a Section on Support Groups, a Glossary, and Resource Listings

Edited by Joyce Brennfleck Shannon. 591 pages. 2000. 0-7808-0383-3. $78.

"A valuable resource."
—American Reference Books Annual, 2001

"This title is recommended for health sciences and public libraries with consumer health collections."
—E-Streams, Oct '00

"Recommended reference source."
—Booklist, American Library Association, Jun '00

■

Lung Disorders Sourcebook

Basic Consumer Health Information about Emphysema, Pneumonia, Tuberculosis, Asthma, Cystic Fibrosis, and Other Lung Disorders, Including Facts about Diagnostic Procedures, Treatment Strategies, Disease Prevention Efforts, and Such Risk Factors as Smoking, Air Pollution, and Exposure to Asbestos, Radon, and Other Agents

Along with a Glossary and Resources for Additional Help and Information

Edited by Dawn D. Matthews. 678 pages. 2002. 0-7808-0339-6. $78.

"Highly recommended for academic and medical reference collections." *— Library Bookwatch, Sep '02* [Pain SB, 2nd ed.]

"A source of valuable information. . . . This book offers help to nonmedical people who need information about pain and pain management. It is also an excellent reference for those who participate in patient education."
— Doody's Review Service, Sep '02

"Highly recommended for academic and medical reference collections." *— Library Bookwatch, Sep '02*

■

Medical Tests Sourcebook

Basic Consumer Health Information about Medical Tests, Including Periodic Health Exams, General Screening Tests, Tests You Can Do at Home, Findings of the U.S. Preventive Services Task Force, X-ray and Radiology Tests, Electrical Tests, Tests of Blood and Other Body Fluids and Tissues, Scope Tests, Lung Tests, Genetic Tests, Pregnancy Tests, Newborn Screening Tests, Sexually Transmitted Disease Tests, and Computer Aided Diagnoses

Along with a Section on Paying for Medical Tests, a Glossary, and Resource Listings

Edited by Joyce Brennfleck Shannon. 691 pages. 1999. 0-7808-0243-8. $78.

"Recommended for hospital and health sciences libraries with consumer health collections."
—E-Streams, Mar '00

"This is an overall excellent reference with a wealth of general knowledge that may aid those who are reluctant to get vital tests performed."
—Today's Librarian, Jan 2000

"A valuable reference guide."
—American Reference Books Annual, 2000

■

Men's Health Concerns Sourcebook

Basic Information about Health Issues That Affect Men, Featuring Facts about the Top Causes of Death in Men, Including Heart Disease, Stroke, Cancers, Prostate Disorders, Chronic Obstructive Pulmonary Disease, Pneumonia and Influenza, Human Immunodeficiency Virus and Acquired Immune Deficiency Syndrome, Diabetes Mellitus, Stress, Suicide, Accidents and Homicides; and Facts about Common Concerns for Men, Including Impotence, Contraception, Circumcision, Sleep Disorders, Snoring, Hair Loss, Diet, Nutrition, Exercise, Kidney and Urological Disorders, and Backaches

Edited by Allan R. Cook. 738 pages. 1998. 0-7808-0212-8. $78.

"This comprehensive resource and the series are highly recommended."
—American Reference Books Annual, 2000

"Recommended reference source."
— Booklist, American Library Association, Dec '98

■

Mental Health Disorders Sourcebook, 1st Edition

Basic Information about Schizophrenia, Depression, Bipolar Disorder, Panic Disorder, Obsessive-Compulsive Disorder, Phobias and Other Anxiety Disorders, Paranoia and Other Personality Disorders, Eating Disorders, and Sleep Disorders

Along with Information about Treatment and Therapies

Edited by Karen Bellenir. 548 pages. 1995. 0-7808-0040-0. $78.

"This is an excellent new book . . . written in easy-to-understand language."
— Booklist Health Sciences Supplement, American Library Association, Oct '97

". . . useful for public and academic libraries and consumer health collections."
— Medical Reference Services Quarterly, Spring '97

"The great strengths of the book are its readability and its inclusion of places to find more information. Especially recommended." *— Reference Quarterly, American Library Association, Winter '96*

". . . a good resource for a consumer health library."
—Bulletin of the Medical Library Association, Oct '96

Mental Health Disorders Sourcebook, 2nd Edition

Basic Consumer Health Information about Anxiety Disorders, Depression and Other Mood Disorders, Eating Disorders, Personality Disorders, Schizophrenia, and More, Including Disease Descriptions, Treatment Options, and Reports on Current Research Initiatives

Along with Statistical Data, Tips for Maintaining Mental Health, a Glossary, and Directory of Sources for Additional Help and Information

Edited by Karen Bellenir. 605 pages. 2000. 0-7808-0240-3. $78.

Mental Retardation Sourcebook

Basic Consumer Health Information about Mental Retardation and Its Causes, Including Down Syndrome, Fetal Alcohol Syndrome, Fragile X Syndrome, Genetic Conditions, Injury, and Environmental Sources

Along with Preventive Strategies, Parenting Issues, Educational Implications, Health Care Needs, Employment and Economic Matters, Legal Issues, a Glossary, and a Resource Listing for Additional Help and Information

Edited by Joyce Brennfleck Shannon. 642 pages. 2000. 0-7808-0377-9. $78.

Movement Disorders Sourcebook

Basic Consumer Health Information about Neurological Movement Disorders, Including Essential Tremor, Parkinson's Disease, Dystonia, Cerebral Palsy, Huntington's Disease, Myasthenia Gravis, Multiple Sclerosis, and Other Early-Onset and Adult-Onset Movement Disorders, Their Symptoms and Causes, Diagnostic Tests, and Treatments

Along with Mobility and Assistive Technology Information, a Glossary, and a Directory of Additional Resources

Edited by Joyce Brennfleck Shannon. 655 pages. 2003. 0-7808-0628-X. $78.

Obesity Sourcebook

Basic Consumer Health Information about Diseases and Other Problems Associated with Obesity, and Including Facts about Risk Factors, Prevention Issues, and Management Approaches

Along with Statistical and Demographic Data, Information about Special Populations, Research Updates, a Glossary, and Source Listings for Further Help and Information

Edited by Wilma Caldwell and Chad T. Kimball. 376 pages. 2001. 0-7808-0333-7. $78.

Ophthalmic Disorders Sourcebook, 1st Edition

Basic Information about Glaucoma, Cataracts, Macular Degeneration, Strabismus, Refractive Disorders, and More

Along with Statistical and Demographic Data and Reports on Current Research Initiatives

Edited by Linda M. Ross. 631 pages. 1996. 0-7808-0081-8. $78.

SEE ALSO *Eye Care Sourcebook, 2nd Edition*

Oral Health Sourcebook, 1st Edition

Basic Information about Diseases and Conditions Affecting Oral Health, Including Cavities, Gum Disease, Dry Mouth, Oral Cancers, Fever Blisters, Canker Sores, Oral Thrush, Bad Breath, Temporomandibular Disorders, and other Craniofacial Syndromes

Along with Statistical Data on the Oral Health of Americans, Oral Hygiene, Emergency First Aid, Information on Treatment Procedures and Methods of Replacing Lost Teeth

Edited by Allan R. Cook. 558 pages. 1997. 0-7808-0082-6. $78.

"Unique source which will fill a gap in dental sources for patients and the lay public. A valuable reference tool even in a library with thousands of books on dentistry. Comprehensive, clear, inexpensive, and easy to read and use. It fills an enormous gap in the health care literature." — Reference and User Services Quarterly, American Library Association, Summer '98

"Recommended reference source." — Booklist, American Library Association, Dec '97

Osteoporosis Sourcebook

Basic Consumer Health Information about Primary and Secondary Osteoporosis and Juvenile Osteoporosis and Related Conditions, Including Fibrous Dysplasia, Gaucher Disease, Hyperthyroidism, Hypophosphatasia, Myeloma, Osteopetrosis, Osteogenesis Imperfecta, and Paget's Disease

Along with Information about Risk Factors, Treatments, Traditional and Non-Traditional Pain Management, a Glossary of Related Terms, and a Directory of Resources

Edited by Allan R. Cook. 584 pages. 2001. 0-7808-0239-X. $78.

"This would be a book to be kept in a staff or patient library. The targeted audience is the layperson, but the therapist who needs a quick bit of information on a particular topic will also find the book useful." — Physical Therapy, Jan '02

"This resource is recommended as a great reference source for public, health, and academic libraries, and is another triumph for the editors of Omnigraphics." — American Reference Books Annual 2002

"Recommended for all public libraries and general health collections, especially those supporting patient education or consumer health programs." — E-Streams, Nov '01

"Will prove valuable to any library seeking to maintain a current, comprehensive reference collection of health resources. . . . From prevention to treatment and associated conditions, this provides an excellent survey." — The Bookwatch, Aug '01

"Recommended reference source." — Booklist, American Library Association, July '01

SEE ALSO Women's Health Concerns Sourcebook

Pain Sourcebook, 1st Edition

Basic Information about Specific Forms of Acute and Chronic Pain, Including Headaches, Back Pain, Muscular Pain, Neuralgia, Surgical Pain, and Cancer Pain

Along with Pain Relief Options Such as Analgesics, Narcotics, Nerve Blocks, Transcutaneous Nerve Stimulation, and Alternative Forms of Pain Control, Including Biofeedback, Imaging, Behavior Modification, and Relaxation Techniques

Edited by Allan R. Cook. 667 pages. 1997. 0-7808-0213-6. $78.

"The text is readable, easily understood, and well indexed. This excellent volume belongs in all patient education libraries, consumer health sections of public libraries, and many personal collections." — American Reference Books Annual, 1999

"A beneficial reference." — Booklist Health Sciences Supplement, American Library Association, Oct '98

"The information is basic in terms of scholarship and is appropriate for general readers. Written in journalistic style . . . intended for non-professionals. Quite thorough in its coverage of different pain conditions and summarizes the latest clinical information regarding pain treatment." — Choice, Association of College and Research Libraries, Jun '98

"Recommended reference source." — Booklist, American Library Association, Mar '98

Pain Sourcebook, 2nd Edition

Basic Consumer Health Information about Specific Forms of Acute and Chronic Pain, Including Muscle and Skeletal Pain, Nerve Pain, Cancer Pain, and Disorders Characterized by Pain, Such as Fibromyalgia, Shingles, Angina, Arthritis, and Headaches

Along with Information about Pain Medications and Management Techniques, Complementary and Alternative Pain Relief Options, Tips for People Living with Chronic Pain, a Glossary, and a Directory of Sources for Further Information

Edited by Karen Bellenir. 670 pages. 2002. 0-7808-0612-3. $78.

Pediatric Cancer Sourcebook

Basic Consumer Health Information about Leukemias, Brain Tumors, Sarcomas, Lymphomas, and Other Cancers in Infants, Children, and Adolescents, Including Descriptions of Cancers, Treatments, and Coping Strategies

Along with Suggestions for Parents, Caregivers, and Concerned Relatives, a Glossary of Cancer Terms, and Resource Listings

Edited by Edward J. Prucha. 587 pages. 1999. 0-7808-0245-4. $78.

"An excellent source of information. Recommended for public, hospital, and health science libraries with consumer health collections." — E-Streams, Jun '00

Physical & Mental Issues in Aging Sourcebook

Basic Consumer Health Information on Physical and Mental Disorders Associated with the Aging Process, Including Concerns about Cardiovascular Disease, Pulmonary Disease, Oral Health, Digestive Disorders, Musculoskeletal and Skin Disorders, Metabolic Changes, Sexual and Reproductive Issues, and Changes in Vision, Hearing, and Other Senses

Along with Data about Longevity and Causes of Death, Information on Acute and Chronic Pain, Descriptions of Mental Concerns, a Glossary of Terms, and Resource Listings for Additional Help

Edited by Jenifer Swanson. 660 pages. 1999. 0-7808-0233-0. $78.

SEE ALSO *Healthy Aging Sourcebook*

Podiatry Sourcebook

Basic Consumer Health Information about Foot Conditions, Diseases, and Injuries, Including Bunions, Corns, Calluses, Athlete's Foot, Plantar Warts, Hammertoes and Clawtoes, Clubfoot, Heel Pain, Gout, and More

Along with Facts about Foot Care, Disease Prevention, Foot Safety, Choosing a Foot Care Specialist, a Glossary of Terms, and Resource Listings for Additional Information

Edited by M. Lisa Weatherford. 380 pages. 2001. 0-7808-0215-2. $78.

Pregnancy & Birth Sourcebook

Basic Information about Planning for Pregnancy, Maternal Health, Fetal Growth and Development, Labor and Delivery, Postpartum and Perinatal Care, Pregnancy in Mothers with Special Concerns, and Disorders of Pregnancy, Including Genetic Counseling, Nutrition and Exercise, Obstetrical Tests, Pregnancy Discomfort, Multiple Births, Cesarean Sections, Medical Testing of Newborns, Breastfeeding, Gestational Diabetes, and Ectopic Pregnancy

Edited by Heather E. Aldred. 737 pages. 1997. 0-7808-0216-0. $78.

SEE ALSO *Congenital Disorders Sourcebook, Family Planning Sourcebook*

Prostate Cancer Sourcebook

Basic Consumer Health Information about Prostate Cancer, Including Information about the Associated Risk Factors, Detection, Diagnosis, and Treatment of Prostate Cancer

Along with Information on Non-Malignant Prostate Conditions, and Featuring a Section Listing Support and Treatment Centers and a Glossary of Related Terms

Edited by Dawn D. Matthews. 358 pages. 2001. 0-7808-0324-8. $78.

Public Health Sourcebook

Basic Information about Government Health Agencies, Including National Health Statistics and Trends, Healthy People 2000 Program Goals and Objectives, the Centers for Disease Control and Prevention, the Food and Drug Administration, and the National Institutes of Health

Along with Full Contact Information for Each Agency

Edited by Wendy Wilcox. 698 pages. 1998. 0-7808-0220-9. $78.

Reconstructive & Cosmetic Surgery Sourcebook

Basic Consumer Health Information on Cosmetic and Reconstructive Plastic Surgery, Including Statistical Information about Different Surgical Procedures, Things to Consider Prior to Surgery, Plastic Surgery Techniques and Tools, Emotional and Psychological Considerations, and Procedure-Specific Information

Along with a Glossary of Terms and a Listing of Resources for Additional Help and Information

Edited by M. Lisa Weatherford. 374 pages. 2001. 0-7808-0214-4. $78.

"An excellent reference that addresses cosmetic and medically necessary reconstructive surgeries. . . . The style of the prose is calm and reassuring, discussing the many positive outcomes now available due to advances in surgical techniques."
— *American Reference Books Annual 2002*

"Recommended for health science libraries that are open to the public, as well as hospital libraries that are open to the patients. This book is a good resource for the consumer interested in plastic surgery."
—*E-Streams, Dec '01*

"Recommended reference source."
—*Booklist, American Library Association, July '01*

Rehabilitation Sourcebook

Basic Consumer Health Information about Rehabilitation for People Recovering from Heart Surgery, Spinal Cord Injury, Stroke, Orthopedic Impairments, Amputation, Pulmonary Impairments, Traumatic Injury, and More, Including Physical Therapy, Occupational Therapy, Speech/ Language Therapy, Massage Therapy, Dance Therapy, Art Therapy, and Recreational Therapy

Along with Information on Assistive and Adaptive Devices, a Glossary, and Resources for Additional Help and Information

Edited by Dawn D. Matthews. 531 pages. 1999. 0-7808-0236-5. $78.

"This is an excellent resource for public library reference and health collections."
—*American Reference Books Annual, 2001*

"Recommended reference source."
— *Booklist, American Library Association, May '00*

Respiratory Diseases & Disorders Sourcebook

Basic Information about Respiratory Diseases and Disorders, Including Asthma, Cystic Fibrosis, Pneumonia, the Common Cold, Influenza, and Others, Featuring Facts about the Respiratory System, Statistical and Demographic Data, Treatments, Self-Help Management Suggestions, and Current Research Initiatives

Edited by Allan R. Cook and Peter D. Dresser. 771 pages. 1995. 0-7808-0037-0. $78.

"Designed for the layperson and for patients and their families coping with respiratory illness. . . . an extensive array of information on diagnosis, treatment, management, and prevention of respiratory illnesses for the general reader."
— *Choice, Association of College and Research Libraries, Jun '96*

"A highly recommended text for all collections. It is a comforting reminder of the power of knowledge that good books carry between their covers."
— *Academic Library Book Review, Spring '96*

"A comprehensive collection of authoritative information presented in a nontechnical, humanitarian style for patients, families, and caregivers."
— *Association of Operating Room Nurses, Sep/Oct '95*

Sexually Transmitted Diseases Sourcebook, 1st Edition

Basic Information about Herpes, Chlamydia, Gonorrhea, Hepatitis, Nongonoccocal Urethritis, Pelvic Inflammatory Disease, Syphilis, AIDS, and More

Along with Current Data on Treatments and Preventions

Edited by Linda M. Ross. 550 pages. 1997. 0-7808-0217-9. $78.

Sexually Transmitted Diseases Sourcebook, 2nd Edition

Basic Consumer Health Information about Sexually Transmitted Diseases, Including Information on the Diagnosis and Treatment of Chlamydia, Gonorrhea, Hepatitis, Herpes, HIV, Mononucleosis, Syphilis, and Others

Along with Information on Prevention, Such as Condom Use, Vaccines, and STD Education; And Featuring a Section on Issues Related to Youth and Adolescents, a Glossary, and Resources for Additional Help and Information

Edited by Dawn D. Matthews. 538 pages. 2001. 0-7808-0249-7. $78.

"Recommended for consumer health collections in public libraries, and secondary school and community college libraries."
— *American Reference Books Annual 2002*

"Every school and public library should have a copy of this comprehensive and user-friendly reference book."
— *Choice, Association of College & Research Libraries, Sep '01*

"This is a highly recommended book. This is an especially important book for all school and public libraries." — *AIDS Book Review Journal, Jul-Aug '01*

"Recommended reference source."
— *Booklist, American Library Association, Apr '01*

"Recommended pick both for specialty health library collections and any general consumer health reference collection." — *The Bookwatch, Apr '01*

Skin Disorders Sourcebook

Basic Information about Common Skin and Scalp Conditions Caused by Aging, Allergies, Immune Reactions, Sun Exposure, Infectious Organisms, Parasites, Cosmetics, and Skin Traumas, Including Abrasions, Cuts, and Pressure Sores

Along with Information on Prevention and Treatment

Edited by Allan R. Cook. 647 pages. 1997. 0-7808-0080-X. $78.

". . . comprehensive, easily read reference book."
— *Doody's Health Sciences Book Reviews, Oct '97*

SEE ALSO *Burns Sourcebook*

Sleep Disorders Sourcebook

Basic Consumer Health Information about Sleep and Its Disorders, Including Insomnia, Sleepwalking, Sleep Apnea, Restless Leg Syndrome, and Narcolepsy

Along with Data about Shiftwork and Its Effects, Information on the Societal Costs of Sleep Deprivation, Descriptions of Treatment Options, a Glossary of Terms, and Resource Listings for Additional Help

Edited by Jenifer Swanson. 439 pages. 1998. 0-7808-0234-9. $78.

"This text will complement any home or medical library. It is user-friendly and ideal for the adult reader."
—*American Reference Books Annual, 2000*

"A useful resource that provides accurate, relevant, and accessible information on sleep to the general public. Health care providers who deal with sleep disorders patients may also find it helpful in being prepared to answer some of the questions patients ask."
— *Respiratory Care, Jul '99*

"Recommended reference source."
— *Booklist, American Library Association, Feb '99*

Sports Injuries Sourcebook, 1st Edition

Basic Consumer Health Information about Common Sports Injuries, Prevention of Injury in Specific Sports, Tips for Training, and Rehabilitation from Injury

Along with Information about Special Concerns for Children, Young Girls in Athletic Training Programs, Senior Athletes, and Women Athletes, and a Directory of Resources for Further Help and Information

Edited by Heather E. Aldred. 624 pages. 1999. 0-7808-0218-7. $78.

"While this easy-to-read book is recommended for all libraries, it should prove to be especially useful for public, high school, and academic libraries; certainly it should be on the bookshelf of every school gymnasium."
— *E-Streams, Mar '00*

"Public libraries and undergraduate academic libraries will find this book useful for its nontechnical language."
—*American Reference Books Annual, 2000*

Sports Injuries Sourcebook, 2nd Edition

Basic Consumer Health Information about the Diagnosis, Treatment, and Rehabilitation of Common Sports-Related Injuries in Children and Adults

Along with Suggestions for Conditioning and Training, Information and Prevention Tips for Injuries Frequently Associated with Specific Sports and Special Populations, a Glossary, and a Directory of Additional Resources

Edited by Joyce Brennfleck Shannon. 614 pages. 2002. 0-7808-0604-2. $78.

Stress-Related Disorders Sourcebook

Basic Consumer Health Information about Stress and Stress-Related Disorders, Including Stress Origins and Signals, Environmental Stress at Work and Home, Mental and Emotional Stress Associated with Depression, Post-Traumatic Stress Disorder, Panic Disorder, Suicide, and the Physical Effects of Stress on the Cardiovascular, Immune, and Nervous Systems

Along with Stress Management Techniques, a Glossary, and a Listing of Additional Resources

Edited by Joyce Brennfleck Shannon. 610 pages. 2002. 0-7808-0560-7. $78.

"I am impressed by the amount of information. It offers a thorough overview of the causes and consequences of stress for the layperson. . . . A well-done and thorough reference guide for professionals and nonprofessionals alike." — *Doody's Review Service, Dec '02*

Stroke Sourcebook

Basic Consumer Health Information about Stroke, Including Ischemic, Hemorrhagic, Transient Ischemic Attack (TIA), and Pediatric Stroke, Stroke Triggers and Risks, Diagnostic Tests, Treatments, and Rehabilitation Information

Along with Stroke Prevention Guidelines, Legal and Financial Information, a Glossary, and a Directory of Additional Resources

Edited by Joyce Brennfleck Shannon. 606 pages. 2003. 0-7808-0630-1. $78.

Substance Abuse Sourcebook

Basic Health-Related Information about the Abuse of Legal and Illegal Substances Such as Alcohol, Tobacco, Prescription Drugs, Marijuana, Cocaine, and Heroin; and Including Facts about Substance Abuse Prevention Strategies, Intervention Methods, Treatment and Recovery Programs, and a Section Addressing the Special Problems Related to Substance Abuse during Pregnancy

Edited by Karen Bellenir. 573 pages. 1996. 0-7808-0038-9. $78.

"A valuable addition to any health reference section. Highly recommended."
— *The Book Report, Mar/Apr '97*

". . . a comprehensive collection of substance abuse information that's both highly readable and compact. Families and caregivers of substance abusers will find the information enlightening and helpful, while teachers, social workers and journalists should benefit from the concise format. Recommended."
— *Drug Abuse Update, Winter '96/'97*

SEE ALSO *Alcoholism Sourcebook, Drug Abuse Sourcebook*

Surgery Sourcebook

Basic Consumer Health Information about Inpatient and Outpatient Surgeries, Including Cardiac, Vascular, Orthopedic, Ocular, Reconstructive, Cosmetic, Gynecologic, and Ear, Nose, and Throat Procedures and More

Along with Information about Operating Room Policies and Instruments, Laser Surgery Techniques, Hospital Errors, Statistical Data, a Glossary, and Listings of Sources for Further Help and Information

Edited by Annemarie S. Muth and Karen Bellenir. 596 pages. 2002. 0-7808-0380-9. $78.

Transplantation Sourcebook

Basic Consumer Health Information about Organ and Tissue Transplantation, Including Physical and Financial Preparations, Procedures and Issues Relating to Specific Solid Organ and Tissue Transplants, Rehabilitation, Pediatric Transplant Information, the Future of Transplantation, and Organ and Tissue Donation

Along with a Glossary and Listings of Additional Resources

Edited by Joyce Brennfleck Shannon. 628 pages. 2002. 0-7808-0322-1. $78.

"Recommended for libraries with an interest in offering consumer health information." — *E-Streams, Jul '02*

"This is a unique and valuable resource for patients facing transplantation and their families."
— *Doody's Review Service, Jun '02*

Traveler's Health Sourcebook

Basic Consumer Health Information for Travelers, Including Physical and Medical Preparations, Transportation Health and Safety, Essential Information about Food and Water, Sun Exposure, Insect and Snake Bites, Camping and Wilderness Medicine, and Travel with Physical or Medical Disabilities

Along with International Travel Tips, Vaccination Recommendations, Geographical Health Issues, Disease Risks, a Glossary, and a Listing of Additional Resources

Edited by Joyce Brennfleck Shannon. 613 pages. 2000. 0-7808-0384-1. $78.

"Recommended reference source."
— *Booklist, American Library Association, Feb '01*

"This book is recommended for any public library, any travel collection, and especially any collection for the physically disabled."
— *American Reference Books Annual, 2001*

Vegetarian Sourcebook

Basic Consumer Health Information about Vegetarian Diets, Lifestyle, and Philosophy, Including Definitions of Vegetarianism and Veganism, Tips about Adopting Vegetarianism, Creating a Vegetarian Pantry, and Meeting Nutritional Needs of Vegetarians, with Facts Regarding Vegetarianism's Effect on Pregnant and Lactating Women, Children, Athletes, and Senior Citizens

Along with a Glossary of Commonly Used Vegetarian Terms and Resources for Additional Help and Information

Edited by Chad T. Kimball. 360 pages. 2002. 0-7808-0439-2. $78.

Women's Health Concerns Sourcebook

Basic Information about Health Issues That Affect Women, Featuring Facts about Menstruation and Other Gynecological Concerns, Including Endometriosis, Fibroids, Menopause, and Vaginitis; Reproductive Concerns, Including Birth Control, Infertility, and Abortion; and Facts about Additional Physical, Emotional, and Mental Health Concerns Prevalent among Women Such as Osteoporosis, Urinary Tract Disorders, Eating Disorders, and Depression

Along with Tips for Maintaining a Healthy Lifestyle

Edited by Heather E. Aldred. 567 pages. 1997. 0-7808-0219-5. $78.

"Handy compilation. There is an impressive range of diseases, devices, disorders, procedures, and other physical and emotional issues covered . . . well organized, illustrated, and indexed." — *Choice, Association of College and Research Libraries, Jan '98*

SEE ALSO *Breast Cancer Sourcebook, Cancer Sourcebook for Women, 1st and 2nd Editions, Healthy Heart Sourcebook for Women, Osteoporosis Sourcebook*

Workplace Health & Safety Sourcebook

Basic Consumer Health Information about Workplace Health and Safety, Including the Effect of Workplace Hazards on the Lungs, Skin, Heart, Ears, Eyes, Brain, Reproductive Organs, Musculoskeletal System, and Other Organs and Body Parts

Along with Information about Occupational Cancer, Personal Protective Equipment, Toxic and Hazardous Chemicals, Child Labor, Stress, and Workplace Violence

Edited by Chad T. Kimball. 626 pages. 2000. 0-7808-0231-4. $78.

660

Worldwide Health Sourcebook

Basic Information about Global Health Issues, Including Malnutrition, Reproductive Health, Disease Dispersion and Prevention, Emerging Diseases, Risky Health Behaviors, and the Leading Causes of Death

Along with Global Health Concerns for Children, Women, and the Elderly, Mental Health Issues, Research and Technology Advancements, and Economic, Environmental, and Political Health Implications, a Glossary, and a Resource Listing for Additional Help and Information

Edited by Joyce Brennfleck Shannon. 614 pages. 2001. 0-7808-0330-2. $78.

Teen Health Series

*Helping Young Adults Understand, Manage,
and Avoid Serious Illness*

Diet Information for Teens

Health Tips about Diet and Nutrition

*Including Facts about Nutrients, Dietary Guidelines,
Breakfasts, School Lunches, Snacks, Party Food, Weight
Control, Eating Disorders, and More*

Edited by Karen Bellenir. 399 pages. 2001. 0-7808-0441-4. $58.

"Full of helpful insights and facts throughout the book.
. . . An excellent resource to be placed in public libraries
or even in personal collections."
—*American Reference Books Annual 2002*

"Recommended for middle and high school libraries
and media centers as well as academic libraries that
educate future teachers of teenagers. It is also a suitable
addition to health science libraries that serve patrons
who are interested in teen health promotion and education." —*E-Streams, Oct '01*

"This comprehensive book would be beneficial to collections that need information about nutrition, dietary
guidelines, meal planning, and weight control. . . . This
reference is so easy to use that its purchase is recommended." —*The Book Report, Sep-Oct '01*

"This book is written in an easy to understand format
describing issues that many teens face every day, and
then provides thoughtful explanations so that teens can
make informed decisions. This is an interesting book
that provides important facts and information for
today's teens." —*Doody's Health Sciences
Book Review Journal, Jul-Aug '01*

"A comprehensive compendium of diet and nutrition.
The information is presented in a straightforward,
plain-spoken manner. This title will be useful to those
working on reports on a variety of topics, as well as to
general readers concerned about their dietary health."
—*School Library Journal, Jun '01*

Drug Information for Teens

Health Tips about the Physical and Mental Effects of Substance Abuse

*Including Facts about Alcohol, Anabolic Steroids, Club
Drugs, Cocaine, Depressants, Hallucinogens, Herbal
Products, Inhalants, Marijuana, Narcotics, Stimulants,
Tobacco, and More*

Edited by Karen Bellenir. 452 pages. 2002. 0-7808-0444-9. $58.

"This is an excellent resource for teens and their parents. Education about drugs and substances is key to
discouraging teen drug abuse and this book provides
this much needed information in a way that is interesting and factual." —*Doody's Review Service, Dec '02*

Mental Health Information for Teens

Health Tips about Mental Health and Mental Illness

*Including Facts about Anxiety, Depression, Suicide,
Eating Disorders, Obsessive-Compulsive Disorders,
Panic Attacks, Phobias, Schizophrenia, and More*

Edited by Karen Bellenir. 406 pages. 2001. 0-7808-0442-2. $58.

"In both language and approach, this user-friendly entry
in the *Teen Health Series* is on target for teens needing
information on mental health concerns." —*Booklist,
American Library Association, Jan '02*

"Readers will find the material accessible and informative, with the shaded notes, facts, and embedded glossary insets adding appropriately to the already interesting and succinct presentation."
—*School Library Journal, Jan '02*

"This title is highly recommended for any library that
serves adolescents and parents/caregivers of adolescents." —*E-Streams, Jan '02*

"Recommended for high school libraries and young
adult collections in public libraries. Both health professionals and teenagers will find this book useful."
—*American Reference Books Annual 2002*

"This is a nice book written to enlighten the society,
primarily teenagers, about common teen mental health
issues. It is highly recommended to teachers and parents as well as adolescents."
—*Doody's Review Service, Dec '01*

Sexual Health Information for Teens

Health Tips about Sexual Development, Human Reproduction, and Sexually Transmitted Diseases

*Including Facts about Puberty, Reproductive Health,
Chlamydia, Human Papillomavirus, Pelvic Inflammatory Disease, Herpes, AIDS, Contraception, Pregnancy, and More*

Edited by Deborah A. Stanley. 400 pages. 2003. 0-7808-0445-7. $58.

Health Reference Series

Adolescent Health Sourcebook
AIDS Sourcebook, 1st Edition
AIDS Sourcebook, 2nd Edition
AIDS Sourcebook, 3rd Edition
Alcoholism Sourcebook
Allergies Sourcebook, 1st Edition
Allergies Sourcebook, 2nd Edition
Alternative Medicine Sourcebook,
    1st Edition
Alternative Medicine Sourcebook,
    2nd Edition
Alzheimer's, Stroke & 29 Other
    Neurological Disorders Sourcebook,
    1st Edition
Alzheimer's Disease Sourcebook,
    2nd Edition
Arthritis Sourcebook
Asthma Sourcebook
Attention Deficit Disorder Sourcebook
Back & Neck Disorders Sourcebook
Blood & Circulatory Disorders
    Sourcebook
Brain Disorders Sourcebook
Breast Cancer Sourcebook
Breastfeeding Sourcebook
Burns Sourcebook
Cancer Sourcebook, 1st Edition
Cancer Sourcebook (New), 2nd Edition
Cancer Sourcebook, 3rd Edition
Cancer Sourcebook for Women,
    1st Edition
Cancer Sourcebook for Women,
    2nd Edition
Cardiovascular Diseases & Disorders
    Sourcebook, 1st Edition
Caregiving Sourcebook
Childhood Diseases & Disorders
    Sourcebook
Colds, Flu & Other Common Ailments
    Sourcebook
Communication Disorders
    Sourcebook

Congenital Disorders Sourcebook
Consumer Issues in Health Care
    Sourcebook
Contagious & Non-Contagious
    Infectious Diseases Sourcebook
Death & Dying Sourcebook
Depression Sourcebook
Diabetes Sourcebook, 1st Edition
Diabetes Sourcebook, 2nd Edition
Diabetes Sourcebook, 3rd Edition
Diet & Nutrition Sourcebook,
    1st Edition
Diet & Nutrition Sourcebook,
    2nd Edition
Digestive Diseases & Disorder
    Sourcebook
Disabilities Sourcebook
Domestic Violence & Child Abuse
    Sourcebook
Drug Abuse Sourcebook
Ear, Nose & Throat Disorders
    Sourcebook
Eating Disorders Sourcebook
Emergency Medical Services
    Sourcebook
Endocrine & Metabolic Disorders
    Sourcebook
Environmentally Induced Disorders
    Sourcebook
Ethnic Diseases Sourcebook
Eye Care Sourcebook, 2nd Edition
Family Planning Sourcebook
Fitness & Exercise Sourcebook,
    1st Edition
Fitness & Exercise Sourcebook,
    2nd Edition
Food & Animal Borne Diseases
    Sourcebook
Food Safety Sourcebook
Forensic Medicine Sourcebook
Gastrointestinal Diseases & Disorders
    Sourcebook